Pediatric Hematology

Editors

RACHAEL F. GRACE
RUSSELL E. WARE

HEMATOLOGY/ONCOLOGY CLINICS OF NORTH AMERICA

www.hemonc.theclinics.com

Consulting Editors
GEORGE P. CANELLOS
H. FRANKLIN BUNN

June 2019 • Volume 33 • Number 3

ELSEVIER

1600 John F. Kennedy Boulevard • Suite 1800 • Philadelphia, Pennsylvania, 19103-2899

http://www.theclinics.com

HEMATOLOGY/ONCOLOGY CLINICS OF NORTH AMERICA Volume 33, Number 3
June 2019 ISSN 0889-8588, ISBN 13: 978-0-323-67333-4

Editor: Stacy Eastman
Developmental Editor: Kristen Helm

Hematology/Oncology Clinics (ISSN 0889-8588) is published bimonthly by Elsevier Inc., 360 Park Avenue South, New York, NY 10010-1710. Months of issue are February, April, June, August, October, and December. Business and Editorial Offices: 1600 John F. Kennedy Blvd., Ste. 1800, Philadelphia, PA 19103—2899. Customer Service Office: 3251 Riverport Lane, Maryland Heights, MO 63043. Periodicals postage paid at New York, NY and at additional mailing offices. Subscription prices are $430.00 per year (domestic individuals), $830.00 per year (domestic institutions), $100.00 per year (domestic students/residents), $480.00 per year (Canadian individuals), $1028.00 per year (Canadian institutions) $547.00 per year (international individuals), $1028.00 per year (international institutions), and $255.00 per year (international and Canadian students/residents). International air speed delivery is included in all *Clinics* subscription prices. All prices are subject to change without notice. **POSTMASTER:** Send address changes to *Hematology/Oncology Clinics of North America*, Elsevier Health Sciences Division, Subscription Customer Service, 3251 Riverport Lane, Maryland Heights, MO 63043. Customer Service (orders, claims, online, change of address): Elsevier Health Sciences Division, Subscription **Customer Service, 3251 Riverport Lane, Maryland Heights, MO 63043. Tel: 1-800-654-2452 (U.S. and Canada); 314-447-8871 (outside U.S. and Canada). Fax: 314-447-8029. E-mail: journalscustomerservice-usa@elsevier.com (for print support); journalsonlinesupport-usa@elsevier.com (for online support).**

Reprints. For copies of 100 or more, of articles in this publication, please contact the Commercial Reprints Department, Elsevier Inc., 360 Park Avenue South, New York, New York 10010-1710; Tel.: 212-633-3874, Fax: 212-633-3820, E-mail: reprints@elsevier.com.

Hematology/Oncology Clinics of North America is covered in *MEDLINE/PubMed (Index Medicus), EMBASE/ Excerpta Medica, and BIOSIS.*

Printed in the United States of America.

Contributors

CONSULTING EDITORS

GEORGE P. CANELLOS, MD
William Rosenberg Professor of Medicine, Department of Medical Oncology, Dana-Farber Cancer Institute, Boston, Massachusetts, USA

H. FRANKLIN BUNN, MD
Professor of Medicine, Division of Hematology, Brigham and Women's Hospital, Harvard Medical School, Boston, Massachusetts, USA

EDITORS

RACHAEL F. GRACE, MD, MMSc
Department of Pediatric Hematology/Oncology, Dana-Farber/Boston Children's Cancer and Blood Disorders Center, Assistant Professor, Harvard Medical School, Boston, Massachusetts, USA

RUSSELL E. WARE, MD, PhD
Marjory Johnson Chair of Hematology Translational Research, Director, Division of Hematology, Cincinnati Children's Hospital Medical Center, Professor, University of Cincinnati College of Medicine, Cincinnati, Ohio, USA

AUTHORS

DENISE M. ADAMS, MD
Division of Hematology and Oncology, Vascular Anomalies Center, Boston Children's Hospital, Harvard Medical School, Boston, Massachusetts, USA

MARISOL BETENSKY, MD, MPH
Department of Pediatrics, Johns Hopkins School of Medicine, Baltimore, Maryland, USA; Pediatric Thrombosis Program, Johns Hopkins All Children's Cancer and Blood Disorder Institute, Johns Hopkins Medicine, St Petersburg, Florida, USA

GEORGE R. BUCHANAN, MD
Professor Emeritus of Pediatrics, Pediatric Hematology-Oncology, UT Southwestern Medical Center, Dallas, Texas, USA

MANUEL D. CARCAO, MD, MSc
Division of Haematology/Oncology, Department of Paediatrics, University of Toronto, Child Health Evaluative Sciences, Research Institute, The Hospital for Sick Children, Toronto, Canada

JAMES A. CONNELLY, MD
Assistant Professor, Pediatric Hematopoietic Stem Cell Transplant, Department of Pediatrics, Vanderbilt University Medical Center, Nashville, Tennessee, USA

JENNY M. DESPOTOVIC, DO
Associate Professor, Pediatric Hematology/Oncology, Baylor College of Medicine, Texas Children's Cancer and Hematology Center, Houston, Texas, USA

MYESA EMBERESH, MD
Hematology/Oncology Fellow, Cancer and Blood Diseases Institute, Cincinnati Children's Hospital Medical Center, Cincinnati, Ohio, USA

NEIL A. GOLDENBERG, MD, PhD
Departments of Pediatrics and Medicine, Division of Hematology, Johns Hopkins School of Medicine, Johns Hopkins Children's Center, Baltimore, Maryland, USA; Pediatric Thrombosis Program, Johns Hopkins All Children's Hospital, Johns Hopkins All Children's Cancer and Blood Disorder Institute, Johns Hopkins Medicine, St Petersburg, Florida, USA

CAROLYN HOPPE, MD
Associate Hematologist/Oncologist, Department of Pediatrics, Division of Hematology/Oncology, UCSF Benioff Children's Hospital Oakland, Oakland, California, USA

CYRIL JACQUOT, MD, PhD
Associate Medical Director for Blood Donor Center, Divisions of Laboratory Medicine and Hematology, Children's National Health System, Assistant Professor of Pediatrics and Pathology, George Washington University School of Medicine and Health Sciences, Washington, DC, USA

THEODOSIA A. KALFA, MD, PhD
Associate Professor and Co-director of the Erythrocyte Diagnostic Laboratory, Cancer and Blood Diseases Institute, Cincinnati Children's Hospital Medical Center, Department of Pediatrics, University of Cincinnati College of Medicine, Cincinnati, Ohio, USA

EUGENE KHANDROS, MD, PhD
Division of Hematology, Children's Hospital of Philadelphia, Department of Pediatrics, Perelman School of Medicine, University of Pennsylvania, Philadelphia, Pennsylvania, USA

TAYLOR OLMSTED KIM, MD
Instructor, Pediatric Hematology/Oncology, Baylor College of Medicine, Texas Children's Cancer and Hematology Center, Houston, Texas, USA

JANET L. KWIATKOWSKI, MD, MSCE
Director, Thalassemia Program, Division of Hematology, Children's Hospital of Philadelphia, Professor, Department of Pediatrics, Perelman School of Medicine, University of Pennsylvania, Philadelphia, Pennsylvania, USA

MICHELE P. LAMBERT, MD, MSTR
Associate Professor, Department of Pediatrics, Perelman School of Medicine, University of Pennsylvania, Clinical Director, Special Coagulation Laboratory, Associate Clinical Director, Frontier Program in Immune Dysregulation, Attending Physician, Division of Hematology, The Children's Hospital of Philadelphia, Philadelphia, Pennsylvania, USA

ENRICO LOPRIORE, MD, PhD
Department of Pediatrics, Division of Neonatology, Leiden University Medical Center, Leiden, Zuid-Holland, The Netherlands

NAOMI L.C. LUBAN, MD
Vice Chair of Academic Affairs, Medical Director of the Office of Human Subjects
Protection, Children's National Health System, Professor of Pediatrics and Pathology,
George Washington University School of Medicine and Health Sciences, Washington,
DC, USA

ARASH MAHAJERIN, MD, MSCr
CHOC Children's Specialists, Division of Hematology, Orange, California, USA

YUNCHUAN DELORES MO, MD, MSc
Associate Medical Director for Blood Bank, Divisions of Laboratory Medicine and
Hematology Children's National Health System, Assistant Professor of Pediatrics and
Pathology, George Washington University School of Medicine and Health Sciences,
Washington, DC, USA

LYNNE NEUMAYR, MD
Administrative Medical Director, Department of Pediatrics, Division of Hematology/
Oncology, UCSF Benioff Children's Hospital Oakland, Oakland, California, USA

SARAH H. O'BRIEN, MD
Division of Pediatric Hematology/Oncology, Nationwide Children's Hospital, The Ohio
State University College of Medicine, Center for Innovation in Pediatric Practice, The
Research Institute at Nationwide Children's Hospital, Columbus, Ohio, USA

MARIE-CLAUDE PELLAND-MARCOTTE, MD
Division of Haematology/Oncology, Department of Paediatrics, The Hospital for Sick
Children, University of Toronto, Toronto, Canada

JACQUELYN M. POWERS, MD, MS
Assistant Professor of Pediatrics, Section of Hematology-Oncology, Baylor College of
Medicine, Texas Children's Cancer and Hematology Centers, Houston, Texas, USA

ISABELLE M.C. REE, MD
Department of Pediatrics, Division of Neonatology, Leiden University Medical Center,
Leiden, Zuid-Holland, The Netherlands; Center for Clinical Transfusion Research,
Sanquin Research, Leiden, The Netherlands

KIERSTEN W. RICCI, MD
Division of Hematology, Hemangioma and Vascular Malformation Center, Cincinnati
Children's Hospital Medical Center, University of Cincinnati College of Medicine,
Cincinnati, Ohio, USA

MARY RISINGER, PhD
Assistant Professor, College of Nursing, University of Cincinnati, Cincinnati, Ohio, USA

SURBHI SAINI, MD
Division of Pediatric Hematology/Oncology, Penn State Health Children's Hospital, Penn
State College of Medicine, Hershey, Pennsylvania, USA

KELLY WALKOVICH, MD
Associate Professor, Pediatric Hematology/Oncology, Department of Pediatrics,
University of Michigan Medical School, Ann Arbor, Michigan, USA

Contents

> Beta thalassemias are a significant global health problem. Globin chain imbalance leads to a complex physiologic cascade of hemolytic anemia, ineffective erythropoiesis, and iron overload. Management of the broad spectrum of phenotypes requires the careful use of red blood transfusions, supportive care, monitoring, and management of iron overload. In this article, the authors discuss recommendations for monitoring of individuals with thalassemia, as well as ongoing preclinical and clinical trials of therapies targeting different aspects of thalassemia pathophysiology.

> Screening and early detection of organ injury, as well as expanded use of red cell transfusion and hydroxyurea in children have changed best practices for clinical care in sickle cell disease. The current standard of care for children with sickle cell disease is discussed through a review of screening recommendations, disease monitoring, and approach to treatment. Novel pharmacologic agents under investigation in clinical trials are also reviewed.

> Hereditary hemolytic anemias (HHAs) comprise a heterogeneous group of anemias caused by mutations in genes coding the globins, red blood cell (RBC) membrane proteins, and RBC enzymes. Congenital dyserythropoietic anemias (CDAs) are rare disorders of erythropoiesis characterized by binucleated and multinucleated erythroblasts in bone marrow. CDAs typically present with a hemolytic phenotype, as the produced RBCs have structural defects and decreased survival and should be considered in the differential of HHAs. This article discusses the clinical presentation, laboratory findings, and management considerations for rare HHAs arising from unstable hemoglobins, RBC hydration defects, the less common RBC enzymopathies, and CDAs.

> Iron deficiency anemia is the leading cause of anemia worldwide and affects many young children and adolescent girls in the United States.

Its signs and symptoms are subtle despite significant clinical effects. Iron deficiency anemia is diagnosed clinically by the presence of risk factors and microcytic anemia. Improvement following a trial of oral iron therapy is confirmative. An array of iron laboratory tests is available with variable indications. Clinical trial and iron absorption data support a shift to lower-dose oral iron therapy. Intravenous iron should be considered in children who fail oral iron or who have more complex disorders.

The mainstay of hemophilia management has been the regular, prophylactic infusion of missing coagulation factors VIII/IX. This approach is limited by the need for frequent intravenous infusions, high cost, limited availability, and the development of inhibitory antibodies to factors VIII/IX. Numerous recent breakthroughs are addressing many of these limitations. These include the development of extended half-life factors that require less frequent infusions and the development of various novel agents that can be given subcutaneously and infrequently, including FVIII-mimetic antibody and downregulators of natural anticoagulants. Finally, gene therapy is set to offer patients a possibility for a cure.

Advances in the use of standardized bleeding assessment tools, functional laboratory assays, and genetic testing have all improved the ability of hematologists to more accurately diagnose von Willebrand disease (VWD) in patients presenting with easy bruising or bleeding. This article reviews these recent advances, as well as currently available treatment options, including desmopressin, antifibrinolytics, and both plasma-based and recombinant von Willebrand factor products. The diagnosis of VWD remains complex and this article provides an understanding of the various subtypes and phenotypes of VWD, as well as the appropriateness and interpretation of the many available laboratory tests.

Pediatric venous thromboembolism (VTE) is increasing in incidence but minimal data exist for best practices regarding therapy, use of thrombophilia testing, and management of long-term complications. Classification schema use anatomic location and presence of clinical or thrombophilic inciting factors. There are a small number of risk-assessment and risk-modeling systems for incident VTE, but all suffer from low numbers, single-institution design, and lack of prospective validation. Acute treatment is limited to heparin products and thrombolysis may be indicated in specific situations. In addition, chronic postthrombotic comorbidities are expected to increase in incidence and lack evidence-based treatment paradigms.

Vascular anomalies consist of a diverse group of disorders that are broadly categorized as tumors and malformations. Recently, there has been significant genomic discovery allowing phenotype/genotype correlation of disease. An increasing number of pediatric hematologists/oncologists are caring for individuals with vascular anomalies as these patients require chronic care and have high medical acuity needs. The advent of new medical therapy options, along with ongoing and upcoming clinical trials, makes the involvement of hematologists/oncologists essential. This article highlights diagnosis and management of complicated vascular anomalies as well as important new treatment options and discoveries.

The inherited platelet disorders are a heterogeneous group of disorders that can be pleotropic in their clinical presentations. They may present with variable platelet counts and bleeding, making their diagnosis difficult. New diagnostic tools range from flow cytometric platelet function assessments to next-generation sequencing. Several platelet disorders may now be treated with gene therapy or bone marrow transplant. Improved understanding of the molecular and biologic mechanisms of the inherited platelet disorders may lead to novel targeted therapies.

This review summarizes the evaluation and management of the autoimmune cytopenias, a heterogeneous group of conditions including, but not limited to, autoimmune hemolytic anemia, immune thrombocytopenia, and multilineage disorders in Evans syndrome. These diseases can be challenging to treat and there are limited data comparing second-line therapeutics. The understanding of the molecular cause of these conditions is improving with the goal of advancing therapies and making them more targeted.

Blood transfusions are frequently lifesaving, but there is growing awareness of their associated infectious and noninfectious adverse events. Patient blood management advocates for judicious use of transfusions and considerations of alternatives to correct anemia or achieve hemostasis. Several transfusion practices, either already implemented or under investigation, aim to further improve the safety of transfusions. An enduring challenge in pediatric and neonatal transfusion practice is that studies typically focus on adults, and findings are extrapolated to younger patients. This article aims to summarize some of the newer developments in transfusion medicine with a focus on the neonatal and pediatric population.

> Anemia and thrombocytopenia occur frequently in preterm neonates. Anemia can be physiologic, but is mostly caused by iatrogenic blood sampling. Thrombocytopenia may be present at birth due to intrauterine disorders, but is most commonly detected after birth following bacterial infection. There is no consensus regarding optimal hemoglobin and platelet thresholds for transfusion. An increasing number of studies suggest that restrictive transfusion guidelines may be preferable to liberal guidelines. Better markers to assess the need of transfusions are needed as well as the implementation of effective preventive measures, such as delayed cord clamping and minimization of iatrogenic blood loss.

> Both profound neutropenia and functional phagocyte disorders render patients susceptible to recurrent, unusual, and/or life-threatening infections. Many disorders also have nonhematologic manifestations and a substantial risk of leukemogenesis. Diagnosis relies on clinical suspicion and interrogation of the complete blood count with differential/bone marrow examination coupled with immunologic and genetic analyses. Treatment of the quantitative neutrophil disorders depends on granulocyte colony-stimulating factor, whereas management of functional phagocyte disease is reliant on antimicrobials and/or targeted therapies. Hematopoietic stem cell transplant remains the only curative option for most disorders but is not used on a routine basis.

HEMATOLOGY/ONCOLOGY CLINICS OF NORTH AMERICA

SERIES OF RELATED INTEREST

Surgical Oncology Clinics of North America

THE CLINICS ARE AVAILABLE ONLINE!
Access your subscription at:
www.theclinics.com

Preface

Pediatric Hematology

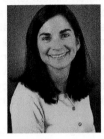
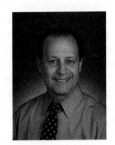

Rachael F. Grace MD, MMSc   Russell E. Ware, MD, PhD
Editors

This issue of *Hematology/Oncology Clinics of North America* focuses on Pediatric Hematology as an important and timely topic for the clinician and the researcher. The articles collectively provide an overview of many important hematologic conditions with an emphasis on recent developments in the diagnosis, monitoring, and novel approaches to treatment. We are in a new era for pediatric hematology that features accessible genetic and genomic diagnostics, unprecedented efforts toward targeted therapies, and expanded clinical trials.

The issue first focuses on erythrocyte disorders with articles from Kwiatkowski and Khandros and also from Hoppe and Neumayr, who together provide an overview of the current monitoring and treatment approaches for hemoglobinopathies, including fetal hemoglobin induction and strategies in gene therapy. Kalfa, Risinger, and Emberesh then provide a review of rare congenital hemolytic anemias, particularly focused on the modern approach to functional and genetic diagnostic testing and managing complications, including non-transfusion-related iron loading. Powers and Buchanan comprehensively report on disorders leading to iron deficiency with an updated approach to iron repletion.

The issue then concentrates on disorders of hemostasis and thrombosis. The article from Carcao and Pelland-Marcotte walks us through the changing approach to hemophilia, including the role of new extended half-life factor products, novel inhibitors of natural anticoagulants, and the promise of gene therapy. O'Brien and Saini then provide a timely update on the diagnosis, classification, and current management of von Willebrand disease. Goldenberg, Betensky, and Mahajerin share their practical approach to diagnosis and management of pediatric thrombosis, discussing the role of risk-assessment models and prophylaxis in high-risk children, as well as the types and length of treatment anticoagulation for children. In their article, Adams and Ricci explain the role of the hematologist/oncologist in the multidisciplinary team caring for patients with vascular anomalies, and they share an updated look at the diagnosis

Hematol Oncol Clin N Am 33 (2019) xiii–xiv
https://doi.org/10.1016/j.hoc.2019.02.001
0889-8588/19/© 2019 Published by Elsevier Inc.   hemonc.theclinics.com

and medical management of this increasing patient population. Lambert then provides an overview of the expanding phenotypic spectrum of patients with platelet disorders and the modern approach to diagnosis.

The topics shift next to cytopenias with Despotovic and Kim succinctly summarizing the manifestations and treatment of immune cytopenias in children, with emphasis on how elucidating the type of immune dysregulation in some children directs targeted treatment. Luban, Jacquot, and Mo then update the reader on new transfusion approaches and therapies in development, which aim to decrease the risks associated with transfusion products and practices. The issue then provides a timely update on hematologic problems in neonates, particularly focusing on optimal transfusion practices for these youngest patients, from Lopriore and Ree. The final article by Walkovich and Connelly focuses on the diagnosis and treatment of neutropenia and leukocyte disorders, including the expanding list of causative genes and the therapeutic role of growth factors and stem cell transplant.

An improved understanding of the phenotypic spectrum and diagnostic testing in pediatric hematologic disorders has led to more accurate diagnoses and helped to optimize management. The list of novel therapies is expanding at an exhilarating rate and will push practicing hematologists/oncologists to modify and refine their treatment approach. For many of these conditions, multiple treatment options will soon be available and, given the spectrum of patient phenotypes, individualized approaches will be necessary with shared decision making between informed clinicians and patients.

This issue provides an accurate, timely, and detailed view of the extraordinary advances in the diagnostic and treatment approach to hematologic conditions affecting children. We are indebted to the authors for their remarkable contributions to this issue.

Rachael F. Grace, MD, MMSc
Department of Pediatric Hematology/Oncology
Dana-Farber/Boston Children's Cancer and
Blood Disorders Center
Harvard Medical School
450 Brookline Avenue, Dana 3-106
Boston, MA 02215, USA

Russell E. Ware, MD, PhD
Division of Hematology
Cincinnati Children's Hospital Medical Center
University of Cincinnati College of Medicine
3333 Burnet Avenue, R3.3306
Cincinnati, OH 45229, USA

E-mail addresses:
Rachael.Grace@childrens.harvard.edu (R.F. Grace)
Russell.Ware@cchmc.org (R.E. Ware)

Beta Thalassemia
Monitoring and New Treatment Approaches

Eugene Khandros, MD, PhD[a,b], Janet L. Kwiatkowski, MD, MSCE[a,b,*]

KEYWORDS

- Beta thalassemia • Iron overload • Chelation • Gene therapy

KEY POINTS

- Individuals with thalassemia should be monitored for disease and treatment-related complications, adequacy and safety of transfusions, iron overload, and adverse effects of iron chelation.
- Ongoing preclinical and clinical trials target globin chain imbalance, fetal hemoglobin reactivation, signaling pathways in ineffective erythropoiesis, and mechanisms of iron overload.
- In this article, the authors discuss recommendations for monitoring of individuals with thalassemia, as well as ongoing preclinical and clinical trials of therapies targeting different aspects of thalassemia pathophysiology.

INTRODUCTION

Beta thalassemias represent a class of disorders with a high global prevalence and significant health and economic impact.[1] Since the elucidation of the molecular mechanism in the 1960s, there has been significant progress in treatment of disease complications. With increasing use of transfusion therapy, iron overload has become a pressing problem, and chelation therapy is a key component of treatment. The first part of this review focuses on monitoring of disease complications, transfusion therapy, iron overload, and chelator toxicity. In the second part, the authors review new developments in therapy for beta thalassemia.

BETA THALASSEMIA PATHOPHYSIOLOGY

Thalassemias are a class of disorders caused by imbalance of the alpha (α) and beta (β) globin chains that make up the principal adult oxygen transporter hemoglobin

Disclosure Statement: E. Khandros has nothing to disclose. J.L. Kwiatkowski has participated as a site investigator in studies sponsored by Novartis, Apopharma, bluebird bio, Agios, and Terumo BCT. She has consulted for bluebird bio, Agios, and Celgene.
[a] Division of Hematology, Children's Hospital of Philadelphia, 3401 Civic Center Boulevard, Colket Translational Research Building, Room 11024, Philadelphia, PA 19104, USA;
[b] Department of Pediatrics, Perelman School of Medicine of the University of Pennsylvania, Philadelphia, PA, USA
* Corresponding author. Division of Hematology, Children's Hospital of Philadelphia, 3401 Civic Center Boulevard, Colket Translational Research Building, Room 11024, Philadelphia, PA 19104.
E-mail address: kwiatkowski@email.chop.edu

Hematol Oncol Clin N Am 33 (2019) 339–353
https://doi.org/10.1016/j.hoc.2019.01.003
0889-8588/19/© 2019 Elsevier Inc. All rights reserved.

A ($\alpha_2\beta_2$). Beta thalassemias result from a relative excess of α chains due to reduced production of β globin chains and, in some instances, increased dosage of α globin genes.[2] In addition to reduced functional hemoglobin production, red blood cells (RBCs) and their precursors are damaged by α globin, which is unstable in the absence of a binding partner. Free α globin forms precipitates, leads to formation of reactive oxygen species, and damages RBC membranes leading to hemolysis and abnormal erythroid maturation. The beta thalassemia phenotype is determined by the degree of the imbalance and ranges from minimal effects in beta thalassemia trait to severe transfusion-dependent anemia.

Symptoms in beta thalassemia are due to a combination of anemia and ineffective erythropoiesis. Increased erythropoietin levels due to anemia drive erythroblast proliferation through JAK2-STAT5 signaling; additional RBC extrinsic and intrinsic factors have been implicated in this process and are reviewed elsewhere.[3] Complications of beta thalassemia are numerous and include growth failure, bone disease, cardiac abnormalities (pulmonary hypertension, heart failure, arrhythmias), predisposition to thrombosis, extramedullary hematopoiesis (splenomegaly, masses with compression), and a broad range of endocrinopathies.

BETA THALASSEMIA THERAPY

Beta thalassemias were previously classified as thalassemia major, thalassemia intermedia, and thalassemia minor (trait), but a more useful classification is one of transfusion-dependent thalassemia (TDT) or non-transfusion-dependent thalassemia (NTDT). The decision to initiate regular transfusions includes objective laboratory data as well as clinical findings. Transfusions are recommended if the steady-state hemoglobin level is less than 7 g/dL. Poor growth, the development of frontal bossing or maxillary hyperplasia or other symptoms of anemia and ineffective erythropoiesis, even in the absence of severe anemia, should prompt initiation of transfusions. The goals of regular RBC transfusion therapy are relief of anemia symptoms (allowing for normal growth) as well as suppression of endogenous ineffective erythropoiesis. This generally is accomplished by administering transfusions every 3 to 5 weeks to maintain the hemoglobin level greater than 9.5 g/dL before transfusion.[4]

IRON OVERLOAD AND CHELATION

Beta thalassemia is characterized by abnormal iron metabolism through increased erythroferrone production by erythroid precursors and downregulation of hepatic hepcidin production, resulting in increased iron absorption.[5,6] Patients with NTDT can develop iron overload even in the absence of transfusions through increased dietary absorption, whereas TDT patients invariably have more rapid iron loading because of the high content of iron within transfused cells. Iron deposition in the liver, heart, and endocrine organs causes the most significant morbidity. Heart disease, the leading cause of death from iron overload,[7] includes left ventricular dysfunction, heart failure, and arrhythmias. Iron deposition in endocrine organs causes hypothyroidism, hypoparathyroidism, growth failure, delayed puberty, and diabetes. Hepatic fibrosis, cirrhosis, and hepatocellular carcinoma related to cumulative iron exposure usually do not manifest until later in life. Monitoring and management of iron overload are therefore an essential part of thalassemia treatment.

Iron chelation therapy is administered with the goal of providing as much chelator exposure per 24-h period as possible to reduce the toxic effects of non-transferrin bound iron (NTBI). Three iron chelators are approved for use in the United States—deferoxamine, deferasirox, and deferiprone. Deferoxamine, the first approved agent, is administered by intravenous or subcutaneous infusion. Deferiprone and deferasirox are administered orally, and both have pediatric-friendly forms. Deferiprone is available in tablet and solution forms, with 3 times daily administration. Currently, it is approved as a second-line agent in the United States. Deferasirox, available as a dispersible tablet, film-coated tablet, and granule formulation, provides good chelation coverage with once daily dosing. Combination therapy may be beneficial for some patients with severe iron overload. The properties of iron chelators have been extensively reviewed elsewhere.[8]

Initiation of iron chelation in children is usually delayed until after age 2 years and when there is evidence of significant iron loading (10–20 transfusions, ferritin >1000 ng/mL and liver iron concentration >5–7 mg/g dry weight [dw]). This practice stems from concerns about growth delay and bone toxicity when deferoxamine was used in young children with low iron burden, which might not apply to the newer oral chelators. A recent pilot study assessed the earlier use of low-dose deferiprone in infants and toddlers with serum ferritin levels of 400 to less than 1000 ng/mL.[9] This approach delayed development of iron overload and reduced exposure to toxic labile plasma iron without unexpected, serious, or severe adverse effects. Larger confirmatory studies, and studies with deferasirox, are needed before routinely recommending earlier chelation initiation.

ALLOGENEIC STEM CELL TRANSPLANT

Correction of the underlying genetic defect through stem cell transplantation is currently the only curative therapy for beta thalassemia (reviewed elsewhere[10]). Unfortunately, access to this therapy is limited by the resources of the local medical system as well as by availability of optimal donors. In addition, the patients who benefit most are younger patients whose transfusion and chelation have been well managed and who have good organ function. Outcomes are better in younger patients (preferably under 14 years old), and predictors of increased transplant mortality have been described, including hepatomegaly, portal fibrosis, and history of inadequate iron chelation therapy.[11] A large part of transplant-associated toxicity is due to myeloablative conditioning regimens; as mixed donor-recipient chimerism can still produce transfusion independence, reduced intensity conditioning is currently being explored to improve outcomes.[12] Transplant outcomes are best with a fully HLA-matched related donor; cord blood from a matched related donor can also potentially provide good outcome in young patients.[13,14] HLA-matched unrelated donors are available for approximately 40% to 50% of patients of caucasian background, and although in past studies these patients had worse outcomes than with matched related donors, this has improved with better matching, donor cell processing, and graft versus host disease prophylaxis. Finally, HLA haploidentical parent donors are a more easily available option, but with higher risks of graft-versus-host disease, mortality, and graft failure, and currently should be used in clinical trial setting only. Therefore, it is important to carefully weigh the risks associated with the transplant versus the known complications of thalassemia.

MONITORING

Monitoring recommendations can be divided into several categories. Assessment for known complications of thalassemia due to anemia and ineffective erythropoiesis allows for appropriate decision-making regarding the need for and efficacy of transfusions (**Table 1**). For patients with TDT, monitoring is necessary to optimize transfusion therapy and to evaluate for infectious, immunologic, and iron-related complications of

Table 1
Routine monitoring for individuals with thalassemia

Test	Frequency of Monitoring
Alpha and beta globin genotyping	Once at diagnosis
High-resolution HLA typing	At diagnosis, when transplant is being considered
Growth parameters: height, truncal height, weight, head circumference, growth velocity	Every 3–6 mo[a]
Pain assessment	Every 3–6 mo
CBC with differential	Every 6 mo if no transfusions[b]
Comprehensive metabolic panel	Every 6 mo
Iron panel	Every 6 mo
Ferritin	Every 3 mo (monthly if on intensive chelation or low iron burden)
Echocardiogram and EKG	Annually starting at 10–14 y
Tanner staging and menstrual assessment	Every 6 months starting at 8–10 y.
TSH and free T_4	Annually starting at 6 y
FSH, LH, estradiol, prolactin (women) Testosterone (men)	Annually starting at 10 y
Vitamin D	Annually
PTH	Annually, starting at age 10 - 12 y
Bone density by DXA scan	Annually starting at 10 y
Fasting glucose, fructosamine	Annually starting at 10 y

Abbreviations: CBC, complete blood count; DXA, dual enegy x-ray absorptiometry; EKG, electrocardiogram; FSH, follicle-stimulating hormone; LH, luteinizing hormone; PTH, parathyroid hormone; TSH, thyrotropin; T4 thyroxine.

[a] Endocrine evaluation should be undertaken if there is a fall-off on the growth curve or decreased height velocity.

[b] At least monthly CBC should be performed in infants when determining if regular transfusions are indicated.

transfusion therapy (**Table 2**). Both TDT and NTDT patients must be routinely evaluated for degree of iron overload to guide the need for chelation, as well as to assess the efficacy of ongoing chelation therapy (**Table 3**). Finally, patients receiving chelation therapy must be assessed for known chelator toxicities (**Table 4**).

Monitoring for Complications of Thalassemia and Iron Overload

The clinical complications of thalassemia have been extensively outlined previously.[7,15] The first step is to determine whether a patient will need transfusions; a combination of molecular genotyping, serial hemoglobin levels, and close monitoring of growth parameters, symptoms of anemia, and signs of ineffective erythropoiesis are necessary to make this decision.

Growth and bone health

In pediatric patients, height, weight, head circumference, and growth velocity should be assessed at least annually, and ideally every 3 months. Truncal (sitting) height should be obtained in older children. Osteopenia and osteoporosis are common in TDT and NTDT, and develop early, with spine bone mineral density Z score less than –2 SD reported in 9% of 6 to 10 year olds and 44% of 11 to 19 year olds.[16] Annual dual energy x-ray absorptiometry scan is recommended beginning by age 10 years old.

Table 2 Monitoring of transfusions and related complications	
Test	**Frequency of Monitoring**
Red blood cell genotype/phenotype	Once at start of transfusions
Pre-transfusion CBC	Every 3–5 wk
Transfusion history assessment (volume transfused, presence of red cell antibody, IV access)	Every 3–5 wk
Hepatitis A, B, C serology (PCR as indicated) HIV testing	Annually

Abbreviations: CBC, complete blood count; HIV, human immunodeficiency virus; IV, intravenous; PCR, polymerase chain reaction.

Endocrine

Iron deposition in the pituitary, pancreas, and other endocrine organs leads to significant morbidity in TDT. The prevalence of hypothyroidism and hypoparathyroidism is about 10% and 2%, respectively.[17] Patients should undergo annual screening for thyroid function (thyrotropin and thyroxine), and 25-hydroxyvitamin D levels, and possibly also parathyroid hormone levels and urinary calcium. North American TDT patients have a 14% prevalence of diabetes mellitus.[17] At a minimum, patients should be screened annually for fasting levels of glucose and fructosamine (hemoglobin A1C is unreliable in transfused patients) beginning around adolescence. Several groups also recommend annual oral glucose tolerance tests. Hypogonadism is common, occurring in about 50% to 60% of patients with TDT.[17] Adolescent patients should be screened for onset of menarche and progression through puberty with careful history and Tanner staging every 6 months. Serum gonadotropins should be monitored annually for male and female adolescents. If abnormalities are detected, early referral to an endocrinologist is recommended.

Pain and quality of life

Pain is a frequent symptom in both TDT and NTDT, and negatively affects quality of life. In the Thalassemia Longitudinal Cohort, 69% of adolescents and adults and 56% of children reported pain over a 4-week period, most commonly in the back, knees, and head and neck.[18] Importantly, pain reports were similar in TDT and

Table 3 Monitoring for Iron overload		
Test	**Frequency of Monitoring**	**Starting Time**
Serum ferritin	Every 3 mo (TDT) Monthly for TDT with low iron burden or on aggressive chelation At least annually (NTDT)	With start of transfusions in TDT
Liver iron concentration by MRI	Annually in TDT Every 6 mo if LIC >10 mg/g dw	1–2 y after start of transfusions or at start of chelation in TDT[a] When ferritin level reaches 500 ng/mL in NTDT
Cardiac T2* MRI	Annually Every 6 mo if T2* <10 ms	By 10 y of age if appropriately chelated

[a] For young children, risks of sedation need to be weighed against the value of the information to be obtained. Initial MRI may be deferred if transfusion and chelation history are known and ferritin is well controlled.

Table 4	
Monitoring for adverse effects of iron chelation	
Test	**Frequency of Monitoring**
All chelators	
Visual acuity and dilated ophthalmology examination	Annually
Audiology examination	Annually
Vitamin C level	Annually
Zinc level	Annually
Deferasirox	
Urinalysis for proteinuria	Every 3 mo
Liver function testing	Every 2 wk × 2 after initiation, then monthly
Renal and tubular function—creatinine, potassium, phosphorus, bicarbonate	Monthly
Deferiprone	
Complete blood count with differential	Weekly
Liver function testing	Every 3 mo

NTDT. The cause of the pain is unclear but may be related to intramedullary or extra-medullary hematopoiesis or bone pathology. Patients should therefore be assessed for pain at all visits.

Monitoring Patients on Chronic Transfusions

Patients on chronic transfusions must be regularly assessed both to optimize trans-fusion therapy and to minimize transfusion risks. At initiation of transfusions, an RBC antigen profile (genotype or phenotype) should be obtained to facilitate appropriate RBC product choice and evaluation of any new RBC antibodies that develop. Allo-antibodies in patients with hemoglobinopathies are most commonly directed toward C, E, and Kell, and, at a minimum, these antigens should be matched beyond the typical ABO and RhD matching.[19] A goal pre-transfusion hemoglobin of 9.5 to 10.5 g/dL usually is recommended because this level suppresses ineffective erythro-poiesis[4] and relieves symptoms of anemia, allowing for normal growth. Typically this can be achieved with every 3- to 5-week transfusions. Higher pre-transfusion hemo-globin levels may be needed in the setting of heart disease or other complications. Patients should be asked about symptoms before transfusion to determine if a higher hemoglobin goal is appropriate. Pre-transfusion hemoglobin levels and vol-ume of RBCs administered should be routinely tracked to allow adjustment of trans-fusion regimens and assessment of iron loading. Unexpectedly low pre-transfusion hemoglobin levels may indicate a hemolytic transfusion reaction or hypersplenism. Although the rates of infection in modern blood-banking systems are low, patients should have annual testing for human immunodeficiency virus, hepatitis A, hepatitis B, and hepatitis C.

Iron Overload Monitoring

Monitoring of iron overload is an essential aspect of care and several different tests are used. Initial observational studies in TDT showed higher rates of complications and mortality in patients with severe iron overload, indicated by serum ferritin greater than 2500 ng/L or liver iron concentration (LIC) greater than 15 mg/g dw.[20,21] Although serum ferritin is a readily available and inexpensive test, it has multiple limitations. Ferritin provides a global reflection of iron stores and trends are helpful, but it does not correlate well with organ-specific iron deposition.[22,23] NTBI and labile plasma iron may provide alternative serum markers to ferritin but are not routinely available or fully validated. The LIC provides a reliable estimate of total body iron stores[24]; use of MRI techniques has generally replaced the more invasive liver biopsy. Cardiac iron estimation by MRI allows accurate prediction of risk of heart failure and arrhythmias.[25] Liver and cardiac iron imaging by MRI are the standard of care, although iron quantification in other organs is currently under investigation.

Spin echo (R2) and gradient echo (R2*) are the 2 most widely used validated MRI techniques for LIC. These methods report iron loading as mg iron per gram dry weight, as they are based on correlation curves with liver biopsy iron quantification. R2 and R2* measurements generally correlate well, but variability in quantification between methods exists and most validation has been done on LIC values less than 30 mg/g dw.[26,27] Although both methods have good accuracy and reproducibility, individual patients ideally should be monitored with the same method longitudinally.

Cardiac iron is typically measured with T2* images with electrocardiogram gating, and this technique is widely available and highly reproducible.[28–30] Results are usually presented in milliseconds, with T2* of greater than 20 ms being adequate. Mild cardiac iron overload is defined as T2* of 10 to 20 ms, and severe iron overload is less than 10 ms. In a large study, nearly half of patients with T2* less than 6 ms developed heart failure within 1 year.[25]

Guidelines for monitoring of iron overload are shown in **Table 3**. Serum ferritin should be assessed at least every 3 months in TDT, with more frequent monitoring in the setting of intensive chelation or with ferritin levels less than 1000 ng/mL to avoid overchelation. Most centers aim to keep the ferritin in a range of 500 to 1500 ng/mL in TDT. LIC should first be measured after 1 to 2 years of transfusions in TDT. For young children, the value of information gained from MRI should be weighed against the risks of sedation, and imaging may be deferred if the serum ferritin is in an appropriate range. Annual liver MRI is generally recommended; imaging every 6 months is useful in patients with high LIC undergoing aggressive chelation. Cardiac iron monitoring should begin by 10 years of age based on studies of timing of cardiac iron loading, but, as one study reported, 5% of 2- to 5.5-year-old children had T2* of less than 20 ms, an earlier start is reasonable, especially if chelation is inadequate or history unknown.[27,31] Cardiac MRI should then be monitored annually; high-risk patients should have T2* assessed every 6 months, whereas well-chelated, low-risk patients may have assessment spaced to every 2 years.

Monitoring for Complications of Chelator Therapy

Iron chelators have varying potential adverse effects, depending on the agent used. Patients receiving chelation should be regularly assessed for symptoms and laboratory signs of these toxicities to select the best chelator, reduce barriers to adherence, and minimize potential for irreversible damage (see **Table 4**). Iron chelation may cause ophthalmologic and audiologic adverse effects, including reduced visual acuity, impaired color vision, night blindness, tinnitus, and high-frequency sensorineural hearing loss.[32] These risks are greatest with deferoxamine, particularly when the chelator dose is high relative to the total body iron load.[32,33] Patients should be assessed for these symptoms at all visits and should undergo annual ophthalmology and audiology evaluations. Zinc deficiency can develop with any of the 3 chelators, and zinc levels should be checked annually. Iron overload can cause vitamin C deficiency, which adversely affects iron excretion and bone health so levels should be routinely checked.[34]

Patients on deferoxamine should be regularly assessed for adherence and any potential barriers, such as injection site reactions. Bone dysplasia and growth failure can occur in young children,[35] and all patients should be monitored for growth velocity.

Gastrointestinal side effects such as abdominal pain, emesis, and diarrhea occur in approximately 16% of pediatric patients receiving the dispersible tablet form of deferasirox and may limit adherence.[36] These adverse effects may be lessened with the newer film-coated tablet and granule forms, which do not contain lactose, which is thought to contribute to this effect. Renal side effects including elevated creatinine and proteinuria occur in 8.8%; renal Fanconi syndrome occurs less commonly.[36] Risk factors for renal complications include pre-existing kidney disease, dehydration, ferritin less than 1000 ng/mL, and concomitant use of nephrotoxic agents; more frequent monitoring of renal function and appropriate dose adjustment are recommended in these situations. Elevation of liver transaminases also can commonly occur. In one large 5-year study of deferasirox, 3.4% of patients had a serious adverse event, 21% of patients experienced an elevation in alanine aminotransferase, and 3.8% of patients had an elevation in creatinine.[37] All patients on deferasirox should have a monthly complete metabolic panel and urinalysis checked.

The most concerning adverse event of deferiprone is reversible agranulocytosis (absolute neutrophil count <500/µL), with an incidence of 0.2 to 0.43 per 100 patient-years, most commonly in the first year of therapy; milder, often reversible, neutropenia also occurs.[38–40] A complete blood count with differential should be assessed weekly to monitor for neutropenia/agranulocytosis. The drug should be held and a complete blood count with differential checked for all febrile illnesses. Elevation in serum alanine aminotransferase are reported in 2.8% to 10.4% of patients,[38–40] and this should be monitored every 3 months. Arthralgia and arthropathy also are common, occurring in 3.9% to 11.8% of patients and leading to drug discontinuation in 2% to 8.4%, so all patients should be asked about these symptoms.[38,39]

NEW THERAPEUTIC APPROACHES
Pharmacologic Fetal Hemoglobin Induction

Patients with NTDT may benefit from reactivation of gamma globin expression to produce fetal hemoglobin (HbF, $\alpha_2\gamma_2$) as a replacement for β globin and improve the α-/β-like globin chain imbalance. Hydroxyurea has established efficacy in sickle cell disease in part through induction of HbF through still poorly understood pathways, but no rigorous randomized trials have been done to assess its potential in beta thalassemia. Observational studies have demonstrated some benefit in TDT and NTDT.[41–43] Metformin is a well-tolerated US Food and Drug Administration-approved medication used for management of type 2 diabetes mellitus. Recent preclinical studies have demonstrated that metformin induces expression of fetal hemoglobin in primary erythroid cell cultures and is additive with hydroxyurea.[44] There is currently a phase I study of metformin in sickle cell disease and NTDT (NCT02981329) that includes children 12 years old and older.[45] Both hydroxyurea and metformin may be especially beneficial in resource-poor settings and further studies are warranted.

Gene Therapy

Beta globin replacement

The first human gene therapy trial for beta thalassemia was published in 2010.[46] Using a lentiviral vector expressing β globin with a T87Q mutation that mimics the anti-sickling properties of gamma globin (HPV569) in a patient with β_E/β_0 thalassemia, transfusion independence was achieved, but this study also demonstrated risks of potential integration-dependent clonal hematopoiesis. Subsequently, a phase 1/2 trial was carried out using the LentiGlobin BB305 vector, which was modified from the HPV569 vector. Following myeloablative conditioning with busulfan, BB305 transduced autologous hematopoietic stem cells were infused. The results of 22 treated patients ranging from 12 to 35 years old, with median follow-up of 26 months recently were published.[47] Of 13 patients with a non-β_0/β_0 genotype, 12 achieved transfusion independence with hemoglobin levels ranging from 8.2 to 13.7 g/dL. Of 9 patients with β_0/β_0 genotypes, 3 became transfusion-independent and the median annual transfusion volume decreased by 73% in the others. Importantly, the authors demonstrated good expression of vector-derived hemoglobin, no clonal predominance in patient hematopoiesis, no evidence of replication-competent virus production, and an adverse event profile no worse than that of routine myeloablative conditioning. Two phase III trials are currently enrolling patients, for TDT with non-β_0/β_0 genotypes (NCT02906202)[48] and with β_0/β_0 genotypes (NCT03207009).[49] Preliminary data from these studies were recently presented and of patients with at least 6 months of follow-up, 7 out of 8 treated with non-β_0/β_0 genotypes were able to stop transfusions.[50]

Preliminary data also were recently reported from another phase 1/2 trial using the GLOBE lentiviral vector expressing human β globin, with myeloablative conditioning, and intraosseus infusion of the modified hematopoietic stem cells.[51] Three adults and 4 children (age 6–13 years) were treated, with no adverse events beyond those expected from an autologous stem cell transplant and no evidence of clonal viral integrations. Outcomes for the pediatric patients were better, with 3 of 4 pediatric patients achieving transfusion independence; the adult patients had a reduction in transfusion requirements but still require transfusions. Enrollment is ongoing (NCT02453477).[52]

An additional phase I trial of a TNS9.3 lentiviral vector with wild-type human β globin following a reduced intensity conditioning regimen has also been initiated, but data are not yet available (NCT01639690).[53]

Fetal globin reactivation

Bcl11a is a recently discovered repressor of fetal hemoglobin that is being studied as a therapeutic target in beta thalassemia[54] as loss of Bcl11a activity leads to robust expression of HbF. Tissue-specific expression of Bcl11a is driven by an erythroid-specific upstream enhancer element.[55] Genetic targeting of this enhancer allows for disruption of Bcl11a specifically in erythroid cells. One approach uses a zinc-finger nuclease that is delivered by lentiviral transduction of stem cells and specifically disrupts the Bcl11a erythroid enhancer; a phase I/II study in adult patients with TDT is ongoing (NCT03432364).[56] Another approach utilizes CRISPR-Cas9 gene editing of the Bcl11a erythroid enhancer, which is being studied in a phase I/II study in adults with non-β_0/β_0 TDT (NCT03655678).[57]

Ineffective Erythropoiesis Signaling Modulators

Signaling molecules in the transforming growth factor beta family, such as BMP4, GDF11, and GDF15 contribute to ineffective erythropoiesis.[58,59] Luspatercept (ACE-536) and sotatercept (ACE-011) target this pathway by competing with the extracellular domain of the activin receptor for circulating ligand; both are produced as human IgG1 Fc domain fusions and are administered subcutaneously every 3 weeks. They were initially developed to treat osteoporosis in postmenopausal women but were found to transiently increase hemoglobin in a dose-dependent fashion.[60] These findings, as well as clinical safety, were confirmed for both drugs in phase I trials.[61,62] A phase II study of luspatercept (NCT01749540) in adults with beta thalassemia showed a reduction in transfusion burden in TDT patients (by one-third in 83% of patients), and a sustained hemoglobin increase of ≥ 1 g/dL in 50% of NTDT patients in the highest dose group.[63] A phase II study of sotatercept (NCT01571635) showed similar improvements in hemoglobin level and decreased transfusion burden in NTDT and TDT patients, respectively.[64] Luspatercept is being assessed in phase III studies in TDT (BELIEVE, NCT02604433) and phase II in NTDT (BEYOND, NCT03342404).[65,66] Recently presented preliminary data from the BELIEVE trial showed that 21.4% of patients receiving luspatercept achieved the primary endpoint of at least a 33% reduction in RBC transfusion compared to baseline over weeks 13 to 24 versus 4.5% of placebo-treated patients.[67]

Erythropoietin signaling through the Jak2 receptor and the STAT kinases is critical for erythroid precursor survival and maturation. Mice with beta thalassemia intermedia recapitulate ineffective erythropoiesis and have high levels of erythropoietin and activated Jak2 signaling.[68] Jak2 inhibition in this mouse model results in a decrease in spleen size.[69] A single-arm open-label phase IIa study of the Jak2 inhibitor, ruxolitinib, in 30 TDT patients with splenomegaly showed a decrease in spleen size and a modest decrease in transfusion requirements of 5.9% from baseline, and was overall well tolerated.[70] There are no current plans for phase III studies.

Targeting Hepcidin to Reduce Iron Overload

Hepcidin is a 25-amino acid peptide hormone that blocks iron absorption, recycling, and storage through downregulation of the cellular iron exporter ferroportin 1. Hepcidin is produced by the liver in response to inflammation and increased iron stores, and, in the case of thalassemia, is suppressed by erythroferrone produced by erythroid precursors. Ineffective erythropoiesis in thalassemia therefore leads to a state of low hepcidin and high iron absorption.[71] Increasing hepcidin expression ameliorates iron overload in a mouse model of beta thalassemia intermedia.[72] Phase I and II trials are currently ongoing for several classes of hepcidin-targeting drugs, including hepcidin mimetics (LJPC-401, La Jolla Pharmaceutical-NCT03395704[73]; PTG-300, Protagonist Therapeutics), agonists of the hepcidin regulator Tmprss6 (Ionis-TMPRSS6-LRx, Ionis Pharmaceuticals), and ferroportin inhibitors (VIT-2763, Vifor Pharma).

Reducing Cardiac Iron

Animal studies have suggested that iron enters cardiomyocytes through L-type calcium channels.[74] Amlodipine is a calcium channel blocker broadly used in adults and children, and a recent small phase III randomized trial examined whether addition of amlodipine to standard chelation therapy would reduce cardiac iron deposition.[75] This trial enrolled patients from 8 to 49 years old, with a mean age of 22.5 years. In subgroup analysis, patients with high cardiac iron burden had a greater 12-month reduction in cardiac iron with the addition of amlodipine (0.26 mg/g) versus standard therapy alone (0.01 mg/g). Although larger trials are needed for follow-up, this is a potentially promising use of a well-tolerated and studied medication.

SUMMARY

Advances in monitoring and treatment of children and adults with beta thalassemia have led to increased survival and decreased morbidity, but challenges still remain.

New therapies under investigation offer promise of improvements in current standards of care as well as revolutionary curative approaches.

REFERENCES

1. Weatherall DJ. The inherited diseases of hemoglobin are an emerging global health burden. Blood 2010;115(22):4331–6.
2. Mettananda S, Higgs DR. Molecular basis and genetic modifiers of thalassemia. Hematol Oncol Clin North Am 2018;32(2):177–91.
3. Gupta R, Musallam KM, Taher AT, et al. Ineffective erythropoiesis: anemia and iron overload. Hematol Oncol Clin North Am 2018;32(2):213–21.
4. Cazzola M, Borgna-Pignatti C, Locatelli F, et al. A moderate transfusion regimen may reduce iron loading in beta-thalassemia major without producing excessive expansion of erythropoiesis. Transfusion 1997;37(2):135–40.
5. Kautz L, Jung G, Valore EV, et al. Identification of erythroferrone as an erythroid regulator of iron metabolism. Nat Genet 2014;46(7):678–84.
6. Oikonomidou PR, Casu C, Rivella S. New strategies to target iron metabolism for the treatment of beta thalassemia. Ann N Y Acad Sci 2016;1368(1):162–8.
7. Borgna-Pignatti C, Cappellini MD, De Stefano P, et al. Survival and complications in thalassemia. Ann N Y Acad Sci 2005;1054:40–7.
8. Kwiatkowski JL. Current recommendations for chelation for transfusion-dependent thalassemia. Ann N Y Acad Sci 2016;1368(1):107–14.
9. Elalfy MS, Adly A, Awad H, et al. Safety and efficacy of early start of iron chelation therapy with deferiprone in young children newly diagnosed with transfusion-dependent thalassemia: a randomized controlled trial. Am J Hematol 2018; 93(2):262–8.
10. Strocchio L, Locatelli F. Hematopoietic stem cell transplantation in thalassemia. Hematol Oncol Clin North Am 2018;32(2):317–28.
11. Lucarelli G, Galimberti M, Polchi P, et al. Bone marrow transplantation in patients with thalassemia. N Engl J Med 1990;322(7):417–21.
12. Andreani M, Nesci S, Lucarelli G, et al. Long-term survival of ex-thalassemic patients with persistent mixed chimerism after bone marrow transplantation. Bone Marrow Transplant 2000;25(4):401–4.
13. Baronciani D, Angelucci E, Potschger U, et al. Hemopoietic stem cell transplantation in thalassemia: a report from the European Society for Blood and Bone Marrow Transplantation Hemoglobinopathy Registry, 2000-2010. Bone Marrow Transplant 2016;51(4):536–41.
14. Locatelli F, Kabbara N, Ruggeri A, et al. Outcome of patients with hemoglobinopathies given either cord blood or bone marrow transplantation from an HLA-identical sibling. Blood 2013;122(6):1072–8.
15. Marcon A, Motta I, Taher AT, et al. Clinical complications and their management. Hematol Oncol Clin North Am 2018;32(2):223–36.
16. Vogiatzi MG, Macklin EA, Fung EB, et al. Bone disease in thalassemia: a frequent and still unresolved problem. J Bone Miner Res 2009;24(3):543–57.
17. Vogiatzi MG, Macklin EA, Trachtenberg FL, et al. Differences in the prevalence of growth, endocrine and vitamin D abnormalities among the various thalassaemia syndromes in North America. Br J Haematol 2009;146(5):546–56.
18. Trachtenberg F, Foote D, Martin M, et al. Pain as an emergent issue in thalassemia. Am J Hematol 2010;85(5):367–70.

19. Vichinsky E, Neumayr L, Trimble S, et al. Transfusion complications in thalassemia patients: a report from the Centers for Disease Control and Prevention. Transfusion 2014;54(4):972–81.

20. Olivieri NF, Nathan DG, MacMillan JH, et al. Survival in medically treated patients with homozygous beta-thalassemia. N Engl J Med 1994;331(9):574–8.

21. Telfer PT, Prestcott E, Holden S, et al. Hepatic iron concentration combined with long-term monitoring of serum ferritin to predict complications of iron overload in thalassaemia major. Br J Haematol 2000;110(4):971–7.

22. Porter JB, Elalfy M, Taher A, et al. Limitations of serum ferritin to predict liver iron concentration responses to deferasirox therapy in patients with transfusion-dependent thalassaemia. Eur J Haematol 2017;98(3):280–8.

23. Puliyel M, Sposto R, Berdoukas VA, et al. Ferritin trends do not predict changes in total body iron in patients with transfusional iron overload. Am J Hematol 2014; 89(4):391–4.

24. Angelucci E, Brittenham GM, McLaren CE, et al. Hepatic iron concentration and total body iron stores in thalassemia major. N Engl J Med 2000;343(5):327–31.

25. Kirk P, Roughton M, Porter JB, et al. Cardiac T2* magnetic resonance for prediction of cardiac complications in thalassemia major. Circulation 2009;120(20): 1961–8.

26. Garbowski MW, Carpenter J-P, Smith G, et al. Biopsy-based calibration of T2* magnetic resonance for estimation of liver iron concentration and comparison with R2 Ferriscan. J Cardiovasc Magn Reson 2014;16:40.

27. Wood JC. Estimating tissue iron burden: current status and future prospects. Br J Haematol 2015;170(1):15–28.

28. Anderson LJ, Holden S, Davis B, et al. Cardiovascular T2-star (T2*) magnetic resonance for the early diagnosis of myocardial iron overload. Eur Heart J 2001;22(23):2171–9.

29. Kirk P, He T, Anderson LJ, et al. International reproducibility of single breathhold T2* MR for cardiac and liver iron assessment among five thalassemia centers. J Magn Reson Imaging 2010;32(2):315–9.

30. Westwood MA, Firmin DN, Gildo M, et al. Intercentre reproducibility of magnetic resonance T2* measurements of myocardial iron in thalassaemia. Int J Cardiovasc Imaging 2005;21(5):531–8.

31. Berdoukas V, Nord A, Carson S, et al. Tissue iron evaluation in chronically transfused children shows significant levels of iron loading at a very young age. Am J Hematol 2013;88(11):E283–5.

32. Botzenhardt S, Li N, Chan EW, et al. Safety profiles of iron chelators in young patients with haemoglobinopathies. Eur J Haematol 2017;98(3):198–217.

33. Olivieri NF, Buncic JR, Chew E, et al. Visual and auditory neurotoxicity in patients receiving subcutaneous deferoxamine infusions. N Engl J Med 1986;314(14): 869–73.

34. Elalfy MS, Saber MM, Adly AAM, et al. Role of vitamin C as an adjuvant therapy to different iron chelators in young β-thalassemia major patients: efficacy and safety in relation to tissue iron overload. Eur J Haematol 2016;96(3):318–26.

35. De Sanctis V, Pinamonti A, Di Palma A, et al. Growth and development in thalassaemia major patients with severe bone lesions due to desferrioxamine. Eur J Pediatr 1996;155(5):368–72.

36. Cappellini MD, Bejaoui M, Agaoglu L, et al. Iron chelation with deferasirox in adult and pediatric patients with thalassemia major: efficacy and safety during 5 years' follow-up. Blood 2011;118(4):884–93.

37. Vichinsky E, El-Beshlawy A, Al Zoebie A, et al. Long-term safety and efficacy of deferasirox in young pediatric patients with transfusional hemosiderosis: results from a 5-year observational study (ENTRUST). Pediatr Blood Cancer 2017; 64(9). https://doi.org/10.1002/pbc.26507.
38. Botzenhardt S, Felisi M, Bonifazi D, et al. Long-term safety of deferiprone treatment in children from the Mediterranean region with beta-thalassemia major: the DEEP-3 multi-center observational safety study. Haematologica 2018; 103(1):e1–4.
39. Ceci A, Baiardi P, Felisi M, et al. The safety and effectiveness of deferiprone in a large-scale, 3-year study in Italian patients. Br J Haematol 2002;118(1):330–6.
40. Cohen AR, Galanello R, Piga A, et al. Safety and effectiveness of long-term therapy with the oral iron chelator deferiprone. Blood 2003;102(5):1583–7.
41. Algiraigri AH, Wright NAM, Paolucci EO, et al. Hydroxyurea for nontransfusion-dependent β-thalassemia: a systematic review and meta-analysis. HematoL Oncol Stem Cell Ther 2017;10(3):116–25.
42. Algiraigri AH, Wright NAM, Paolucci EO, et al. Hydroxyurea for lifelong transfusion-dependent β-thalassemia: a meta-analysis. Pediatr Hematol Oncol 2017;34(8):435–48.
43. Foong WC, Ho JJ, Loh CK, et al. Hydroxyurea for reducing blood transfusion in non-transfusion dependent beta thalassaemias. Cochrane Database Syst Rev 2016;(10):CD011579.
44. Zhang Y, Paikari A, Sumazin P, et al. Metformin induces FOXO3-dependent fetal hemoglobin production in human primary erythroid cells. Blood 2018;132(3): 321–33.
45. NCT02981329: fetal hemoglobin induction treatment metformin (FITMet). 2018. Available at: https://clinicaltrials.gov/ct2/show/NCT02981329. Accessed October 15, 2018.
46. Cavazzana-Calvo M, Payen E, Negre O, et al. Transfusion independence and HMGA2 activation after gene therapy of human β-thalassaemia. Nature 2010; 467(7313):318–22.
47. Thompson AA, Walters MC, Kwiatkowski J, et al. Gene therapy in patients with transfusion-dependent β-thalassemia. N Engl J Med 2018;378(16):1479–93.
48. NCT02906202: a study evaluating the efficacy and safety of the LentiGlobin® BB305 drug product in subjects with transfusion-dependent β-thalassemia, who do not have a β0/β0 genotype. 2018. Available at: https://clinicaltrials.gov/ct2/show/NCT02906202. Accessed October 15, 2018.
49. NCT03207009: a study evaluating the efficacy and safety of the LentiGlobin® BB305 drug product in subjects with transfusion-dependent β-thalassemia, who have a β0/β0 genotype. 2018. Available at: https://clinicaltrials.gov/ct2/show/NCT03207009. Accessed October 15, 2018.
50. Locatelli F, Walters MC, Kwiatkowski JL, et al. Lentiglobin gene therapy for patients with transfusion-dependent β-thalassemia (TDT): results from the phase 3 Northstar-2 and Northstar-3 Studies. Blood 2018;132:1025a.
51. Marktel S, Cicalese MP, Giglio F, et al. Gene therapy for beta thalassemia: preliminary results from the phase I/II Tiget-Bthal trial of autologous hematopoietic stem cells genetically modified with GLOBE lentiviral vector. Blood 2017;130(Suppl 1):355.
52. NCT02453477: gene therapy for transfusion dependent beta-thalassemia (TIGET-BTHAL). 2018. Available at: https://clinicaltrials.gov/ct2/show/NCT02453477. Accessed October 15, 2018.
53. NCT01639690: β-thalassemia major with autologous CD34+ hematopoietic progenitor cells transduced with TNS9.3.55 a Lentiviral vector encoding the normal

human β-globin gene. 2018. Available at: https://clinicaltrials.gov/ct2/show/NCT01639690. Accessed October 15, 2018.

54. Sankaran VG, Menne TF, Xu J, et al. Human fetal hemoglobin expression is regulated by the developmental stage-specific repressor BCL11A. Science 2008;322(5909):1839–42.

55. Bauer DE, Kamran SC, Lessard S, et al. An erythroid enhancer of BCL11A subject to genetic variation determines fetal hemoglobin level. Science 2013;342(6155):253–7.

56. NCT03432364: a study to assess the safety, tolerability, and efficacy of ST-400 for treatment of transfusion-dependent beta-thalassemia (TDT). 2018. Available at: https://clinicaltrials.gov/ct2/show/NCT03432364. Accessed October 15, 2018.

57. NCT03655678: a safety and efficacy study evaluating CTX001 in subjects with transfusion-dependent β-thalassemia. 2018. Available at: https://clinicaltrials.gov/ct2/show/NCT03655678. . Accessed October 15, 2018.

58. Dussiot M, Maciel TT, Fricot AE, et al. An activin receptor IIA ligand trap corrects ineffective erythropoiesis in beta-thalassemia. Nat Med 2014;20(4):398–407.

59. Suragani RNVS, Cadena SM, Cawley SM, et al. Transforming growth factor beta superfamily ligand trap ACE-536 corrects anemia by promoting late-stage erythropoiesis. Nat Med 2014;20(4):408–14.

60. Ruckle J, Jacobs M, Kramer W, et al. Single-dose, randomized, double-blind, placebo-controlled study of ACE-011 (ActRIIA-IgG1) in postmenopausal women. J Bone Miner Res 2009;24(4):744–52.

61. Attie KM, Allison MJ, McClure T, et al. A phase 1 study of ACE-536, a regulator of erythroid differentiation, in healthy volunteers. Am J Hematol 2014;89(7):766–70.

62. Sherman ML, Borgstein NG, Mook L, et al. Multiple-dose, safety, pharmacokinetic, and pharmacodynamic study of sotatercept (ActRIIA-IgG1), a novel erythropoietic agent, in healthy postmenopausal women. J Clin Pharmacol 2013;53(11):1121–30.

63. Piga A, Perrotta S, Gamberini MR, et al. Luspatercept (ACE-536) reduces disease burden, including anemia, iron overload, and leg ulcers, in adults with beta-thalassemia: results from a phase 2 study. Blood 2015;126(23):752.

64. Cappellini MD, Porter J, Origa R, et al. Sotatercept, a novel transforming growth factor beta ligand trap, improves anemia in beta-thalassemia: a phase 2, open-label, dose-finding study. Haematologica 2018. https://doi.org/10.3324/haematol.2018.198887.

65. NCT03342404: a study to determine the efficacy and safety of luspatercept in adults with non transfusion dependent beta (β)-thalassemia (BEYOND). 2018. Available at: https://clinicaltrials.gov/ct2/show/NCT03342404. Accessed October 15, 2018.

66. NCT02604433: an efficacy and safety study of luspatercept (ACE-536) versus placebo in adults who require regular red blood cell transfusions due to beta (β) thalassemia (BELIEVE). 2018. Available at: https://clinicaltrials.gov/ct2/show/NCT02604433. Accessed October 15, 2018.

67. Cappellini MD, Viprakasit V, Taher A, et al. The believe trial: results of a phase 3, randomized, double-blind, placebo-controlled study of luspatercept in adult beta-thalassemia patients who require regular red blood cell (RBC) transfusions. Blood 2018;132:163a.

68. Libani IV, Guy EC, Melchiori L, et al. Decreased differentiation of erythroid cells exacerbates ineffective erythropoiesis in beta-thalassemia. Blood 2008;112(3):875–85.

69. Casu C, Presti VL, Oikonomidou PR, et al. Short-term administration of JAK2 inhibitors reduces splenomegaly in mouse models of β-thalassemia intermedia and major. Haematologica 2018;103(2):e46–9.

70. Taher AT, Karakas Z, Cassinerio E, et al. Efficacy and safety of ruxolitinib in regularly transfused patients with thalassemia: results from a phase 2a study. Blood 2018;131(2):263–5.

71. Casu C, Nemeth E, Rivella S. Hepcidin agonists as therapeutic tools. Blood 2018; 131(16):1790–4.

72. Gardenghi S, Ramos P, Marongiu MF, et al. Hepcidin as a therapeutic tool to limit iron overload and improve anemia in β-thalassemic mice. J Clin Invest 2010; 120(12):4466–77.

73. NCT03395704: a study of LJPC-401 for the treatment of iron overload in adult patients with hereditary hemochromatosis. 2018. Available at: https://clinicaltrials. gov/ct2/show/NCT03395704. Accessed October 15, 2018.

74. Oudit GY, Sun H, Trivieri MG, et al. L-type Ca2+ channels provide a major pathway for iron entry into cardiomyocytes in iron-overload cardiomyopathy. Nat Med 2003;9(9):1187–94.

75. Fernandes JL, Loggetto SR, Verissimo MPA, et al. A randomized trial of amlodipine in addition to standard chelation therapy in patients with thalassemia major. Blood 2016;128(12):1555–61.

Sickle Cell Disease
Monitoring, Current Treatment, and Therapeutics Under Development

Carolyn Hoppe, MD*, Lynne Neumayr, MD

KEYWORDS

- Sickle cell disease • Treatment • Screening • Hydroxyurea • Novel therapeutics

KEY POINTS

- Sickle cell disease is an inherited blood disorder associated with significant morbidity and early mortality.
- Improved survival and quality of life possible with newborn screening and comprehensive care, including penicillin prophylaxis, immunization, education and access to subspecialists; disease-modifying and curative therapies; and clinical research trials.
- Novel pharmacologic agents in development are discussed.

INTRODUCTION

Sickle cell disease (SCD) is a complex, clinically heterogeneous disorder affecting approximately 100,000 individuals in the United States and millions worldwide. The disease is characterized by progressive vascular injury that develops in response to ongoing hemolytic anemia, vasoocclusion, and subsequent ischemia–reperfusion injury. Subclinical ischemic events beginning in early childhood may not be recognized until organ dysfunction or permanent tissue damage has occurred later in life. Specialized comprehensive care, including regular screening assessments and monitoring for disease manifestations, is required from identification by newborn screening through adulthood.

Disclosure Statement: C. Hoppe has consultancies with Bioverativ, Novartis, and Imarais; and is on an Advisory Board for Global Blood Therapeutics. She wrote the article while a faculty member at UCSF Benioff Children's Hospital Oakland, but after the submission, she became an employee at Global Blood Therapeutics Inc. L. Neumayr worked as a consultant for CTD Holdings, and Pfizer; is currently on a DSMB for Apopharma; is a site Principal Investigator for Pfizer, Micelle Biopharma, and PCORI; a co-investigator for Novartis, Bluebird Bio, Sangamo, Global Blood Therapeutics, Silarus, Celgene, and Imara. She also is an investigator on NIHLBI, FDA, HRSA and CDC grants.
Department of Pediatrics, Division of Hematology/Oncology, UCSF Benioff Children's Hospital Oakland, 747 52nd Street, Oakland, CA 94609, USA
* Corresponding author.
E-mail addresses: CHoppe@mail.cho.org; choppe@gbt.com; choppe1230@gmail.com

Hematol Oncol Clin N Am 33 (2019) 355–371
https://doi.org/10.1016/j.hoc.2019.01.014
0889-8588/19/© 2019 Elsevier Inc. All rights reserved.
hemonc.theclinics.com

The recommendations for screening and monitoring in SCD modified from the National Heart, Lung, and Blood Institute consensus panel and are shown in **Table 1** and **Box 1**.[1]

SCREENING FOR SICKLE CELL DISEASE-RELATED DISEASE MANIFESTATIONS
Cerebrovascular Disease

Primary stroke prevention

Overt stroke occurs in up to 11% of children with SCD by age 18% and 24% by age 45.[11] The reported incidence of pediatric stroke ranges from 1.2 to 13.0 cases per 100,000 and is up to 300 times higher than in the general population (**Box 2**).[12]

Transcranial Doppler (TCD) measurements of blood flow velocities in the major cerebral arteries are predictors of stroke risk in HbSS/HbSB^0 at ages 2 to 16.[3] Chronic red cell transfusions (CRT) aimed at decreasing the percent hemoglobin S to less than 30% normalizes TCD velocities in approximately 80% and reduces the risk of primary stroke by 90%.[14] Children withdrawn from CRT after 30 months had higher primary stroke rates.[15] Hydroxyurea (HU) can decrease TCD velocities,[16,17] and the TWITCH trial demonstrated that young children at risk for stroke whose TCDs normalized on CRT could be gradually weaned off of CRT onto HU with stable TCD velocities.[18]

The recommended follow-up and management of TCD[19,20] screening results are shown in **Fig. 1**.

Secondary stroke prevention

CRT decreases the risk of stroke recurrence from 67% to 20%.[14,21–24] HU does not provide the same level of protection for secondary stroke prevention (**Box 3**).[25,26]

Silent cerebral infarcts

Silent cerebral infarcts occur in up to 39% of children with SCD and 43% of adults,[4,29–32] and are associated with neurocognitive deficits[33–35] and increased risk for overt strokes (**Box 4**).[36]

Pulmonary Disease

Asthma is common in SCD[40–43] and is associated with a higher incidence of acute chest syndrome,[44–46] vasoocclusive episodes (VOE), and mortality (**Box 5**).[47–50] Common underlying pathophysiology includes dysregulation of arginine metabolism and nitric oxide.[7,51]

Cardiac Disease

Pulmonary hypertension, defined as a mean pulmonary artery pressure estimated by tricuspid regurgitant jet velocity of 2.5 m/s or greater on Doppler echocardiogram, occurs in more than 30% of adults with SCD and is associated with an increased risk of mortality.[54,55] Estimates of pulmonary hypertension from an echocardiogram may have low positive predictive value compared with right heart catheterization.[56] Pulmonary hypertension is associated with diastolic dysfunction, but both are independent predictors of mortality in adults and are seen less frequently in children (**Box 6**).[57–60] Ischemic heart disease, left ventricular dysfunction, and congestive heart failure are associated with mortality in adults with SCD.[61]

Renal Disease

Sickle cell nephropathy includes hyposthenuria, proteinuria, episodic hematuria and papillary necrosis, renal tubular disorders, glomerulonephropathy, acute renal injury,

Table 1
Novel agents currently in clinical trials

Category	Agent/NCT ID	Mechanism of Action[a]	Phase	Primary Outcome
Inhibits sickling	Voxelotor (GBT440) NCT03036813	Allosteric modulation of Hb S shifts oxyHb curve to left	3	≥1 g/dL increase in Hb level VOE
	NCT02850406		2	Safety and PK in children
Augments Hb F	IMR-687 NCT03401112	PDE-9 inhibitor, upregulates cGMP	2	Dose-finding and safety in adults with SCA
Inhibits cellular adhesion	Crizanlizumab (SELG101B22) NCT03474965	Humanized monoclonal antibody blocks P-selectin	2	Dosing and safety in children with SCD
	Rivipansel (GMI-1070) NCT02187003	Pan-selectin inhibitor	3	Time to readiness for hospital discharge in children with SCA
Inhibits Platelet Aggregation	Ticagrelor HESTIA3 NCT03615924	P2Y12 ADP receptor antagonist	3	Reduction in rate of VOC in children with SCA
Oxidative injury	Altemia NCT02604368	Omega 3-FA Docosahexaenoic acid; stabilizes RBC membrane	3	Annualized rate of sickle cell crisis
NO modulation	IW-1701 Olinciguat NCT03285178	Stimulates soluble guanylate cyclase > restores NO bioavailability	2	Safety and preliminary efficacy in adults with SCD
	Riociguat NCT02633397		2	Safety and preliminary efficacy in adults with SCD

Abbreviations: Hb, hemoglobin; oxyHb, oxyhemoglobin; NO, nitric oxide; PDE-9, phosphodiesterase 9; PK, pharmacokinetics; RBC, red blood cells; SCA, sickle cell anemia; VOE, vasoocclusive episode.
[a] Some agents have multiple mechanisms of action.

Box 1
Screening and monitoring in sickle cell disease

- Comprehensive health maintenance at specialized centers that provide multidisciplinary care using standard guidelines. The frequency of visits depends on education needs, access to primary health care, medication toxicity monitoring, and disease complications.
  ○ Preventive measures
    ■ Antibiotic prophylaxis for prevention of invasive bacterial disease in functionally asplenic patients until at least age 5.[2]
    ■ Folic acid supplementation if diet inadequate.
    ■ Genetic counseling.
    ■ Immunization according to the Centers for Disease Control and Prevention's Advisory Committee on Immunization Practices.
    ■ Education about complications of sickle cell disease: bacteremia, splenic and hepatic sequestration, stroke, priapism, cholelithiasis, avascular necrosis, cardiac dysfunction, retinopathy, nephropathy, symptoms of asthma, obstructive sleep apnea, transition, and treatment options.
  ○ Regular monitoring and periodic comprehensive evaluations for common complications.
    ■ Complete blood count, reticulocyte count, and red blood cell phenotype by age 9 months to provide phenotypically matched transfusions.
    ■ Frequency of visits and laboratory monitoring depends on the genotype, medication, and disease severity.
    ■ Hydroxyurea monitoring visits with a complete blood count, reticulocyte count, and quantitative fetal hemoglobin levels every 2 to 3 months.
    ■ Monthly complete blood count, reticulocyte count, percent hemoglobin S, CMP, and ferritin for patients on chronic transfusion and chelation.
    ■ Monitor vitamin D levels and supplement if <30 IU.
    ■ Blood pressure measurement each visit.
    ■ Transcranial Doppler annually at age 2 through 16 to evaluate stroke risk.[3]
    ■ Annual urinalysis and urine albumin/creatinine ratio after age 10 years.
    ■ Screening MRI to evaluate silent cerebral infarct and cerebral vascular disease at least once at age 10 (without general anesthesia).[4]
    ■ Neurocognitive testing if imaging abnormalities, or school or work performance difficulties.[5]
    ■ Ophthalmology evaluation for retinopathy at age 10 and biannually if normal.
    ■ Echocardiogram to evaluate pulmonary hypertension and diastolic dysfunction at least once at age 10 and 6-minute walk and brain natriuretic peptide if any symptoms of pulmonary hypertension.[6]
    ■ Pulmonary function studies if history, signs, or symptoms of asthma or other respiratory disease.[7]
    ■ Sleep study if history of snoring or other symptoms of obstructive sleep apnea.
    ■ Evaluate bone density at age 10, nutrition consult and reevaluation if abnormal.[8,9]
    ■ Radiographic evaluation of hips to assess femoral avascular necrosis if pain in hips, knees or low back. Avascular necrosis also seen in shoulder and knees.
    ■ Transition screening.
  ○ Follow age-specific guidelines from the US Preventive Service Task Force.[10]

Abbreviation: CMP - complete metabolic panel.

Box 2
Risk factors for stroke

- Elevated cerebral blood flow velocity by transcranial Doppler.[3]
- Obstructive sleep apnea and nocturnal hypoxemia.
- Silent cerebral infarctions.
- Hypertension.
- Patent foramen ovale.[13]
- Atrial fibrillation.

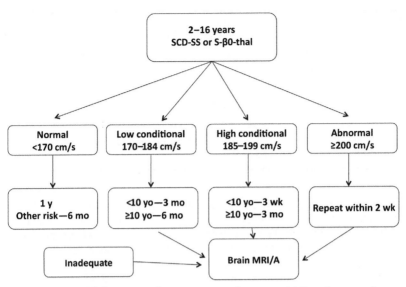

Fig. 1. Recommended follow-up and management of transcranial Doppler screening results. (*Courtesy of* J.L. Kwiatkowski, MD, MSCE, Philadelphia, PA.)

segmental glomerulosclerosis, chronic kidney disease, and chronic renal failure.[64] Sickle cell nephropathy is more common in HbSS than in HbSC genotypes, and contributes to mortality in adults (**Box 7**).[65–72]

CURRENT TREATMENT

Current disease-modifying therapies for SCD remain limited to HU, red blood cell transfusion, stem cell transplantation in selected patients, and, recently, glutamine.[74–77]

Hydroxyurea

HU remains the most effective disease-modifying therapy for SCD and is now approved for use in both children and adults. The clinical efficacy and safety of HU has been repeatedly demonstrated,[18,78] and its indications have extended to very young children in the hopes of preventing acute and chronic complications.[78–82]

Box 3
Secondary stroke prevention

- Continue chronic red cell transfusions[15,21] with pretransfusion percent hemoglobin S goal of less than 30% and posttransfusion hemoglobin goal of 9 g/dL or greater.[27] Red blood cell exchange may prevent iron overload.

- Consider daily low-dose aspirin in patients if there is no evidence of Moya Moya or hemorrhagic risk.

- Neurosurgical evaluation for encephaloduroarteriosynangiosis in patients with severe cerebral vasculopathy.[28]

- Assess for headache and obstructive sleep apnea.

> **Box 4**
> **Screening and management of silent cerebral infarcts**
>
> - Baseline cerebral MRI/magnetic resonance angiography at age 10 (without sedation).[35]
> - Neurocognitive testing for any child with difficulties in school, abnormal transcranial Doppler, or MRI.
> - Evaluation and follow-up by a neurologist.
> - Hydroxyurea prophylaxis to decrease white blood cell count and increase total hemoglobin.
> - Offer chronic red cell transfusions to reduce risk for progressive silent cerebral infarcts,[36–39] neurocognitive dysfunction, and stroke.

Although there are lingering concerns about the long-term risks of HU, particularly its effects on fertility and reproduction, results from the multicenter clinical trial of fixed dose HU in children 9 to 18 months of age demonstrated safety and efficacy in reducing SCD-related complications. HU is now recommended for all children with SCD ages 9 months and older, independent of disease severity. In older children, dose intensification of HU is associated with improved clinical and laboratory parameters compared with fixed lower dosing. A study evaluating the added clinical benefit from HU dose intensification in young children 9 to 36 months is now planned (HUG-KISS NCT03020615). HU has not been studied systematically in individuals with HbSC; a clinical efficacy trial in this patient population is now being planned (**Box 8**).

Hydroxyurea Dose Escalation

The laboratory and clinical effects of HU are dose dependent, with greatest benefit shown with dose escalation to the maximum tolerated dose (MTD), defined as an absolute neutrophil count of 1.5 to 3.0×10^9/L, that is, mild neutropenia without an associated risk of infection. At the MTD, the majority of patients with SCD exhibit an increase from baseline in total hemoglobin concentration, as well as the percent fetal hemoglobin. An increase in the mean corpuscular volume is observed; if the patient has S/β^0 thalassemia or a coinherited alpha thalassemia trait, the increase will be relative to the baseline mean corpuscular volume.

> **Box 5**
> **Screening and management of asthma in sickle cell disease**
>
> - Identify history of wheezing, shortness of breath, nighttime cough, and frequent upper respiratory infections.
> - Family history of allergy, asthma, or atopic dermatitis.
> - Identify triggers including allergies, chronic rhinosinusitis, obstructive sleep apnea, and gastroesophageal reflux.
> - Prior documented episodes of acute chest syndrome.
> - Pulmonary function tests at age 8 or older, peak expiratory flow rate in the office or at home; repeat annually if abnormal or clinically symptomatic; periodic screening to monitor for restrictive changes.[52]
>   - Refer to pulmonologist if symptomatic or abnormal pulmonary function tests.
>   - Treat following using multidisciplinary approach and National Institutes of Health guidelines (NIH 08-0451).[53]
>   - Patient education and Asthma Action Plans.

Box 6
Guidelines for diagnosis and treatment of pulmonary hypertension and diastolic dysfunction

- Screening echocardiogram at age 10 and every 2 to 5 years, if normal.
- Evaluate tricuspid regurgitant jet velocity, diastolic dysfunction (mitral valve E/A velocity and lateral left ventricular E/e' ratios) and left ventricular function.[62]
- Evaluate right ventricular function with tricuspid annular plane systolic excursion.
- For repeated measures of tricuspid regurgitant jet velocity of 3.0 m/s or greater at clinical baseline:
  - Obtain a 6-minute walk test, pulmonary function tests, and NT-proBNP.[6]
  - Evaluate for obstructive sleep apnea, hepatic dysfunction, and chronic kidney disease.
  - Refer to cardiologist for right heart catheterization.
  - Tailor treatment modalities to hemodynamic findings on right heart catheterization.[63]
  - Maximize hydroxyurea dose.
  - Consider chronic transfusion.

A standard protocol to safely escalate to the MTD is recommended for patients with SCD.[1] To achieve the MTD, start at 15 mg/kg/d and increase by increments of approximately 5 mg/kg/d every 4 to 8 weeks until a maximum dose of 30 to 35 mg/kg/d or the MTD is achieved (up to a maximum dose of 30–35 mg/kg/d).

Box 7
Guidelines for the prevention, diagnosis, and management of renal disease

- Increase hydration, especially during exercise.
- Limit use of nonsteroidal antiinflammatory medications: ketorolac for only 5 days during vasoocclusive episodes.
- Monitor blood pressure and hemoglobin at all visits.
- Annual urine analysis and urine microalbuminuria/creatinine ratio starting at age 10; if positive, obtain first morning void urine albumin/creatinine ratio.
- If either microalbuminuria or macroalbuminuria is present, obtain a 24-hour urine collection for protein.
- Treat microalbuminuria or macroalbuminuria with an angiotensin-converting enzyme inhibitor; monitor blood pressure and potassium; estimate the glomerular filtration rate and stage of chronic kidney disease.
- Consult a nephrologist for hypertension, proteinuria, a creatinine of greater than 0.7 mg/dL in children and greater than 1.0 mg/dL in adults.
- Gross or microscopic hematuria: obtain a renal ultrasound examination to diagnose papillary necrosis. Hematuria is usually self-limited; treat with hydration, pain relief, and consider antibiotics.
- Consider medullary renal cell carcinoma in the setting of hematuria, flank or abdominal pain, abdominal mass, and symptoms of metastatic disease. Obtain a computed tomography scan.[73]
- Maximize hydroxyurea treatment.
- Rule out other causes of proteinuria and hematuria.
- Erythropoietin may be beneficial in early chronic kidney disease, especially in combination with hydroxyurea.
- Dialysis.
- Transplantation.

> **Box 8**
> **Hydroxyurea indications (clinical and preventive)**
>
> - All children with sickle cell disease (SS or S/β^0 thal) age 9 months or older regardless of disease severity.[1]
> - Clinical symptoms: dactylitis or pain crises, acute chest syndrome, hemolytic crisis requiring transfusion.
> - Conditional transcranial Doppler imaging.
> - Parent preference for primary stroke prevention after transcranial Doppler normalization with chronic transfusion.
> - Parent preference for management of silent cerebral infarct (offer hydroxyurea vs chronic red cell transfusions).
> - Secondary stroke prevention to augment goals of chronic red cell transfusions in patients with significant anemic, progressive vasculopathy with chronic red cell transfusions.
> - Patients where chronic red cell transfusions is not an option: lack of intravenous access, rare blood types, alloimmunization, or severe iron overload.
> - Organ protection and modification of disease complications in adults.

Because of the large interpatient variability in drug exposure, individual dose escalation requires frequent laboratory monitoring, and it can take up to 6 to 12 months to reach a stable maintenance dose. A novel precision dosing strategy that incorporates Bayesian methods to analyze pharmacokinetic measurements and inform patient-specific dosing may overcome the current challenges to achieving MTD.[83,84] This precision dosing approach is being evaluated prospectively.[85]

Hydroxyurea toxicity

The most commonly reported side effects of HU are mild gastrointestinal upset, darkening of the skin or nail beds, and rarely thinning of the hair. An National Institutes of Health Consensus Conference in 2008 found no convincing evidence of increased cancer (**Box 9**).

A new formulation of HU, SIKLOS (100 mg tab), was recently approved by the US Food and Drug Administration (FDA) for the treatment of children with SCD. The main advantage is greater dosing flexibility in children ages 2 years and older.

Glutamine

Glutamine is an amino acid involved in nitrogen transport and as a precursor for the synthesis of glutathione, nicotinamide adenine dinucleotide, and arginine; is theorized to protect sickled red blood cells from oxidative damage. The FDA approved glutamine in 2017 for patients ages 5 years and older with SCD based on findings from a randomized, placebo-controlled, multicenter, phase 3 trial showing small but statistically significant reductions and hospitalizations in acute sickle cell crises.[86] Glutamine is administered orally twice daily in a powder form. There is no information about the optimal dose or specific laboratory monitoring. Continued clarity regarding cost and availability is also needed. Limited safety data and concerns about potential toxicity in patients with hepatic or renal impairment suggest cautious use in this subgroup until more robust safety data become available.[87]

Transfusion Therapy

Indications for acute transfusion therapy in SCD include prophylactic transfusion for surgeries involving general anesthesia with a preoperative hemoglobin goal of

---

Box 9
Hydroxyurea laboratory monitoring

- Baseline: complete blood count/differential (absolute neutrophil count), reticulocyte count, hemoglobin electrophoresis (high-performance liquid chromatography), creatinine, and liver function tests (ALT, bilirubin).

- Baseline percent fetal hemoglobin to monitor adherence and laboratory benefit.

- Monthly toxicity laboratory tests: complete blood count with differential.
  - Hold if the absolute neutrophil count is less than $1 \times 10^9/L$ or the platelet count is less than 100,000.
  - Reduce dose if the absolute neutrophil count is 1 to $1.5 \times 10^9/L$ or the platelet count id less than 150,000.
  - Restart at a lower dose once recovered.

- Once maximum tolerated dose is reached, follow every 2 to 3 months and assess for compliance and toxicity (complete blood count with differential, mean corpuscular volume, creatinine, ALT, reticulocyte count).

- Efficacy assessed by reviewing history (crisis, admissions, and blood transfusions), mean corpuscular volume, white blood cell about, reticulocyte count, bilirubin, lactate dehydrogenase, and measure percent fetal hemoglobin at least twice yearly until % fetal hemoglobin level stable (then measure as needed).

10.0 g/dL in HbSS/Sβ^0.[88] Patients with high baseline hemoglobin levels (HbSC/SB+) may require exchange transfusion. Acute complications that benefit from transfusion include stroke, acute chest syndrome, splenic sequestration, and other SCD-related complications (**Boxes 10 and 11**).

NOVEL PHARMACOLOGIC AGENTS UNDER INVESTIGATION

HU and glutamine are the only FDA-approved drugs for the treatment of SCD. However, these therapies do not completely prevent progression of SCD to a chronic disease.

Legislation to incentivize global drug development in orphan diseases and in children has facilitated the clinical development of novel therapies for SCD. Several investigational agents with different mechanisms of action have been advanced from preclinical studies to multicenter clinical trials.

Box 10
Indications for chronic red cell transfusions

- Abnormal transcranial Doppler (primary stroke prevention).[1]

- Overt stroke (secondary stroke prevention).[1]

- Silent cerebral infarcts (in children whose transcranial Doppler velocities have normalized), chronic red cell transfusions may decrease the risk of silent cerebral infarcts.[18]

- No treatment duration threshold has been established for stopping transfusions for primary or secondary stroke prevention.

- Switching to hydroxyurea with phlebotomy may increase the risk of silent cerebral infarcts and sickle cell disease-related serious adverse events in secondary stroke prevention.[26]

- Other sickle cell disease-related complications (eg, recurrent acute chest syndrome or vasoocclusive episodes).

Box 11
Chronic red cell transfusion monitoring

- Hyperviscosity – avoid hemoglobin levels of greater than 10 g/dL unless the percent hemoglobin S is already low.
- Alloimmunization – red blood cell phenotype before the start of transfusion, monthly screening for alloantibodies.
- Extended phenotypically matched blood (D, Cc, Ee, Kell, Kidd, and Duffy).
- Complete blood count, reticulocyte count, percent hemoglobin S, type and screen before each transfusion.
- Screen for transfusion transmitted infections (hepatitis/human immunodeficiency virus) annually.
- Monitor for central venous catheter-associated thrombosis and infection if symptomatic.
- Iron overload and chelation toxicity monitoring.
  ◦ Initiate chelation when evidence of iron overload.
  ◦ Monthly serum ferritin, renal and hepatic function.
  ◦ Annual audiology and ophthalmology screenings.
  ◦ Measurement of hepatic iron loading and extrahepatic iron deposition in severely iron overloaded patients (ferritin, MRI liver R2 or ferritometer [SQUID] for liver iron deposition and concentration, cardiac MRI T2* for cardiac iron deposition).

Abbreviation: SQUID - Superconducting Quantum Interference Device.

Inhibition of Hemoglobin S Polymerization

Voxelotor (GBT440) is an allosteric modifier of hemoglobin oxygen affinity that, when bound to hemoglobin S, inhibits polymerization and red blood cell sickling. In phase 1/2 studies, once daily oral voxelotor was safe and well-tolerated, resulted in increased hemoglobin levels from baseline and improvement in markers of hemolysis.

The Hemoglobin Oxygen Affinity Modulation to Inhibit Hb S Polymerization (HOPE) study is an ongoing phase 3 randomized, double-blind, placebo-controlled, multi-center study evaluating the efficacy and safety of voxelotor in adults and children with SCD (NCT03036813).[89,90]

Induction of Fetal Hemoglobin

Increasing cGMP with HU or a phosphodiesterase 9 inhibitor is known to increase fetal hemoglobin levels,[91–94] which generally correlate with reduced disease severity in patients with SCD.[69,95,96] IMR-687 is a potent, specific, and highly selective small molecule phosphodiesterase 9 inhibitor that increases cGMP levels and stimulates the production of fetal hemoglobin. IMR-687 increases cGMP via a different mechanism and may be an adjunct to HU, improving outcomes without added toxicity. In preclinical studies, IMR-687 also reduced white blood cell adhesion to the endothelium. The safety, tolerability, pharmacokinetics, pharmacodynamics, and clinical outcomes of IMR-687 are now being evaluated in a phase 2a trial in adults.

Inhibition of Cellular Adhesion

Crizanlizumab (SELG101B22)

Crizanlizumab (SelG1) is a humanized monoclonal antibody that inhibits endothelial adhesion molecules (vascular cell adhesion molecule 1, intercellular cell adhesion molecule 1) and abrogates hypoxia-induced vasoocclusion through P-selectin blockade. In a phase 2, multicenter, placebo-controlled randomized study (SUSTAIN) in adults with SCD, monthly intravenous administration was well-tolerated and demonstrated a dose-dependent decrease in the frequency of VOE and a delay in time to first VOE compared with placebo.[97] A phase 2, open-label dosing study in children is underway.

Rivipansel

Rivipansel (GMI-1070) is a synthetic glycomimetic molecule pan-selectin inhibitor designed to prevent adhesion between red cells and circulating monocytes and neutrophils. A phase 2 trial demonstrating a decrease in time to resolution of vaso-occlusive crisis (VOC) and intravenous opioid use after intravenous administration in hospitalized patients prompted the current multicenter phase 3 trial, "Evaluating Safety, Efficacy and Time to Discharge" or RESET trial (NCT02187003).

Restoration of Bioavailable Nitric Oxide

Olinciguat (Ironwood Pharmaceuticals [Cambridge, MA] IW-1701) is an oral investigational agent that binds to and stimulates soluble guanylate cyclase, and can thereby restore the bioavailability of nitric oxide to improve blood flow and perhaps prevent hemolysis of sickle red blood cells. Based on phase 1 data, olinciguat was recently granted FDA orphan drug status and is currently being evaluated in a phase 2 double-blind, placebo-controlled, dose-ranging study in patients with SCD ages 16 to 70: the STRONG-SCD clinical trial (NCT03285178).

Riociguat has a similar mechanism to olinciguat, and a phase 2 multicenter, randomized, double-blind, placebo-controlled, parallel group study is underway to evaluate its safety, tolerability, and efficacy in patients with SCD.

Inhibition of Platelet Aggregation

Therapies targeting platelet activation and interaction with inflammatory cells may represent another therapeutic avenue to prevent inflammation in SCD.

A randomized phase 3 trial of the platelet P2Y12 ADP receptor antagonist, prasugrel, failed to reach its end point in decreasing the incidence of VOE in children with SCD. Ticagrelor, another platelet P2Y12 ADP receptor antagonist, is currently being evaluated for safety and efficacy in a phase 2 trial in adults and children with SCA: the HESTIA 2 trial (NCT02482298).

Antioxidants

Red blood cell membrane abnormalities observed in patients with SCD include a dysfunctional lipid bilayer with perturbation of the fatty acid composition of membrane phospholipids that is associated with blood cell adhesion, aggregation, blood coagulation and inflammation.[98,99] SC411 (Altemia) is a highly purified docosahexaenoic acid ethyl ester formulation using advanced lipid technologies. The SCOT trial was a phase 2 randomized, double-blind, placebo-controlled, parallel-group, dose-finding study of SC411 in children (NCT02604368). Blood cell membrane, docosahexaenoic acid and eicosapentaenoic acid levels, and adhesion markers E-selectin and D-dimer were significantly reduced. Home analgesic use for sickle cell pain and trends in rates of VOE and hospitalization were reduced. A phase 3 pivotal study is planned.

REFERENCES

1. Yawn BP, Buchanan GR, Afenyi-Annan AN, et al. Management of sickle cell disease: summary of the 2014 evidence-based report by expert panel members. JAMA 2014;312(10):1033–48.

2. Gaston MH, Verter JI, Woods G, et al. Prophylaxis with oral penicillin in children with sickle cell anemia. A randomized trial. N Engl J Med 1986;314(25):1593–9.

3. Adams R, McKie V, Nichols F, et al. The use of transcranial ultrasonography to predict stroke in sickle cell disease. N Engl J Med 1992;326(9):605–10.

4. DeBaun MR, Armstrong FD, McKinstry RC, et al. Silent cerebral infarcts: a review on a prevalent and progressive cause of neurologic injury in sickle cell anemia. Blood 2012;119(20):4587–96.

5. Daly B, Kral MC, Tarazi RA. The role of neuropsychological evaluation in pediatric sickle cell disease. Clin Neuropsychol 2011;25(6):903–25.

6. Klings ES, Machado RF, Barst RJ, et al. An official American Thoracic Society clinical practice guideline: diagnosis, risk stratification, and management of pulmonary hypertension of sickle cell disease. Am J Respir Crit Care Med 2014; 189(6):727–40.

7. Morris CR. Asthma management: reinventing the wheel in sickle cell disease. Am J Hematol 2009;84(4):234–41.

8. Adams-Graves P, Daniels AB, Womack CR, et al. Bone mineral density patterns in vitamin D deficient African American men with sickle cell disease. Am J Med Sci 2014;347(4):262–6.

9. Lal A, Fung EB, Pakbaz Z, et al. Bone mineral density in children with sickle cell anemia. Pediatr Blood Cancer 2006;47(7):901–6.

10. Melnyk BM, Grossman DC, Chou R, et al. USPSTF perspective on evidence-based preventive recommendations for children. Pediatrics 2012;130(2): e399–407.

11. Ohene-Frempong K, Weiner SJ, Sleeper LA, et al. Cerebrovascular accidents in sickle cell disease: rates and risk factors. Blood 1998;91(1):288–94.

12. Tsze DS, Valente JH. Pediatric stroke: a review. Emerg Med Int 2011;2011: 734506.

13. Dowling MM, Quinn CT, Ramaciotti C, et al. Increased prevalence of potential right-to-left shunting in children with sickle cell anaemia and stroke. Br J Haematol 2017;176(2):300–8.

14. Adams RJ, McKie VC, Hsu L, et al. Prevention of a first stroke by transfusions in children with sickle cell anemia and abnormal results on transcranial Doppler ultrasonography. N Engl J Med 1998;339(1):5–11.

15. Adams RJ, Brambilla D. Optimizing primary stroke prevention in sickle cell anemia trial I. Discontinuing prophylactic transfusions used to prevent stroke in sickle cell disease. N Engl J Med 2005;353(26):2769–78.

16. Thornburg CD, Dixon N, Burgett S, et al. A pilot study of hydroxyurea to prevent chronic organ damage in young children with sickle cell anemia. Pediatr Blood Cancer 2009;52(5):609–15.

17. Zimmerman SA, Schultz WH, Burgett S, et al. Hydroxyurea therapy lowers transcranial Doppler flow velocities in children with sickle cell anemia. Blood 2007; 110(3):1043–7.

18. Ware RE, Davis BR, Schultz WH, et al. Hydroxycarbamide versus chronic transfusion for maintenance of transcranial doppler flow velocities in children with sickle cell anaemia-TCD With Transfusions Changing to Hydroxyurea (TWiTCH): a multicentre, open-label, phase 3, non-inferiority trial. Lancet 2016;387(10019): 661–70.

19. McCarville MB, Goodin GS, Fortner G, et al. Evaluation of a comprehensive transcranial doppler screening program for children with sickle cell anemia. Pediatr Blood Cancer 2008;50(4):818–21.

20. Platt OS. Prevention and management of stroke in sickle cell anemia. Hematology Am Soc Hematol Educ Program 2006;54–7.
21. Fortin PM, Hopewell S, Estcourt LJ. Red blood cell transfusion to treat or prevent complications in sickle cell disease: an overview of Cochrane reviews. Cochrane Database Syst Rev 2018;(8):CD012082.
22. Hulbert ML, McKinstry RC, Lacey JL, et al. Silent cerebral infarcts occur despite regular blood transfusion therapy after first strokes in children with sickle cell disease. Blood 2011;117(3):772–9.
23. Powars D, Wilson B, Imbus C, et al. The natural history of stroke in sickle cell disease. Am J Med 1978;65(3):461–71.
24. Scothorn DJ, Price C, Schwartz D, et al. Risk of recurrent stroke in children with sickle cell disease receiving blood transfusion therapy for at least five years after initial stroke. J Pediatr 2002;140(3):348–54.
25. Estcourt LJ, Fortin PM, Hopewell S, et al. Interventions for preventing silent cerebral infarcts in people with sickle cell disease. Cochrane Database Syst Rev 2017;(5):CD012389.
26. Ware RE, Helms RW, Investigators SW. Stroke with transfusions changing to hydroxyurea (SWiTCH). Blood 2012;119(17):3925–32.
27. Sarode R, Ballas SK, Garcia A, et al. Red blood cell exchange: 2015 American Society for Apheresis consensus conference on the management of patients with sickle cell disease. J Clin Apher 2017;32(5):342–67.
28. Yang W, Xu R, Porras JL, et al. Effectiveness of surgical revascularization for stroke prevention in pediatric patients with sickle cell disease and moyamoya syndrome. J Neurosurg Pediatr 2017;20(3):232–8.
29. Bernaudin F, Verlhac S, Arnaud C, et al. Chronic and acute anemia and extracranial internal carotid stenosis are risk factors for silent cerebral infarcts in sickle cell anemia. Blood 2015;125(10):1653–61.
30. DeBaun MR, Sarnaik SA, Rodeghier MJ, et al. Associated risk factors for silent cerebral infarcts in sickle cell anemia: low baseline hemoglobin, sex, and relative high systolic blood pressure. Blood 2012;119(16):3684–90.
31. Jordan LC, Kassim AA, Donahue MJ, et al. Silent infarct is a risk factor for infarct recurrence in adults with sickle cell anemia. Neurology 2018;91(8):e781–4.
32. Rigano P, Pecoraro A, Calvaruso G, et al. Cerebrovascular events in sickle cell-beta thalassemia treated with hydroxyurea: a single center prospective survey in adult Italians. Am J Hematol 2013;88(11):E261–4.
33. Armstrong FD, Thompson RJ Jr, Wang W, et al. Cognitive functioning and brain magnetic resonance imaging in children with sickle Cell disease. Neuropsychology Committee of the Cooperative Study of sickle cell disease. Pediatrics 1996;97(6 Pt 1):864–70.
34. Bernaudin F, Verlhac S, Freard F, et al. Multicenter prospective study of children with sickle cell disease: radiographic and psychometric correlation. J Child Neurol 2000;15(5):333–43.
35. DeBaun MR, Kirkham FJ. Central nervous system complications and management in sickle cell disease. Blood 2016;127(7):829–38.
36. Miller ST, Macklin EA, Pegelow CH, et al. Silent infarction as a risk factor for overt stroke in children with sickle cell anemia: a report from the Cooperative Study of sickle cell disease. J Pediatr 2001;139(3):385–90.
37. Abboud MR, Jackson SM, Barredo J, et al. Neurologic complications following bone marrow transplantation for sickle cell disease. Bone Marrow Transplant 1996;17(3):405–7.

38. DeBaun MR, Rodeghier M, Cohen R, et al. Factors predicting future ACS episodes in children with sickle cell anemia. Am J Hematol 2014;89(11):E212–7.

39. Wang WC, Wynn LW, Rogers ZR, et al. A two-year pilot trial of hydroxyurea in very young children with sickle-cell anemia. J Pediatr 2001;139(6):790–6.

40. Koumbourlis AC, Zar HJ, Hurlet-Jensen A, et al. Prevalence and reversibility of lower airway obstruction in children with sickle cell disease. J Pediatr 2001; 138(2):188–92.

41. Leong MA, Dampier C, Varlotta L, et al. Airway hyperreactivity in children with sickle cell disease. J Pediatr 1997;131(2):278–83.

42. Ozbek OY, Malbora B, Sen N, et al. Airway hyperreactivity detected by methacholine challenge in children with sickle cell disease. Pediatr Pulmonol 2007; 42(12):1187–92.

43. Strunk RC, Brown MS, Boyd JH, et al. Methacholine challenge in children with sickle cell disease: a case series. Pediatr Pulmonol 2008;43(9):924–9.

44. Knight-Madden JM, Forrester TS, Lewis NA, et al. Asthma in children with sickle cell disease and its association with acute chest syndrome. Thorax 2005;60(3): 206–10.

45. Nordness ME, Lynn J, Zacharisen MC, et al. Asthma is a risk factor for acute chest syndrome and cerebral vascular accidents in children with sickle cell disease. Clin Mol Allergy 2005;3(1):2.

46. Sylvester KP, Patey RA, Broughton S, et al. Temporal relationship of asthma to acute chest syndrome in sickle cell disease. Pediatr Pulmonol 2007;42(2):103–6.

47. An P, Barron-Casella EA, Strunk RC, et al. Elevation of IgE in children with sickle cell disease is associated with doctor diagnosis of asthma and increased morbidity. J Allergy Clin Immunol 2011;127(6):1440–6.

48. Boyd JH, Macklin EA, Strunk RC, et al. Asthma is associated with acute chest syndrome and pain in children with sickle cell anemia. Blood 2006;108(9): 2923–7.

49. Boyd JH, Macklin EA, Strunk RC, et al. Asthma is associated with increased mortality in individuals with sickle cell anemia. Haematologica 2007;92(8):1115–8.

50. Strunk RC, Cohen RT, Cooper BP, et al. Wheezing symptoms and parental asthma are associated with a physician diagnosis of asthma in children with sickle cell anemia. J Pediatr 2014;164(4):821–6.e1.

51. Field JJ, DeBaun MR. Asthma and sickle cell disease: two distinct diseases or part of the same process? Hematology Am Soc Hematol Educ Program 2009;45–53. https://doi.org/10.1182/asheducation-2009.1.45.

52. Lunt A, McGhee E, Sylvester K, et al. Longitudinal assessment of lung function in children with sickle cell disease. Pediatr Pulmonol 2016;51(7):717–23.

53. McClain BL, Ivy ZK, Bryant V, et al. Improved guideline adherence with integrated sickle cell disease and asthma care. Am J Prev Med 2016;51(1 Suppl 1):S62–8.

54. Gladwin MT, Sachdev V, Jison ML, et al. Pulmonary hypertension as a risk factor for death in patients with sickle cell disease. N Engl J Med 2004;350(9):886–95.

55. Mehari A, Gladwin MT, Tian X, et al. Mortality in adults with sickle cell disease and pulmonary hypertension. JAMA 2012;307(12):1254–6.

56. Parent F, Bachir D, Inamo J, et al. A hemodynamic study of pulmonary hypertension in sickle cell disease. N Engl J Med 2011;365(1):44–53.

57. Gladwin MT. Cardiovascular complications and risk of death in sickle-cell disease. Lancet 2016;387(10037):2565–74.

58. Caldas MC, Meira ZA, Barbosa MM. Evaluation of 107 patients with sickle cell anemia through tissue Doppler and myocardial performance index. J Am Soc Echocardiogr 2008;21(10):1163–7.

59. Hankins JS, McCarville MB, Hillenbrand CM, et al. Ventricular diastolic dysfunction in sickle cell anemia is common but not associated with myocardial iron deposition. Pediatr Blood Cancer 2010;55(3):495–500.

60. Niss O, Quinn CT, Lane A, et al. Cardiomyopathy with restrictive physiology in sickle cell disease. JACC Cardiovasc Imaging 2016;9(3):243–52.

61. Fitzhugh CD, Lauder N, Jonassaint JC, et al. Cardiopulmonary complications leading to premature deaths in adult patients with sickle cell disease. Am J Hematol 2010;85(1):36–40.

62. Mitter SS, Shah SJ, Thomas JD. A test in context: E/A and E/e' to assess diastolic dysfunction and LV filling pressure. J Am Coll Cardiol 2017;69(11):1451–64.

63. Ataga KI, Klings ES. Pulmonary hypertension in sickle cell disease: diagnosis and management. Hematology Am Soc Hematol Educ Program 2014;2014(1):425–31.

64. Guasch A, Navarrete J, Nass K, et al. Glomerular involvement in adults with sickle cell hemoglobinopathies: prevalence and clinical correlates of progressive renal failure. J Am Soc Nephrol 2006;17(8):2228–35.

65. Elmariah H, Garrett ME, De Castro LM, et al. Factors associated with survival in a contemporary adult sickle cell disease cohort. Am J Hematol 2014;89(5):530–5.

66. Gladwin MT, Barst RJ, Gibbs JS, et al. Risk factors for death in 632 patients with sickle cell disease in the United States and United Kingdom. PLoS One 2014;9(7):e99489.

67. Manci EA, Culberson DE, Yang YM, et al. Causes of death in sickle cell disease: an autopsy study. Br J Haematol 2003;123(2):359–65.

68. Pham PT, Pham PC, Wilkinson AH, et al. Renal abnormalities in sickle cell disease. Kidney Int 2000;57(1):1–8.

69. Platt OS, Brambilla DJ, Rosse WF, et al. Mortality in sickle cell disease. Life expectancy and risk factors for early death. N Engl J Med 1994;330(23):1639–44.

70. Powars DR, Chan LS, Hiti A, et al. Outcome of sickle cell anemia: a 4-decade observational study of 1056 patients. Medicine 2005;84(6):363–76.

71. Powars DR, Elliott-Mills DD, Chan L, et al. Chronic renal failure in sickle cell disease: risk factors, clinical course, and mortality. Ann Intern Med 1991;115(8):614–20.

72. Nath KA, Hebbel RP. Sickle cell disease: renal manifestations and mechanisms. Nat Rev Nephrol 2015;11(3):161–71.

73. Beckermann KE, Sharma D, Chaturvedi S, et al. Renal medullary carcinoma: establishing standards in practice. J Oncol Pract 2017;13(7):414–21.

74. Arnold SD, Brazauskas R, He N, et al. Clinical risks and healthcare utilization of hematopoietic cell transplantation for sickle cell disease in the USA using merged databases. Haematologica 2017;102(11):1823–32.

75. Demirci S, Uchida N, Tisdale JF. Gene therapy for sickle cell disease: an update. Cytotherapy 2018;20(7):899–910.

76. Guilcher GMT, Truong TH, Saraf SL, et al. Curative therapies: allogeneic hematopoietic cell transplantation from matched related donors using myeloablative, reduced intensity, and nonmyeloablative conditioning in sickle cell disease. Semin Hematol 2018;55(2):87–93.

77. Walters MC. Update of hematopoietic cell transplantation for sickle cell disease. Curr Opin Hematol 2015;22(3):227–33.

78. Wang WC, Ware RE, Miller ST, et al. Hydroxycarbamide in very young children with sickle-cell anaemia: a multicentre, randomised, controlled trial (BABY HUG). Lancet 2011;377(9778):1663–72.

79. Lederman HM, Connolly MA, Kalpatthi R, et al. Immunologic effects of hydroxyurea in sickle cell anemia. Pediatrics 2014;134(4):686–95.

80. Rogers ZR, Wang WC, Luo Z, et al. Biomarkers of splenic function in infants with sickle cell anemia: baseline data from the BABY HUG trial. Blood 2011;117(9):2614–7.

81. Strouse JJ, Heeney MM. Hydroxyurea for the treatment of sickle cell disease: efficacy, barriers, toxicity, and management in children. Pediatr Blood Cancer 2012;59(2):365–71.

82. Ware RE. How I use hydroxyurea to treat young patients with sickle cell anemia. Blood 2010;115(26):5300–11.

83. Dong M, Mizuno T, Vinks AA. Opportunities for model-based precision dosing in the treatment of sickle cell anemia. Blood Cells Mol Dis 2017;67:143–7.

84. McGann PT, Dong M, Marahatta A, et al. Individualized dosing of hydroxyurea for children with sickle cell anemia using a population pharmacokinetic-based model: the TREAT study. Blood 2016;128:3652.

85. Kizaki M, Ogawa T, Toyama K. A case of idiopathic thrombocytopenic purpura (ITP) associated with intracranial hemorrhage and hyperthyroidism successfully treated by splenectomy. Rinsho ketsueki 1984;25(2):182–7 [in Japanese].

86. Niihara Y, Miller ST, Kanter J, et al. A phase 3 trial of l-glutamine in sickle cell disease. N Engl J Med 2018;379(3):226–35.

87. Quinn CT. l-Glutamine for sickle cell anemia: more questions than answers. Blood 2018;132(7):689–93.

88. Vichinsky EP, Neumayr LD, Haberkern C, et al. The perioperative complication rate of orthopedic surgery in sickle cell disease: report of the National Sickle Cell Surgery Study Group. Am J Hematol 1999;62(3):129–38.

89. Hoppe CC, Inati AC, Brown C, et al. Initial results from a cohort in a phase 2a study (GBT440-007) evaluating adolescents with sickle cell disease treated with multiple doses of GBT440, a HbS polymerization inhibitor. Blood 2017;130:689.

90. Hoppe CC, Inati AC, Brown C, et al. Initial results from a cohort in a phase 2A Study (GBT440-007) evaluating adolescents with sickle cell disease treated with multiple doses of voxelotor, a sickle hemoglobin polymerization inhibitor. Paper presented at: American Society of Pediatric Hematology/Oncology. Pittsburgh, PA, 2018.

91. Almeida CB, Traina F, Lanaro C, et al. High expression of the cGMP-specific phosphodiesterase, PDE9A, in sickle cell disease (SCD) and the effects of its inhibition in erythroid cells and SCD neutrophils. Br J Haematol 2008;142(5):836–44.

92. Cokic VP, Smith RD, Beleslin-Cokic BB, et al. Hydroxyurea induces fetal hemoglobin by the nitric oxide-dependent activation of soluble guanylyl cyclase. J Clin Invest 2003;111(2):231–9.

93. Ikuta T, Ausenda S, Cappellini MD. Mechanism for fetal globin gene expression: role of the soluble guanylate cyclase-cGMP-dependent protein kinase pathway. Proc Natl Acad Sci U S A 2001;98(4):1847–52.

94. Ikuta T, Sellak H, Odo N, et al. Nitric Oxide-cGMP signaling stimulates erythropoiesis through multiple lineage-specific transcription factors: clinical implications and a novel target for erythropoiesis. PLoS One 2016;11(1):e0144561.

95. Alsultan A, Ngo D, Bae H, et al. Genetic studies of fetal hemoglobin in the Arab-Indian haplotype sickle cell-beta(0) thalassemia. Am J Hematol 2013;88(6):531–2.

96. Platt OS, Thorington BD, Brambilla DJ, et al. Pain in sickle cell disease. Rates and risk factors. N Engl J Med 1991;325(1):11–6.

97. Ataga KI, Kutlar A, Kanter J, et al. Crizanlizumab for the prevention of pain crises in sickle cell disease. N Engl J Med 2017;376(5):429–39.

98. Daak AA, Elderdery AY, Elbashir LM, et al. Omega 3 (n-3) fatty acids down-regulate nuclear factor-kappa B (NF-kappaB) gene and blood cell adhesion molecule expression in patients with homozygous sickle cell disease. Blood Cells Mol Dis 2015;55(1):48–55.

99. Daak AA, Ghebremeskel K, Hassan Z, et al. Effect of omega-3 (n-3) fatty acid supplementation in patients with sickle cell anemia: randomized, double-blind, placebo-controlled trial. Am J Clin Nutr 2013;97(1):37–44.

Rare Hereditary Hemolytic Anemias

Diagnostic Approach and Considerations in Management

Mary Risinger, PhD[a], Myesa Emberesh, MD[b],
Theodosia A. Kalfa, MD, PhD[c,d,*]

KEYWORDS

- Rare hereditary hemolytic anemias • Unstable hemoglobin
- Red cell hydration disorders • Red cell enzymopathies
- Congenital dyserythropoietic anemias

KEY POINTS

- Hereditary hemolytic anemias (HHAs) are a rare heterogeneous group of anemias caused by mutations in genes coding the globins, red blood cell (RBC) membrane proteins, and enzymes.
- Congenital dyserythropoietic anemias (CDAs), rare disorders of erythropoiesis, typically present with a hemolytic phenotype because the produced RBCs have structural defects and decreased survival. Therefore, CDAs should be considered in the differential of HHAs.
- Patients with HHAs/CDAs can present with similar clinical and laboratory findings; however, they may require different therapeutic approaches depending on the cause of the disease.
- Genetic diagnosis with next-generation sequencing panels or whole exome or genome sequencing may be necessary for accurate diagnosis and appropriate management decisions.
- Although splenectomy can be effective in management of patients with hereditary spherocytosis, patients with hereditary xerocytosis or CDA type I do not benefit from splenectomy, which additionally leads to increased risk for thromboembolic disorders. Postsplenectomy vasculopathy and stroke are seen in patients with prooxidant unstable hemoglobins.

Disclosure Statement: The authors have no relevant conflicts of interest to disclose.
[a] College of Nursing, University of Cincinnati, 3110 Vine Street, Cincinnati, OH 45221-0038, USA; [b] Cancer and Blood Diseases Institute, Cincinnati Children's Hospital Medical Center, 3333 Burnet Avenue, MLC 7018, Cincinnati, OH 45229-3039, USA; [c] Cancer and Blood Diseases Institute, Cincinnati Children's Hospital Medical Center, 3333 Burnet Avenue, MLC 7015, Cincinnati, OH 45229-3039, USA; [d] Department of Pediatrics, University of Cincinnati College of Medicine, Cincinnati, OH, USA
* Corresponding author. Cancer and Blood Diseases Institute, Cincinnati Children's Hospital Medical Center, 3333 Burnet Avenue, MLC 7015, Cincinnati, OH 45229-3039.
E-mail address: theodosia.kalfa@cchmc.org

Hematol Oncol Clin N Am 33 (2019) 373–392
https://doi.org/10.1016/j.hoc.2019.01.002
0889-8588/19/© 2019 Elsevier Inc. All rights reserved.

INTRODUCTION

Hemolytic anemia (HA) arises from a shortened red blood cell (RBC) survival caused by extrinsic factors, an intrinsic abnormality of the cell, or a combination of both. The mechanical injury to erythrocytes in microangiopathic HA and immune-mediated conditions are examples of extrinsic factors causing HA. Intrinsic defects are caused by genetic mutations causing hemoglobin disorders (defects in globin chains or heme synthesis), erythrocyte membrane disorders, and RBC enzymopathies, leading to hereditary hemolytic anemia (HHA). The premature RBC destruction may happen intravascularly or extravascularly via the macrophages of the reticuloendothelial system, mainly in the liver or spleen. Patients may present with pallor, jaundice, dark urine, fatigue, splenomegaly, gallstones, and cholecystitis. Characteristic laboratory findings are anemia (decreased hemoglobin), reticulocytosis, elevated unconjugated bilirubin and lactate dehydrogenase (LDH), serum aspartate aminotransferase (AST) disproportionately higher than serum alanine aminotransferase (ALT), and decreased haptoglobin. Congenital dyserythropoietic anemias (CDAs), although pathologically defined as disorders of erythropoiesis, lead to the production of fragile RBCs and may present with clinical characteristics of hemolysis, albeit typically with suboptimal reticulocytosis, splenomegaly, and abnormal osmotic fragility. Therefore, CDAs are included in the differential diagnosis of HHA.

Although presenting with similar clinical and laboratory findings, different HHAs may require radically different approaches in management. At a time when genetic diagnosis with next-generation sequencing (NGS) panels or whole-exome sequencing is available, consideration for the less common HHAs is critical in attaining the correct diagnosis and preventing complications of a "one-size-fits-all" approach. Although splenectomy may be an effective and fairly safe way to limit extravascular hemolysis in most cases of hereditary spherocytosis, it does not improve the intravascular hemolysis in xerocytosis or CDA type I and can precipitate life-threatening complications of thromboembolic disease and pulmonary hypertension.[1–3] In cases of HHA resulting from prooxidant unstable hemoglobins, increased oxidative stress postsplenectomy may lead to vasculopathy and stroke.[4,5] In addition, chronic iron overload may be a more significant issue than the anemia in several of these diseases, and early diagnosis is key in preventing chronic organ damage, morbidity, and early mortality.

This article discusses the clinical presentation, laboratory findings, and management considerations for rare HHAs caused by unstable hemoglobins, RBC hydration defects, the less common RBC enzymopathies (excluding glucose-6-phosphate dehydrogenase [G6PD] and pyruvate kinase [PK] deficiency), and CDAs.

UNSTABLE HEMOGLOBINS

Unstable hemoglobinopathies are caused by mutations in one of the globin-coding genes (*HBA1*, *HBA2*, *HBB*, *HBG2*, and *HBD*), leading to production of abnormal globin chains with altered solubility that precipitate on the inner surface of the erythrocyte membrane as denatured hemoglobin, forming hemichromes.[6] The hemichromes induce clustering of band 3 at their membrane site; these aggregates are called Heinz bodies.[7] Hemichromes, also found in thalassemias and G6PD deficiency, decrease the RBC life-span by oxidative damage of the membrane that impairs the deformability and increases the fragility of RBCs.[8] Additionally the induction of high-molecular-weight band 3 aggregates enhances opsonization by anti–band 3 antibodies, leading to phagocytic removal of the Heinz bodies (splenic pitting) and eventually of the damaged RBCs.[9] Most cases are inherited in an autosomal dominant pattern, but de novo mutations, or rare homozygous and compound heterozygous cases, have also been reported.[6]

Clinical Presentation and Laboratory Findings

The clinical presentation is variable, depending on the causative mutation. Chronic HA may be mild, moderate, or severe, presenting in infancy or early childhood, and may require chronic transfusion therapy.[6] Patients with *HBB* variants producing unstable β-globin typically present after 5 to 6 months of age with microcytic anemia, brisk reticulocytosis, and hemoglobin electrophoresis indicating increased hemoglobin A_2 (HbA_2) and/or hemoglobin F (HbF). Rare cases of neonates with a mutation in *HBG2* producing unstable γ-globin have been reported, presenting with transient neonatal HA and jaundice that typically resolves in early infancy as HbF is replaced by HbA.[10,11] The mildly unstable hemoglobins may not cause symptoms at baseline; the patients experience significant hemolysis only with oxidative stress, owing to exposure to prooxidant medications or infections. Clinically significant unstable hemoglobins demonstrate anisopoikilocytosis, polychromasia, and basophilic stippling on the peripheral blood smear (**Fig. 1**).

Screening tests to examine hemoglobin stability can be performed after incubation with isopropanol or after heat treatment at 50°C for 1 to 2 hours.[6] Although the unstable hemoglobinopathies are also known in the literature as congenital Heinz bodies in HAs, we should note that staining for Heinz bodies is frequently negative in a sample from a nonplenectomized patient with unstable hemoglobin. The spleen removes the damaged cells or just the part of the RBC membrane with the Heinz body formation very efficiently (see **Fig. 1**). Similarly, a normal hemoglobin electrophoresis does not rule out unstable hemoglobins as the cause of a congenital HA because the unstable denatured hemoglobin is frequently degraded rapidly within RBCs, escaping detection as an intact globin chain. Gene sequencing of the globin genes easily leads to diagnosis. More than 200 unstable hemoglobins are listed in the comprehensive hemoglobin variant database (http://globin.cse.psu.edu./hbvar/menu.html).[12,13]

Management

Patients presenting with a mild disorder require only supportive care. With some unstable hemoglobins,[14] oxidative triggers such as sulfa-containing antibiotics have been observed to cause hemolytic crisis[15,16]; therefore, avoidance of such agents is recommended. Transfusion may be required during episodes of hemolysis and on a chronic basis in patients with severe disease. Splenectomy has been used in patients with severe disease and improves anemia; however, it may lead to vasculopathy and stroke, likely arising from increased oxidative stress and damage to the endothelium.[4,5]

RED CELL MEMBRANE DISORDERS

Several genetically and phenotypically heterogeneous inherited red cell membrane disorders reduce RBC survival and result in HA. The more common of these disorders are those that involve altered membrane structural organization. Weakening of vertical linkages between the lipid bilayer and the spectrin-based cytoskeleton by defects or deficiencies in ankyrin, spectrin, band 3, or band 4.2 result in hereditary spherocytosis (HS), whereas weakening of the horizontal associations of the RBC cytoskeleton by defects or deficiencies in spectrin, or protein 4.1R result in hereditary elliptocytosis or hereditary pyropoikilocytosis (HPP).[17,18] The less commonly diagnosed RBC membrane disorders are those that result from altered membrane transport function and

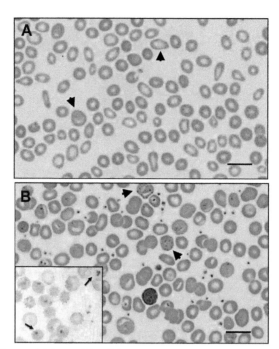

Fig. 1. Unstable hemoglobinopathies. (A) A 7-year-old girl presented with nonimmune hemolytic anemia (HA) at 7 months of age. Baseline hemoglobin at 7 to 8 g/dL, requiring blood transfusions during acute illnesses. Not splenectomized. The patient had a presumed diagnosis of CDA type I, based on dyserythropoiesis seen in bone marrow studies. Genetic workup revealed an unstable β-globin, changing her diagnosis to unstable hemoglobinopathy. The peripheral blood smear of a transfused specimen demonstrates anisopoikilocytosis, polychromasia, occasional basophilic stippling (*arrowheads*), and significant hypochromia between normal transfused cells. Heinz body prep was negative. (B) A 13-year-old girl with unstable hemoglobin Southampton (HBB: c.320T>C, p.L106P) with history of splenectomy. Her course was complicated by cerebral vasculopathy and transient ischemic attacks, subsequently managed with chronic transfusions. Peripheral blood smear demonstrates poikilocytosis, target cells, and extensive basophilic stippling (*arrowheads*). Inset demonstrates Heinz bodies (*arrows*) after staining of her RBCs with a supravital stain (methyl violet). Scale bars, 14 μm.

include primarily hereditary xerocytosis (HX) and overhydrated hereditary stomatocytosis (OHS). In these conditions alterations in membrane cation permeability result in either a decrease (HX) or an increase (OHS) in RBC volume, leading to altered cellular deformability and shortened life-span.[19,20] Although there have been considerable advances in defining the molecular defects responsible for these conditions in recent years, there is still much to be learned about the causative genes, specific variant pathogenicity, and modifying factors involved in these conditions.

Hereditary Xerocytosis

HX is caused by an abnormal RBC K^+ leak not accompanied by a proportional intracellular Na^+ and water gain, leading to osmotic imbalance and decreased deformability, thus contributing to a shortened life-span. It is a dominantly inherited condition and, in most cases, is caused by mutations in the mechanosensitive nonselective cation channel, PIEZO1. As RBCs travel through small capillaries and sinusoids, mechanical stimuli may activate PIEZO1 and increase intracellular Ca^{2+}, which may then activate the Gardos channel, a calcium-sensitive potassium channel encoded by the *KCNN4* gene, causing K^+ loss and water loss.[21,22] Most HX-associated PIEZO1 mutations are missense mutations in the highly conserved COOH-terminal pore region.[23–25] HX-associated PIEZO1 mutations demonstrate a partial gain-of-function phenotype, with many demonstrating a slower rate of inactivation.[26,27] Other mechanisms including alterations in channel kinetics, response to osmotic stress, and membrane trafficking may worsen or ameliorate RBC hydration in HX and contribute to the phenotypic heterogeneity.[28] Some of the HX patients with normal PIEZO1 were found to exhibit gain-of-function mutations in the Gardos channel.[29–32]

There are indications that HX is an underdiagnosed condition. Recent prevalence estimates based on a search of a large United States commercial laboratory database for complete blood counts results consistent with HX suggest an incidence several times higher than the estimate of approximately 1 in 50,000 births that is based on reported cases.[20,33] Minor allele frequencies of major HX-associated mutations are also consistent with a higher incidence (exac.broadinstitute.org).[34] Surprisingly, a recently identified human PIEZO1 gain-of-function mutation, E756del, is estimated to be present in at least one copy in approximately one-third of the African population.[35] Mice with this mutation demonstrated an HX-like syndrome and protection from cerebral malaria. RBCs from humans with one copy of E756del are dehydrated and demonstrate a reduced susceptibility to *Plasmodium* infection. However, a full clinical evaluation of individuals carrying this mutation has not yet been reported.

Clinical presentation and laboratory findings

The HX phenotype is variable, probably owing to a number of factors including differences in the causative variants, differences in transporters and other proteins that mediate compensatory responses, and coinheritance of other variants that cause red cell membrane disorders. Patients with HX typically present with mild to moderate HA or fully compensated hemolysis; some do not come to medical attention until adulthood or later in life. Patients with KCNN4 mutations typically experience more severe anemia than PIEZO1-mutant HX patients. Aplastic crises, thrombosis, and gallstones secondary to hemolysis can occur. Some patients have a history of transient perinatal edema and nonimmune hydrops fetalis; pseudohyperkalemia has also been reported.[20,36] Iron overload disproportionate to transfusion history can be significant, requiring chelation treatment, and is sometimes the first finding of the disease in adulthood. Ferritin and transferrin saturation should be monitored and when iron overload is suspected, T2* MRI of the liver and heart is indicated.[37–40] The mean corpuscular hemoglobin concentration (MCHC) is elevated, as also is the case in HS; however the osmotic fragility is decreased in HX, reflecting RBC dehydration. Peripheral blood smears of HX patients are often relatively normal with few target cells and variable numbers of stomatocytes (**Fig. 2**A). Reflecting cellular dehydration, the osmotic gradient ektacytometry shows a leftward shift (**Fig. 2**B) and intracellular cation determinations reveal a reduced K^+ content without a corresponding increase in Na^+ content.[41]

Management

Management is supportive for complications of hemolysis and anemia and should include monitoring for iron overload and iron chelation as needed. Although splenectomy is usually beneficial in the management of HS patients with moderate or severe anemia (with the exception of the most severe cases of complete α-spectrin deficiency), it is not helpful in reducing anemia in HX and is contraindicated because of

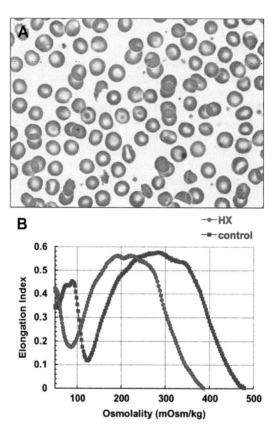

Fig. 2. Hereditary xerocytosis (HX) caused by heterozygous *PIEZO1* mutation. A 10-year-old girl with chronic hemolysis fully compensated with reticulocytosis (hemoglobin 14 g/dL, reticulocytes 16%). The patient was found to have one of the most common PIEZO1 mutations (c.7367G>A; p.R2456H) causing HX. (*A*) Blood smear with macrocytosis (MCV 96 fL) showing occasional stomatocytes, target cells, and dense fragmented cells. (*B*) Osmotic gradient ektacytometry showing the typical HX curve with left shift attributable to decreased O_{min} and O_{hyp}. *Note*: In ektacytometry, O_{min} corresponds to the osmolality at which 50% of the cells hemolyze in the osmotic fragility test, and its value is affected by the surface area to volume ratio. EI_{max} is the maximum elongation that the RBCs can achieve under shear stress and relates specifically to the mechanical properties of the cytoskeleton. The declining portion of the curve is represented by the O_{hyp} value, the osmolality value at which the cell's maximum diameter is half of EI_{max} and correlates with the initial intracellular viscosity of the cell sample. A shift to the left reflects increased intracellular viscosity of the erythrocyte caused by increased intracellular concentration of hemoglobin and/or a dehydration state.[87]

the increased risk of frequently fatal venous and arterial thromboembolic complications.[1,42]

Because the Gardos channel has been shown to be the major determinant/mediator of RBC dehydration in HX,[43] the Gardos channel inhibitor senicapoc has been suggested as a candidate for treatment of HX caused by mutations of either PIEZO1 or the Gardos channel. Senicapoc has been used in a phase III clinical trial to test for effects on clinical manifestations of sickle cell disease. Although it failed to improve the incidence of painful crises, resulting in early termination of the study, it was shown to reduce RBC dehydration and hemolysis and increase hemoglobin levels, and was well tolerated.[44] In vitro studies are promising, indicating that senicapoc inhibits both normal and mutated Gardos channels, although with different sensitivity depending on the mutation, improving the RBC hydration status.[45] Clinical trials will be needed to show whether there will a benefit to the anemia and the associated stress erythropoiesis in patients with HX.

Overhydrated Stomatocytosis

Overhydrated stomatocytosis (OHS) is a very rare autosomal dominant disorder caused by a large net increase in intracellular Na^+ and water with a lesser decrease in intracellular K^+, resulting in increased cell volume without a concomitant increase in membrane surface area.[46] The increased Na^+ content is not adequately compensated despite a significant compensatory increase in Na^+/K^+ ATPase activity. Some patients with OHS demonstrate missense mutations of the Rh-associated glycoprotein (RhAG), which is a component of the band 3 macromolecular complex and functions as an ammonium transporter or a gas channel. The OHS-associated mutations result in decreased ammonium transport and increased cation conductance.[47–49] A rare form of OHS in which there is minimal cation leak at physiologic temperature but a dramatic increase in the cation leak at low temperature (eg, 4°C) is referred to as cryohydrocytosis. In some patients with cryohydrocytosis, heterozygous missense mutations in band 3, the RBC anion exchanger, have been identified. Some of the mutations transform band 3 into a cation conductor at low temperature,[50,51] whereas others may result in the activation of other cation leak pathways.[52] Mutations in GLUT1, the glucose transporter, have also been identified in some patients with cryohydrocytosis.[53,54]

Clinical presentation and laboratory findings

Patients with OHS typically present with moderate to severe, partially compensated HA. The peripheral blood smear reveals numerous stomatocytes and occasional spherocytes. The mean corpuscular volume (MCV) is increased, reflecting macrocytosis, and the MCHC is decreased. Osmotic fragility is highly increased and osmotic gradient ektacytometry curves demonstrate a right shift, indicating overhydration. Intracellular cation determinations reflect a greatly increased Na^+ content with reduced K^+ content.

Management

Management is supportive. Although splenectomy may be partially effective in reducing anemia, it is contraindicated because of the high risk of thromboembolic complications.[1,42]

RED BLOOD CELL ENZYMOPATHIES

Because mitochondria are normally lost during enucleation and reticulocyte maturation, RBCs depend on anaerobic glycolysis for ATP production. In parallel, the pentose phosphate pathway that produces NADPH and reduced glutathione to control oxidative damage is also critical for normal RBC survival (**Fig. 3**). Clearance of the nucleotides after RNA degradation during reticulocyte maturation, performed by pyrimidine 5'-nucleotidase, is also necessary. Hereditary RBC enzymopathies, causing congenital nonspherocytic hemolytic anemia (CNSHA), arise from deficiency of the enzymes involved in any of these pathways.[6] Examples of the CNSHA morphology in peripheral blood smears are shown in **Fig. 4**. The severity of hemolysis, pattern of inheritance, and associated findings for the rare RBC enzyme disorders (excluding G6PD and

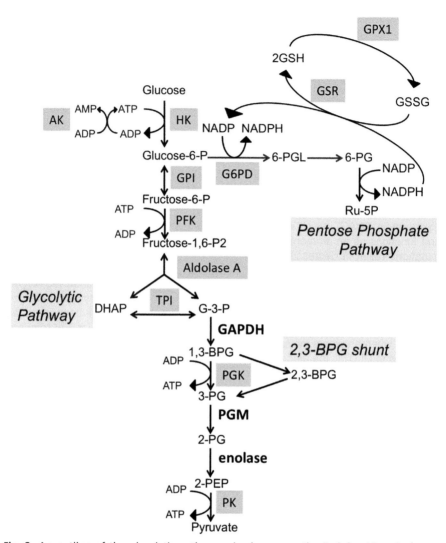

Fig. 3. An outline of the glycolytic pathway, also known as the Embden-Meyerhof enzymatic pathway, along with the pentose phosphate pathway and the 2,3-BPG (2,3-bisphosphoglycerate) shunt. Deficiency of the enzymes shown in orange boxes causes HA. AK, adenylate kinase; G6PD, glucose-6-phosphate dehydrogenase; GPI, glucose-6-phosphate isomerase; GPX1, glutathione peroxidase; GSR, glutathione reductase; HK, hexokinase; PFK, phosphofructokinase; PGK, phosphoglycerate kinase; PK, pyruvate kinase; TPI, triosephosphate isomerase.

PK deficiency) are summarized in **Table 1**. These enzymes are frequently important for the intracellular metabolism in other tissues; in such cases, the associated symptoms and signs may be the ones mainly responsible for morbidity and early mortality in these inborn errors of metabolism. There is significant variability in the phenotype that may be due to the variable mutations causing disease and/or additional recessive disorders that may coincide in patients with history of consanguinity.[55] Treatment is usually supportive, especially given that the anemia frequently improves after early

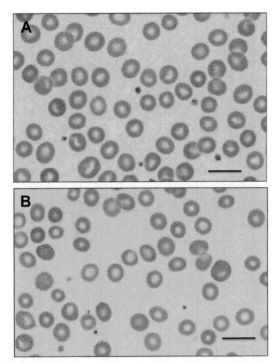

Fig. 4. Rare RBC enzymopathies. (*A*) A 15-year-old European-American youth with chronic HA, reticulocytosis, and progressive neuromuscular disease. He was diagnosed with triose-phosphate isomerase (TPI) deficiency after finding decreased TPI enzymatic activity in his RBCs in early childhood. Significant macrocytosis (MCV 110 fL) is noted. NextGen sequencing revealed homozygosity for a known *TPI1* mutation. (*B*) Peripheral blood smear of a 5-year-old European-American boy with pyrimidine-5′-nucleotidase deficiency. Marked basophilic stippling is characteristic. Scale bars, 14 mm.

childhood. Splenectomy may be helpful in some patients with transfusion-dependent CNSHA; it is contraindicated in triosephosphate isomerase (TPI) deficiency because it does not significantly decrease hemolysis and increases the risk of infections.[6]

CONGENITAL DYSERYTHROPOIETIC ANEMIAS

CDAs are a group of rare heterogeneous genetic disorders causing ineffective eryth-ropoiesis with distinct morphologic abnormalities involving the late erythroblasts in the bone marrow.[56] Clinically the presentation is nonspecific and overlaps with various more common hemolytic disorders such as RBC membrane disorders and thalasse-mias. In addition, HAs caused by globin, membrane, or enzyme disorders with a brisk erythropoietic response may demonstrate erythroid dysplasia in bone marrow studies. This overlap can make the diagnosis challenging and lead to mistargeted treatments.[3] The classification of CDAs has been largely based on bone marrow pathology findings using the working morphologic classification proposed by Heimpel and Weindt in 1968, in which 3 major types of CDA were identified and grouped based on morpho-logic similarities.[57] More subgroups and variants of CDA have been recently identified and added to the classification.[58,59] In 2002, *CDAN1* mutations were identified as the autosomal recessive genetic cause in most cases of CDA-I.[60] Since that time, genetic

Table 1
Rare RBC enzyme disorders

Enzyme	Gene	Pattern of Inheritance	Degree of Hemolysis	Associated Findings
Hexokinase	HK1	AR	Mild to moderate	Different HK1 mutations cause neuropathy (Russe type)
Adenylate kinase	AK1	AR	Mild to moderate	
Glucose-6-phosphate isomerase	GPI	AR	Mild to severe	Certain mutations affecting the monomer (neuroleukin) cause neurologic symptoms
Phosphofructokinase M	PFKM	AR	Mild to moderate	Glycogen storage disease VII: exertional myopathy in the nonhemolytic form
Aldolase A	ALDOA	AR	Mild to moderate	Glycogen storage disease XII: exertional myopathy
Triosephosphate isomerase 1	TPI1	AR	Mild to moderate	White blood cells, rhabdomyocytes, cardiomyocytes, and cerebellum also affected; increased susceptibility to infections; myopathy progressing to respiratory muscles
Phosphoglycerate kinase	PGK1	XLR	Mild to moderate	± Myopathy or neurologic involvement
γ-Glutamylcysteine synthetase deficiency	GCLC	AR	Mild	± Myopathy, late-onset spinocerebellar degeneration, and peripheral neuropathy
Glutathione synthetase	GSS	AR	Hemolysis induced by oxidative stress; chronic hemolysis in some cases	5-Oxoprolinuria, metabolic acidosis, mental retardation
Glutathione peroxidase	GPX1	AR	Hemolysis induced by oxidative stress	
Glutathione reductase	GSR	AR	Hemolysis induced by oxidative stress	
Pyrimidine 5'-nucleotidase	NT5C3A	AR	Mild to moderate	± Learning difficulties

Abbreviations: AR, autosomal recessive; XLR, X-linked recessive.

defects in *SEC23B*, *KIF23*, *KLF1*, and *GATA1* have been found to cause the pathologically classified CDA types II to V, respectively, suggesting that there is a phenotype-genotype correlation.[59,61–64] *C15ORF41* mutations were found to be causative in a few families with CDA-I, indicating that more than one gene may be responsible for the same pathology in bone marrow erythroblasts.[65,66]

CDA-III has the most clearly defined pathogenetic mechanism for multinuclearity among the various types of CDA, caused by mutations of *KIF23*, the gene that encodes mitotic kinesin-like protein 1 (MKLP1), a key component of the midbody.[63,64] The midbody is a transient structure formed between two daughter cells at the end of cytokinesis, with the principal function of "marking" the site of abscission, which physically separates two daughter cells.[67] Codanin 1, encoded by *CDAN1*, which is mutated in most of the cases of CDA-I, is a poorly understood protein that may facilitate histone assembly into chromatin and regulate the cell cycle.[68] *C15ORF41*, the gene associated with CDA-Ib, is predicted to encode a divalent metal ion-dependent restriction endonuclease, with a yet unknown function.[65] *SEC23B*, responsible for CDA-II, encodes a protein involved in endoplasmic reticulum (ER) vesicle trafficking.[62] *KLF1* and *GATA1* genes encode essential erythroid transcription factors; certain missense mutations have been associated with CDA types IV and V, respectively.[69–71]

Because of the rarity of the disease, many gaps still exist in our understanding of the molecular mechanisms. The European registries of CDA types I and II have provided information on the natural history of these 2 CDA types.[72–74] The CDA Registry (CDAR), a registry for patients with any type of CDA in North America (ClinicalTrials.gov Identifier: NCT02964494), has been created with the goal of providing a longitudinal database and associated biorepository to facilitate natural history studies and research on the molecular pathways involved in the pathogenesis of CDAs.

Clinical Presentation and Laboratory Findings

CDA patients present with a variable degree of anemia, with laboratory findings consistent with hemolysis, although typically with suboptimal reticulocyte response, splenomegaly, jaundice, and iron overload disproportionate to the history of RBC transfusions.[56,60,75] The CDA types with their causative genes, pattern of inheritance, and description of the bone marrow findings are summarized in **Table 2**.

CDA-I presents frequently in the newborn period with macrocytic anemia; the degree of the anemia may vary even among siblings with the same *CDAN1* mutations.[73] Some patients with CDA-I also have skeletal and limb abnormalities (eg, syndactyly in hands and feet, supernumerary toes) (**Fig. 5**).

CDA-II is typically milder than CDA-I and often presents later in life.[72] Decreased glycosylation and faster migration of the RBC membrane proteins band 3 and band 4.5 is noted, which contributes to increased RBC hemolysis and to the clinical-picture overlap with HS.[76] CDA-II patients are typically found to have mutations in *SEC23B*.[77] Thirteen percent of the patients have only one mutation in *SEC23B*, and a few patients with morphologic diagnosis of CDA-II still lack a genetic defect, demonstrating that not all mutations underlying CDA-II have yet been identified (**Fig. 6**).[75]

CDA-III is a rare subtype of CDA with 2 identified forms, familial and sporadic. The familial form is an autosomal dominant disease described in 4 families so far worldwide (1 in the United States, 2 in Sweden, and 1 in Argentina). It is characterized by mild anemia, lack of splenomegaly or iron overload, and predominance of intravascular hemolysis. Patients with familial CDA-III may also have retinal angioid streaks and the propensity for monoclonal gammopathy and multiple myeloma. The sporadic cases are autosomal recessive, clinically variable, and characterized by severe

Table 2
Congenital dyserythropoietic anemias

CDA Type	Gene	Pattern of Inheritance	Bone Marrow Pathology Findings	
			Light Microscopy	Electron Microscopy
Ia	CDAN1	AR	3%–7% binucleated erythroblasts, occasional thin chromatin bridges between nuclei of divided erythroblasts	Spongy appearance ("Swiss cheese") of erythroblast heterochromatin
Ib	C15orf41	AR		
II	SEC23B	AR	10%–30% binucleated and occasional multinucleated erythroblasts	Erythroblast plasma membrane appears at sites duplicated. Peripheral cisternae loaded with ER protein
III				
Familial	KIF23	AD	Giant multinucleated erythroblasts with up to 12 nuclei (gigantoblasts)	Intranuclear clefts into heterochromatin, autophagic vacuoles
Sporadic	TBD	AR		
IV	KLF1	AD	Binucleated and multinucleated erythroblasts, karyorrhexis, and nuclear pyknosis	Invagination of nuclear membrane and nuclear blebbing
V (X-linked thrombocytopenia and dyserythropoietic anemia)	GATA1	XLR	Small dysplastic megakaryocytes and giant platelets; erythroblasts megaloblastic with bi- and multinucleation and nuclear irregularities	Megakaryocytes with abundance of smooth endoplasmic reticulum; decreased α granules in platelets
Nontypable variants	TBD	TBD	Variable dyserythropoiesis findings including bi- and multinucleated erythroblasts, nuclear lobation or fragmentation, cytoplasmic bridges between divided erythroblasts	

Abbreviations: AD, autosomal dominant; AR, autosomal recessive; TBD, to be determined; XLR, X-linked recessive.

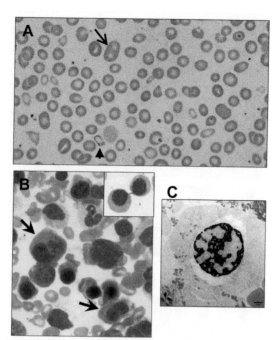

Fig. 5. CDA type Ia caused by biallelic *CDAN1* mutations. A 5-year-old old European-American boy diagnosed with CDA-I after presenting with transfusion-dependent, nonimmune HA with suboptimal reticulocytosis and skeletal deformities involving fingers and toes. Hemoglobin nadir was 8 g/dL before starting peripheral RBC transfusions. (*A*) Blood smear showing the patient's RBCs, between the normal transfused RBCs, demonstrating marked anisopoikilocytosis, dacryocytes, red cell fragments, impressive macrocytes with "double-dimple," (*arrow*) and basophilic stippling (*arrowhead*). (*B*) Bone marrow aspirate revealed erythroblasts with prominent dyserythropoiesis with megaloblastoid maturation, binucleation (*arrows*), and nuclear contour irregularities. A chromatin bridge between nuclei in erythroblasts, typical for CDA type I, is shown in the inset. (*C*) Spongy appearance of heterochromatin, also called "Swiss cheese appearance," is seen in intermediate and late erythroblasts by electron microscopy and is considered pathognomonic.[88] Scale bar, 1μm.

erythroid hyperplasia. Patients with this form of CDA-III may also have skeletal disorders, mental retardation, and hepatosplenomegaly.[78]

CDA-IV, attributable to KLF1 p.E325K, presents with a variable phenotype, with anemia ranging from hydrops fetalis and transfusion dependency to a moderate anemia with occasional transfusion needs. Growth effects and cardiac abnormalities are also noted in these patients, and increased HbF is a fairly consistent finding.[69,79]

CDA-V is also named XLTDA (for X-linked thrombocytopenia and dyserthyropoiesis) and has been associated so far with 2 missense mutations (p.V205M and p.G208R) in the N-terminal zinc-finger domain of *GATA1*, a transcription factor essential for the erythroid and megakaryocytic lineage differentiation. Patients with CDA-V present with significant bleeding tendency and variable degrees of anemia.[70,71]

Nontypable CDA variants

Families and individuals with disease that meets the diagnostic criteria of CDA but do not fit in any of the aforementioned 5 CDA types, either because of different bone marrow morphologic findings or because none of the known CDA-associated genes

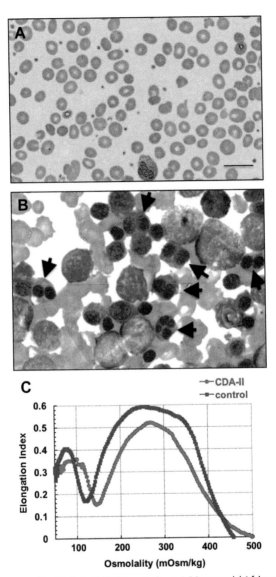

Fig. 6. CDA type II caused by biallelic *SEC23B* mutations. A 39-year-old African-American woman diagnosed with CDA-II at 4 years of age. Clinical course has been benign with only mild anemia (hemoglobin ~10 g/dL with normal absolute reticulocyte count) with no transfusion requirement despite an active life including a normal pregnancy and delivery. (*A*) Blood smear showing spherocytes, marked poikilocytosis, and inadequate reticulocytosis. Scale bar, 14 mm. (*B*) Bone marrow studies revealing binucleated and occasional multinucleated erythroblasts (indicated by *arrows*). (*C*) Ektacytometry for this patient shows a curve that resembles HS, compatible with the known fact that RBCs in CDA-II patients have a secondary membrane defect.

were found mutated, are grouped under "nontypable CDA variants" (see **Table 2**). Based on the authors' experience with the patients enrolled in CDAR and the relatively low frequency of a positive result in NGS CDA panels performed for patients with clinical diagnosis of CDA,[80,81] novel gene mutations may be responsible for up to 50% of patients with congenital dyserythropoietic anemia.

Management

Treatment of CDA is primarily supportive and targeted toward preventing the consequences of anemia and iron overload. Supportive blood transfusions and iron chelation are the 2 most commonly used therapies. Iron overload is variable and disproportionate to the history of blood transfusions. Therefore, careful monitoring of body iron and early management of iron overload, even in patients not receiving regular blood transfusions, is very important for the prevention of chronic organ damage. However, there is limited experience with the use of oral iron chelators in patients with CDA, with a question of unusual side effects in this population. Splenectomy has been performed in some CDA-II patients and found to be beneficial in decreasing the transfusion requirement; however, it does not prevent iron overload, which increases the long-term morbidity and mortality if not closely monitored and treated.[74] In CDA-I, splenectomy is not helpful and may precipitate life-threatening thromboembolic complications and pulmonary hypertension.[3] Interferon-α (IFN-α) was incidentally found to improve the anemia and iron overload (likely because of improvement in erythropoiesis efficiency) in a patient with CDA-I treated for hepatitis C; more patients with CDA-I have since responded to such treatment but the mechanism of therapeutic action is not known.[82–84] Other CDA subtypes do not show similar response to IFN-α. Cholecystectomy is often needed in CDA patients because of the increased prevalence of gallstone formation, especially in patients with concurrent Gilbert syndrome. There are few reports of successful stem cell transplantation (SCT) in severe cases of CDA. No systematic analysis has been performed to evaluate long-term outcomes after SCT[85,86] and the potential risks of pre-SCT conditioning for a disease that appears to be strongly associated with mitosis and cytokinesis defects. The CDAR has the goal of providing answers to these questions and eventually leading to organized clinical trials for this group of diseases.

SUMMARY

The rare hereditary hemolytic and dyserythropoietic anemias present with clinical and laboratory findings similar to their most common counterparts such as G6PD deficiency and HS. A high index of suspicion is necessary to proceed to specialized testing, such as osmotic gradient ektacytometry and genetic analysis, to achieve accurate diagnosis and apply safe therapeutic approaches depending on the cause of the disease. Chronic iron overload may be significant and out of proportion to the transfusion history in several of these disorders; monitoring of iron status and treatment, when necessary, with chelation is essential in preventing chronic organ damage, morbidity, and early mortality.

ACKNOWLEGEMENTS

This work was supported by the NHLBI grant R01HL116352 (T.A.K.) and by the National Center for Advancing Translational Sciences of the National Institutes of Health, under Award Number 1UL1TR001425-01. The content is solely the responsibility of the authors and does not necessarily represent the official views of the NIH.

REFERENCES

1. Stewart GW, Amess JA, Eber SW, et al. Thrombo-embolic disease after splenectomy for hereditary stomatocytosis. Br J Haematol 1996;93(2):303–10.
2. Jais X, Till SJ, Cynober T, et al. An extreme consequence of splenectomy in dehydrated hereditary stomatocytosis: gradual thrombo-embolic pulmonary

hypertension and lung-heart transplantation. Hemoglobin 2003;27(3): 139–47.

3. Chonat S, McLemore ML, Bunting ST, et al. Congenital dyserythropoietic anaemia type I diagnosed in a young adult with a history of splenectomy in childhood for presumed haemolytic anaemia. Br J Haematol 2018;182(1):10.

4. Thuret I, Bardakdjian J, Badens C, et al. Priapism following splenectomy in an unstable hemoglobin: hemoglobin Olmsted beta 141 (H19) Leu–>Arg. Am J Hematol 1996;51(2):133–6.

5. Haque A, Quint DJ, Castle VP, et al. Another rare unstable hemoglobinopathy: hemoglobin Casper/Southampton associated with moyamoya disease. Cerebrovasc Dis Extra 2015;5(2):52–4.

6. Gallagher PG. Diagnosis and management of rare congenital nonimmune hemolytic disease. Hematology Am Soc Hematol Educ Program 2015;2015:392–9.

7. Waugh SM, Low PS. Hemichrome binding to band 3: nucleation of Heinz bodies on the erythrocyte membrane. Biochemistry 1985;24(1):34–9.

8. Chiu D, Lubin B. Oxidative hemoglobin denaturation and RBC destruction: the effect of heme on red cell membranes. Semin Hematol 1989;26(2):128–35.

9. Mannu F, Arese P, Cappellini MD, et al. Role of hemichrome binding to erythrocyte membrane in the generation of band-3 alterations in beta-thalassemia intermedia erythrocytes. Blood 1995;86(5):2014–20.

10. Lee-Potter JP, Deacon-Smith RA, Simpkiss MJ, et al. A new cause of haemolytic anaemia in the newborn. A description of an unstable fetal haemoglobin: F Poole, alpha2-G-gamma2 130 tryptophan yields glycine. J Clin Pathol 1975;28(4): 317–20.

11. Pirastru M, Mereu P, Trova S, et al. Hb F-Avellino [(G)gamma41(C7)Phe–> Leu; HBG2: c.124 T > C]: a new hemoglobin variant observed in a healthy newborn. Hemoglobin 2016;40(1):61–3.

12. Hardison RC, Chui DHK, Giardine B, et al. HbVar: a relational database of human hemoglobin variants and thalassemia mutations at the globin gene server. Hum Mutat 2002;19(3):225–33.

13. Giardine B, Borg J, Viennas E, et al. Updates of the HbVar database of human hemoglobin variants and thalassemia mutations. Nucleic Acids Res 2014; 42(Database issue):D1063–9.

14. Williamson D. The unstable haemoglobins. Blood Rev 1993;7(3):146–63.

15. Frick PG, Hitzig WH, Betke K. Hemoglobin Zurich. I. A new hemoglobin anomaly associated with acute hemolytic episodes with inclusion bodies after sulfonamide therapy. Blood 1962;20:261–71.

16. Adams JG, Heller P, Abramson RK, et al. Sulfonamide-induced hemolytic anemia and hemoglobin Hasharon. Arch Intern Med 1977;137(10):1449–51.

17. Narla J, Mohandas N. Red cell membrane disorders. Int J Lab Hematol 2017; 39(Suppl 1):47–52.

18. Niss O, Chonat S, Dagaonkar N, et al. Genotype-phenotype correlations in hereditary elliptocytosis and hereditary pyropoikilocytosis. Blood Cells Mol Dis 2016; 61:4–9.

19. Gallagher PG. Disorders of erythrocyte hydration. Blood 2017;130(25):2699–708.

20. Andolfo I, Russo R, Gambale A, et al. Hereditary stomatocytosis: an underdiagnosed condition. Am J Hematol 2018;93(1):107–21.

21. Dyrda A, Cytlak U, Ciuraszkiewicz A, et al. Local membrane deformations activate Ca^{2+}-dependent K^+ and anionic currents in intact human red blood cells. PLoS One 2010;5(2):e9447.

22. Cahalan SM, Lukacs V, Ranade SS, et al. Piezo1 links mechanical forces to red blood cell volume. eLife 2015;4. https://doi.org/10.7554/eLife.07370.

23. Zarychanski R, Schulz VP, Houston BL, et al. Mutations in the mechanotransduction protein PIEZO1 are associated with hereditary xerocytosis. Blood 2012; 120(9):1908–15.

24. Andolfo I, Alper SL, De Franceschi L, et al. Multiple clinical forms of dehydrated hereditary stomatocytosis arise from mutations in PIEZO1. Blood 2013;121(19): 3925–35. S1–12.

25. Albuisson J, Murthy SE, Bandell M, et al. Dehydrated hereditary stomatocytosis linked to gain-of-function mutations in mechanically activated PIEZO1 ion channels. Nat Commun 2013;4:1884.

26. Bagriantsev SN, Gracheva EO, Gallagher PG. Piezo proteins: regulators of mechanosensation and other cellular processes. J Biol Chem 2014;289(46): 31673–81.

27. Bae C, Gnanasambandam R, Nicolai C, et al. Xerocytosis is caused by mutations that alter the kinetics of the mechanosensitive channel PIEZO1. Proc Natl Acad Sci U S A 2013;110(12):E1162–8.

28. Glogowska E, Schneider ER, Maksimova Y, et al. Novel mechanisms of PIEZO1 dysfunction in hereditary xerocytosis. Blood 2017;130(16):1845–56.

29. Glogowska E, Lezon-Geyda K, Maksimova Y, et al. Mutations in the Gardos channel (KCNN4) are associated with hereditary xerocytosis. Blood 2015; 126(11):1281–4.

30. Rapetti-Mauss R, Lacoste C, Picard V, et al. A mutation in the Gardos channel is associated with hereditary xerocytosis. Blood 2015;126(11):1273–80.

31. Andolfo I, Russo R, Manna F, et al. Novel Gardos channel mutations linked to dehydrated hereditary stomatocytosis (xerocytosis). Am J Hematol 2015;90(10): 921–6.

32. Fermo E, Bogdanova A, Petkova-Kirova P, et al. 'Gardos Channelopathy': a variant of hereditary Stomatocytosis with complex molecular regulation. Sci Rep 2017;7(1):1744.

33. Kaufman HW, Niles JK, Gallagher DR, et al. Revised prevalence estimate of possible Hereditary Xerocytosis as derived from a large U.S. Laboratory database. Am J Hematol 2018;93(1):E9–12.

34. Lek M, Karczewski KJ, Minikel EV, et al. Analysis of protein-coding genetic variation in 60,706 humans. Nature 2016;536(7616):285–91.

35. Ma S, Cahalan S, LaMonte G, et al. Common PIEZO1 allele in African populations causes RBC dehydration and attenuates plasmodium infection. Cell 2018;173(2): 443–55.e12.

36. Grootenboer S, Schischmanoff PO, Cynober T, et al. A genetic syndrome associating dehydrated hereditary stomatocytosis, pseudohyperkalaemia and perinatal oedema. Br J Haematol 1998;103(2):383–6.

37. Syfuss PY, Ciupea A, Brahimi S, et al. Mild dehydrated hereditary stomatocytosis revealed by marked hepatosiderosis. Clin Lab Haematol 2006;28(4):270–4.

38. Houston BL, Zelinski T, Israels SJ, et al. Refinement of the hereditary xerocytosis locus on chromosome 16q in a large Canadian kindred. Blood Cells Mol Dis 2011;47(4):226–31.

39. Assis RA, Kassab C, Seguro FS, et al. Iron overload in a teenager with xerocytosis: the importance of nuclear magnetic resonance imaging. Einstein (Sao Paulo) 2013;11(4):528–32.

40. Fermo E, Vercellati C, Marcello AP, et al. Hereditary xerocytosis due to mutations in PIEZO1 gene associated with heterozygous pyruvate kinase deficiency and

beta-thalassemia trait in two unrelated families. Case Rep Hematol 2017;2017: 2769570.

41. Risinger M, Glogowska E, Chonat S, et al. Hereditary xerocytosis: diagnostic considerations. Am J Hematol 2018;93(3):E67–9.

42. Iolascon A, Andolfo I, Barcellini W, et al. Recommendations regarding splenectomy in hereditary hemolytic anemias. Haematologica 2017;102(8):1304–13.

43. Rapetti-Mauss R, Picard V, Guitton C, et al. Red blood cell Gardos channel (KCNN4): the essential determinant of erythrocyte dehydration in hereditary xerocytosis. Haematologica 2017;102(10):e415–8.

44. Ataga KI, Reid M, Ballas SK, et al. Improvements in haemolysis and indicators of erythrocyte survival do not correlate with acute vaso-occlusive crises in patients with sickle cell disease: a phase III randomized, placebo-controlled, double-blind study of the Gardos channel blocker senicapoc (ICA-17043). Br J Haematol 2011;153(1):92–104.

45. Rapetti-Mauss R, Soriani O, Vinti H, et al. Senicapoc: a potent candidate for the treatment of a subset of hereditary xerocytosis caused by mutations in the Gardos channel. Haematologica 2016;101(11):e431–5.

46. Bruce LJ. Hereditary stomatocytosis and cation-leaky red cells—recent developments. Blood Cells Mol Dis 2009;42(3):216–22.

47. Bruce LJ, Guizouarn H, Burton NM, et al. The monovalent cation leak in overhydrated stomatocytic red blood cells results from amino acid substitutions in the Rh-associated glycoprotein. Blood 2009;113(6):1350–7.

48. Genetet S, Ripoche P, Picot J, et al. Human RhAG ammonia channel is impaired by the Phe65Ser mutation in overhydrated stomatocytic red cells. Am J Physiol Cell Physiol 2012;302(2):C419–28.

49. Caner T, Abdulnour-Nakhoul S, Brown K, et al. Mechanisms of ammonia and ammonium transport by rhesus-associated glycoproteins. Am J Physiol Cell Physiol 2015;309(11):C747–58.

50. Bruce LJ, Robinson HC, Guizouarn H, et al. Monovalent cation leaks in human red cells caused by single amino-acid substitutions in the transport domain of the band 3 chloride-bicarbonate exchanger, AE1. Nat Genet 2005;37(11): 1258–63.

51. Guizouarn H, Martial S, Gabillat N, et al. Point mutations involved in red cell stomatocytosis convert the electroneutral anion exchanger 1 to a nonselective cation conductance. Blood 2007;110(6):2158–65.

52. Barneaud-Rocca D, Pellissier B, Borgese F, et al. Band 3 missense mutations and stomatocytosis: insight into the molecular mechanism responsible for monovalent cation leak. Int J Cell Biol 2011;2011:136802.

53. Weber YG, Storch A, Wuttke TV, et al. GLUT1 mutations are a cause of paroxysmal exertion-induced dyskinesias and induce hemolytic anemia by a cation leak. J Clin Invest 2008;118(6):2157–68.

54. Flatt JF, Guizouarn H, Burton NM, et al. Stomatin-deficient cryohydrocytosis results from mutations in SLC2A1: a novel form of GLUT1 deficiency syndrome. Blood 2011;118(19):5267–77.

55. Orosz F, Olah J, Ovadi J. Reappraisal of triosephosphate isomerase deficiency. Eur J Haematol 2011;86(3):265–7.

56. Renella R, Wood WG. The congenital dyserythropoietic anemias. Hematol Oncol Clin North Am 2009;23(2):283–306.

57. Heimpel H, Wendt F. Congenital dyserythropoietic anemia with karyorrhexis and multinuclearity of erythroblasts. Helv Med Acta 1968;34(2):103–15.

58. Wickramasinghe SN, Wood WG. Advances in the understanding of the congenital dyserythropoietic anaemias. Br J Haematol 2005;131(4):431–46.
59. Dgany O, Avidan N, Delaunay J, et al. Congenital dyserythropoietic anemia type I is caused by mutations in codanin-1. Am J Hum Genet 2002;71(6):1467–74.
60. Gambale A, Iolascon A, Andolfo I, et al. Diagnosis and management of congenital dyserythropoietic anemias. Expert Rev Hematol 2016;9(3):283–96.
61. Iolascon A, Delaunay J. Close to unraveling the secrets of congenital dyserythropoietic anemia types I and II. Haematologica 2009;94(5):599–602.
62. Schwarz K, Iolascon A, Verissimo F, et al. Mutations affecting the secretory COPII coat component SEC23B cause congenital dyserythropoietic anemia type II. Nat Genet 2009;41(8):936–40.
63. Liljeholm M, Irvine AF, Vikberg AL, et al. Congenital dyserythropoietic anemia type III (CDA III) is caused by a mutation in kinesin family member, KIF23. Blood 2013;121(23):4791–9.
64. Traxler E, Weiss MJ. Congenital dyserythropoietic anemias: III's a charm. Blood 2013;121(23):4614–5.
65. Babbs C, Roberts NA, Sanchez-Pulido L, et al. Homozygous mutations in a predircted endonuclease are a novel cause of congenital dyserythropoietic anemia type I. Haematologica 2013;98(9):1383–7.
66. Tamary H, Dgany O. Congenital dyserythropoietic anemia Type I. In: Adam MP, Ardinger HH, Pagon RA, et al, editors. GeneReviews® [Internet]. Seattle (WA): University of Washington Seattle; 2016.
67. Hu CK, Coughlin M, Mitchison TJ. Midbody assembly and its regulation during cytokinesis. Mol Biol Cell 2012;23(6):1024–34.
68. Noy-Lotan S, Dgany O, Lahmi R, et al. Codanin-1, the protein encoded by the gene mutated in congenital dyserythropoietic anemia type I (CDAN1), is cell cycle-regulated. Haematologica 2009;94(5):629–37.
69. Arnaud L, Saison C, Helias V, et al. A dominant mutation in the gene encoding the erythroid transcription factor KLF1 causes a congenital dyserythropoietic anemia. Am J Hum Genet 2010;87(5):721–7.
70. Nichols KE, Crispino JD, Poncz M, et al. Familial dyserythropoietic anaemia and thrombocytopenia due to an inherited mutation in GATA1. Nat Genet 2000;24(3):266–70.
71. Del Vecchio GC, Giordani L, De Santis A, et al. Dyserythropoietic anemia and thrombocytopenia due to a novel mutation in GATA-1. Acta Haematol 2005;114(2):113–6.
72. Heimpel H, Anselstetter V, Chrobak L, et al. Congenital dyserythropoietic anemia type II: epidemiology, clinical appearance, and prognosis based on long-term observation. Blood 2003;102(13):4576–81.
73. Heimpel H, Schwarz K, Ebnother M, et al. Congenital dyserythropoietic anemia type I (CDA I): molecular genetics, clinical appearance, and prognosis based on long-term observation. Blood 2006;107(1):334–40.
74. Iolascon A, Delaunay J, Wickramasinghe SN, et al. Natural history of congenital dyserythropoietic anemia type II. Blood 2001;98(4):1258–60.
75. Iolascon A, Heimpel H, Wahlin A, et al. Congenital dyserythropoietic anemias: molecular insights and diagnostic approach. Blood 2013;122(13):2162–6.
76. Scartezzini P, Forni GL, Baldi M, et al. Decreased glycosylation of band 3 and band 4.5 glycoproteins of erythrocyte membrane in congenital dyserythropoietic anaemia type II. Br J Haematol 1982;51(4):569–76.

77. Iolascon A, Esposito MR, Russo R. Clinical aspects and pathogenesis of congenital dyserythropoietic anemias: from morphology to molecular approach. Haematologica 2012;97(12):1786–94.

78. Sandstrom H, Wahlin A. Congenital dyserythropoietic anemia type III. Haematologica 2000;85(7):753–7.

79. Ravindranath Y, Johnson RM, Goyette G, et al. KLF1 E325K-associated congenital dyserythropoietic anemia type IV: insights into the variable clinical severity. J Pediatr Hematol Oncol 2018;40(6):e405–9.

80. Lesmana H, Christakopoulos GE, Seu KG, et al. Clinical application of massively parallel sequencing in the diagnosis of hereditary hemolytic and dyserythropoietic anemias. Blood 2016;128(22):4786 [abstract].

81. Niss O, Lorsbach RB, Christakopoulos GE, et al. The first registry for patients with congenital dyserythropoietic anemia in North America: design and preliminary results. Blood 2017;130(Suppl 1):2210.

82. Shamseddine A, Taher A, Jaafar H, et al. Interferon alpha is an effective therapy for congenital dyserythropoietic anaemia type I. Eur J Haematol 2000;65(3): 207–9.

83. Lavabre-Bertrand T, Ramos J, Delfour C, et al. Long-term alpha interferon treatment is effective on anaemia and significantly reduces iron overload in congenital dyserythropoiesis type I. Eur J Haematol 2004;73(5):380–3.

84. Lavabre-Bertrand T, Blanc P, Navarro R, et al. alpha-Interferon therapy for congenital dyserythropoiesis type I. Br J Haematol 1995;89(4):929–32.

85. Ayas M, al-Jefri A, Baothman A, et al. Transfusion-dependent congenital dyserythropoietic anemia type I successfully treated with allogeneic stem cell transplantation. Bone Marrow Transplant 2002;29(8):681–2.

86. Remacha AF, Badell I, Pujol-Moix N, et al. Hydrops fetalis-associated congenital dyserythropoietic anemia treated with intrauterine transfusions and bone marrow transplantation. Blood 2002;100(1):356–8.

87. Mohandas N, Clark MR, Health BP, et al. A technique to detect reduced mechanical stability of red cell membranes: relevance to elliptocytic disorders. Blood 1982;59(4):768–74.

88. Heimpel H, Forteza-Vila J, Queisser W, et al. Electron and light microscopic study of the erythroblasts of patients with congenital dyserythropoietic anemia. Blood 1971;37(3):299–310.

Disorders of Iron Metabolism
New Diagnostic and Treatment Approaches to Iron Deficiency

Jacquelyn M. Powers, MD, MS[a],*, George R. Buchanan, MD[b]

KEYWORDS

- Iron • Ferritin • Hepcidin • Oral • Intravenous • Therapy

KEY POINTS

- Iron deficiency in the United States affects approximately 15% of children 1 to 2 years of age and 11% of adolescent girls.
- Signs and symptoms of iron deficiency anemia, such as pica, fatigue, and pallor, may be present, but their absence does not minimize its clinical significance.
- The presence of microcytic anemia with clinical risk factors, response to a therapeutic trial of oral iron therapy, and/or low serum ferritin are among the most well-established markers for the diagnosis of iron deficiency anemia.
- Recent developments in laboratory testing, such as soluble transferrin receptor, hepcidin, and erythroferrone, may be helpful in characterizing certain subpopulations of children affected by iron deficiency anemia in the future.
- The use and success of low-dose oral iron therapy are supported by recent clinical trials of iron absorption and clinical response. Intravenous iron administration has proven safe and beneficial for children who have failed oral iron therapy and therefore warrants further clinical trial exploration.

INTRODUCTION
Role of Iron

Iron is a vitally important element in all living organisms. It is omnipresent, constituting 4.5% of the earth's crust. However, iron constitutes only 0.005% of the body weight in humans. Total body iron content in men and women is 4 and 3 g, respectively, but only 300 mg in newborn infants. Iron in the human body represents a paradox. Insufficient

Disclosure: The authors have no conflict of interests.
[a] Department of Pediatrics, Section of Hematology-Oncology, Baylor College of Medicine, Texas Children's Cancer and Hematology Centers, 6701 Fannin Street, Suite 1580, Houston, TX 77030, USA; [b] Pediatric Hematology-Oncology, UT Southwestern Medical Center, 5323 Harry Hines Boulevard, H3.104A, Dallas, TX 75390-9063, USA
* Corresponding author.
E-mail addresses: jmpowers@texaschildrens.org; Jacquelyn.Powers@bcm.edu

iron is deleterious, causing myriad nonhematologic effects and anemia in its most severe form. However, protective mechanisms exist, such as the high efficiency and tight regulation of iron absorption and recycling and minimal loss of iron from the body. Conversely, too much iron is detrimental. Excessive iron causes free radical generation, and the resultant oxidant injury to damaged cells can be lethal. Protection from iron overload includes regulation and limitation of iron absorption as well as the binding of iron to proteins, such as transferrin, ferritin, and hemoglobin. It is therefore not surprising that iron deficiency is a multisystem disorder with innumerable effects, including behavioral abnormalities, cognitive deficits, and biochemical alterations (**Table 1**).

Epidemiology

Iron deficiency, with or without frank anemia, is an extremely common condition worldwide and is the most common cause of anemia globally.[1] The highest burden occurs in children aged 1 to 4 years and women of reproductive age. In lower-income countries, iron deficiency is common in all age groups as a result of malnutrition, including limited meat intake, gastrointestinal bleeding due to hookworms and other parasites, and limited availability of iron supplementation. Confounders of iron deficiency anemia include concomitant infections and other causes of anemia, such as sickle cell disease, thalassemia, and other nutritional deficiencies. In the United States and other developed countries, the prevalence of iron deficiency in infants and young children increased during the 1940s, resulting in part from recommendations to switch from breast feeding to cow milk–based formula, which at that time was not appropriately iron fortified. Over the subsequent decades, the addition of iron-fortified formulas, development of the WIC (Women, Infants, and Children) program, promotion of breastfeeding, and universal screening in young children have resulted in decreased rates of iron deficiency. However, approximately 15% of children aged 1 to 2 years are iron deficient and approximately 3% have frank iron deficiency anemia.[2,3]

Adolescent girls are also at high risk of developing iron deficiency with an estimated 11% being iron deficient and 5% having frank iron deficiency anemia.[2] Despite such prevalence rates, this group fails to benefit from universal laboratory screening. Risk-based questionnaires commonly used in practice poorly correlate with iron deficiency and anemia in adolescent girls.[4] In many such women with unrecognized menstrual

Table 1 Nonhematologic effects of iron deficiency	
Effect	**Role of Iron**
Biochemical	Oxidative metabolism
	DNA synthesis
	Neurotransmitter metabolism
	Energy metabolism
	Impaired myelination
Cognitive	Impaired verbal learning, memory
	Visual and motor functioning
Physical	Pica
	Breath-holding spells
	Restless legs
	Fatigue/diminished work performance
	Impaired cardiac function
	Stroke

blood loss, acute or chronic, complications, such as severe anemia requiring emergent care or inpatient hospitalization, occur.[5,6]

CAUSE BY AGE GROUP
Infants

In developed countries, the prevalence of iron deficiency is low at birth because of the in utero transfer of iron from mother to fetus during the third trimester. Premature and low-birth-weight infants are vulnerable to early iron deficiency because of their lower iron endowment at birth and more rapid growth rate postnatally. Depleted iron stores are accordingly problematic in premature infants as early as 2 to 3 months of age yet uncommon before 6 months in term infants.[7] Suboptimal maternal iron status can also contribute to iron deficiency during the neonatal period.

Young Children

In early childhood, "toddlers" aged 12 to 24 months are at highest risk because of their rapid growth coupled with diets containing insufficient iron.[3] **Table 2** summarizes the risk factors for and underlying causes of iron deficiency in this age group.[8,9] These young children are often otherwise healthy. However, specific questioning generally elicits a history of the child as a "picky" eater who prefers to drink milk, often by bottle rather than cup. A detailed history typically reveals that the child's diet is deficient in iron due to grossly excess cow milk intake, pica, irritability, and little appetite for meat, vegetables, and other iron-containing foods.[10] Excessive cow milk intake, in particular, is a strong predictor for iron deficiency because of its low iron content (<1 mg/L), the poor absorption of iron from cow milk (<10% compared with approximately 50% of iron in breast milk), reduced intake of other foods, suboptimal

Table 2	
Iron deficiency risk factors in children by age group	
Age Group	**Clinical or Demographic Risk Factor**
Neonate to 6 mo	Low maternal iron status Prematurity; lack of iron supplementation if premature Low-iron formula
6–12 mo[a]	Exclusive breastfeeding without iron supplementation Introduction of cow milk before 12 mo
12–48 mo[a]	Excessive cow milk intake (>24 ounces per day) Bottle fed Overweight/obese Latino/Hispanic ethnicity or Asian race Low socioeconomic status
School-aged children	Low iron diet Obesity Gastrointestinal conditions
Adolescents	Heavy menstrual bleeding[b] Low-iron diet Obesity High-endurance sports participation/running Blood donation Latino/Hispanic ethnicity or African American race[b] Low socioeconomic status[b]

[a] Risk factors from earlier time periods remain relevant in children aged 6 to 48 mo of age.
[b] Established risk factor in adolescent girls.

absorption of medicinal iron supplements taken with milk, and, in severe cases, occult gastrointestinal blood loss and milk-protein enteropathy.[11,12]

School-Aged Children

In middle school–aged children, the prevalence of iron deficiency is quite low, with external blood loss the most common underlying cause. Epistaxis or gastrointestinal blood loss due to inflammatory bowel disease,[13] parasitic infections, or other anatomic lesions should be assessed. Rarely, occult intrapulmonary or renal blood loss may be causative.

Adolescent Girls

In this population, menstrual blood loss, especially heavy menstrual bleeding, is the most common cause of iron deficiency. Rapid growth and iron-poor diet are also contributory. Evaluation, management, and follow-up of such patients are often variable, falling short of expert recommendations and established guidelines, which repeatedly indicate their higher likelihood for persistent or recurrent iron deficiency anemia.[14] Female athletes are at further risk for the development of iron deficiency because of contributors, such as trace gastrointestinal bleeding, "foot-strike" hemolysis, and exercised-induced inflammation.[15–17]

Rare Causes

Malabsorption of iron is infrequently the primary cause during childhood. However, in children with celiac disease or other gastrointestinal disorders, malabsorption in addition to blood loss may be contributory.[18,19] Children receiving therapy for gastrointestinal reflux, such as proton pump inhibitors or H2-receptor antagonists, may also have impaired absorption because of inability to reduce non–heme iron from the ferric ($+3$) to the preferred ferrous ($+2$) form. Concomitant inflammation from any acute or chronic condition will also impair absorption as a consequence of the regulatory effects of hepcidin on iron described later.[20] An isolated autosomal recessive defect of the TMPRSS6 gene causing iron refractory iron deficiency anemia (IRIDA) results from a sustained overproduction of hepcidin and has been described in familial cohorts[21] but is exceedingly rare.[22]

DIAGNOSIS OF IRON DEFICIENCY
Clinical History

The clinical history is critical for not only making the diagnosis of iron deficiency but also appropriately identifying the underlying cause. Iron deficiency, with or without frank anemia, is often clinically "silent" with signs and symptoms not fully appreciated until the successful institution of iron therapy. Careful and systematic assessment of the diet, sources, and characterization of potential bleeding, malabsorption, and underlying inflammation should be performed. Physical examination should evaluate and characterize tachycardia, presence of a heart murmur, pallor, and absence of the jaundice and hepatosplenomegaly not typical of iron deficiency anemia. Symptoms, such as irritability, fatigue, and decreased activity, are quite often present in more severely affected children with iron deficiency anemia. **Table 2** summarizes the risk factors for and underlying causes of iron deficiency in children as well as their most common clinical signs and symptoms.

Pica

The first clinical manifestation in many patients with iron deficiency is pica, an intense craving for and ingestion of a nonfood item.[23,24] Many such items are crunchy and

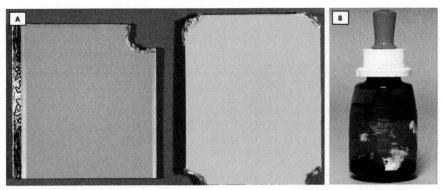

Fig. 1. Manifestations of pica in young children with iron deficiency anemia. (*A*) Cardboard books with chewed corners. (*B*) A full (unconsumed) bottle of ferrous sulfate with label removed and eaten.

often have limited or no nutritional value. Although its true incidence is unknown, in a clinical trial of young children with nutritional iron deficiency anemia whose parents were prospectively asked about pica, 49% of respondents reported such symptoms.[25] **Fig. 1** depicts striking examples of pica in which the corners of books and the label of a bottle containing iron drops were repetitively ingested by 2 affected children. **Table 3** lists the most commonly chosen items that are repetitively chewed and often swallowed. Pagophagia, or intense craving for ice, is a common complaint in affected adolescents. Although sometimes the chief complaint, pica may be underreported as a result of embarrassment. Pica has cultural variations with clay or dirt being more common in certain parts of the world. In an environment contaminated by lead, risk of lead poisoning is heightened due to the combination of enhanced lead absorption in patients with iron deficiency and pica. Testing blood lead level is therefore necessary in all iron-deficient infants and young children with a history of lead exposure.[26]

Laboratory Assessment

The 3 stages of iron deficiency are as follows:

1. Depletion of iron stores,
2. Iron-deficient erythropoiesis,
3. Frank iron deficiency anemia.[27]

Table 3
Items consumed in children and adolescents with pica due to iron deficiency

Age Group	Item
Young children	Dirt
	Rocks
	Cardboard
	Paper
	Baby wipes
Adolescents	Ice (pagophagia)
	Paper (tissue or other)
	Cornstarch
	Laundry detergent/soap
	Clay

Table 4
Laboratory diagnosis of iron deficiency

Iron Compartment	Conventional Tests	Values Suggestive or Diagnostic of Iron Deficiency
Storage	Serum ferritin	<15 mg/L
Plasma	Serum iron (Fe)	<60 mg/dL
	Serum transferrin (TIBC)	>400 μg/dL
	Transferrin saturation (Fe/TIBC)	<15%
Red blood cells	Reticulocyte hemoglobin content or equivalent (CHr, Ret-He)	<26 pg
	Red cell distribution width	>16%
	MCV[a]	<70 fL (young children)
		<80 fL (age ≥10 y)
	Hgb[a]	<11 g/dL (young children)
		<12 g/dL (age ≥10 y)

[a] Lower limit of normal values from MCV and Hgb increase with age and by gender in adolescence.

Accordingly, traditional laboratory measures (**Table 4**) of iron deficiency become abnormal in a stepwise progression with serum ferritin becoming the first abnormal parameter and hemoglobin concentration (Hgb) the last affected marker (in the absence of an acute hemorrhage).

The presence of clinical risk factors along with microcytic anemia (low Hgb, low mean corpuscular volume [MCV]) and elevated red cell distribution width is consistent with the diagnosis of iron deficiency anemia. Review of the peripheral blood smear will demonstrate hypochromic, microcytic red blood cells, often with accompanying thrombocytosis (**Fig. 2**). In such patients, a course of oral iron therapy that elicits a complete hematologic response confirms the diagnosis.[28]

Differential diagnosis of microcytic anemia

The most common causes of microcytic anemia in children are iron deficiency, α- or β-thalassemia, and anemia of inflammation. In the absence of clinical risk factors for iron deficiency, evaluation for other causes should be pursued. A copy of the newborn hemoglobinopathy screening result should be reviewed, when available, for the presence of hemoglobin Bart's as a marker for α-thalassemia trait. Hemoglobin analysis performed in toddlers, and older children can assess for β-thalassemia trait as well

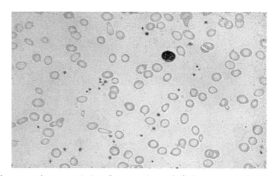

Fig. 2. Peripheral smear characteristic of severe iron deficiency anemia. Hypochromic, microcytic red blood cells are visualized along with thrombocytosis.

as other causes of microcytic anemia, such as hemoglobin C or hemoglobin E disease (but is normal in α-thalassemia trait). Other much more rare causes of microcytic anemia include hereditary pyropoikilocytosis, sideroblastic anemia, copper deficiency, and congenital atransferrinemia.

Novel Laboratory Measures

Soluble/serum transferrin receptor

Additional measures of iron status have emerged as the understanding of iron homeostasis and regulation has broadened. The soluble or serum transferrin receptor (sTfR1) test, which measures a circulating protein derived from cleavage of the membrane transferrin receptor on erythroid precursor cells within the marrow, is inversely proportional to tissue iron availability (ie, the higher the sTfR1 value, the lower the available iron stores).[29] The sTfR/log ferritin index uses these 2 laboratory measures to better distinguish the presence or absence of iron deficiency in persons with anemia of inflammation.[30,31] An elevated sTfR/log ferritin index indicates iron deficiency, whereas a person with a low index has anemia more consistent with inflammation alone. This test is most useful in persons with chronic inflammatory conditions (eg, inflammatory bowel disease) to help determine whether their anemia would benefit from iron therapy.

Hepcidin

The primary regulator of iron homeostasis is the peptide hormone hepcidin, which blocks the action of ferroportin, the only known transmembrane iron transporter.[32] Ferroportin permits the movement of intracellular iron from enterocytes, macrophages, and hepatocytes into the plasma for transport to the bone marrow and other tissues. Hepcidin binding to ferroportin results in its internalization and degradation, the consequence of which is downregulation of both intestinal iron absorption and release of storage iron from macrophages and hepatocytes.[33,34] Hepcidin concentrations are reduced in states of iron deficiency, anemia, and hypoxia, thus enhancing iron absorption and transport as well as releasing storage iron from macrophages and hepatocytes. During states of iron sufficiency, hepcidin limits iron absorption and release. Hepcidin production is increased in states of infection and inflammation via cytokine stimulation, particularly interleukin-6, which decreases iron availability to pathogens. Inherited mutations of the TMPRSS6 gene, which cause IRIDA (described previously), also result in upregulation of hepcidin.[35]

Given hepcidin's role as a major iron regulator, it might become an important diagnostic tool and therapeutic marker to predict treatment success or failure with oral iron.[36,37] Elevated serum hepcidin levels have been shown to predict failure of oral iron treatment in adults with iron deficiency anemia as well as in patients with multifactorial anemia.[38] Studies of children in countries such as Gambia have found that it better differentiates iron deficiency anemia from other causes of anemia and is the major predictor of iron incorporation into red blood cells.[39,40] Currently, there are limited data on the utility of serum hepcidin levels in children with iron deficiency anemia in the United States.

Erythroferrone

Erythroferrone (ERFE) is a protein hormone produced by erythroblasts[41] in response to erythropoietin and episodes of acute blood loss. ERFE inhibits the action of hepcidin, thereby increasing the amount of iron available for hemoglobin synthesis and contributing to the recovery from the anemia of inflammation,[42] ineffective erythropoiesis in thalassemia[43] as well as the anemia of chronic kidney disease.[44] In 1 study of children with iron deficiency anemia, ERFE levels were elevated, and inverse associations were shown between its concentrations and Hgb, transferrin saturation, and serum ferritin.[45] Although ERFE is a commercially available laboratory measure,[46] there is not yet a clear benefit to assessing it over other more common, well-established, and less costly tests in patients with iron deficiency.

TREATMENT APPROACHES

In any patient with iron deficiency anemia, the underlying cause must be identified and corrected. If not, regardless of iron therapy, there is at high likelihood for suboptimal response or persistence or recurrence of anemia. Patients with severe anemia should be assessed for clinical stability and are candidates for receipt of 1 or more packed red blood cell transfusions delivered in small aliquots. Initiation of oral iron therapy and close follow-up are also imperative in the ongoing management of such severely affected patients.

Oral Iron Therapy

Preparations

Myriad oral iron preparations exist. Iron salts, such as ferrous sulfate, ferrous fumarate, and ferrous gluconate, are the most well-known and widely available forms. Iron salts in the ferrous (+2) form are better absorbed than preparations with iron in the ferric (+3) state, which require an acidic environment to ensure reduction to the ferrous state and absorption by the enterocyte. Iron polysaccharide complex preparations, which have been formulated with the aim of improved palatability, are also effective in the treatment of iron deficiency anemia. However, because these preparations contain iron in the ferric form, they are less well absorbed and may require longer duration of therapy overall. The BESTIRON trial randomized 80 young children with nutritional iron deficiency anemia to ferrous sulfate or iron polysaccharide complex and reported a significant difference between groups in the increase in hemoglobin over time (1.0 g/dL [95% confidence interval, 0.4–1.6 g/dL]; $P<.001$), favoring ferrous sulfate. A significant difference in the rate of increase in serum ferritin also favored the ferrous sulfate group. A subgroup analysis of those subjects with mild iron deficiency anemia (Hgb >9 g/dL) showed a similar trend.[47] Carbonyl iron and other forms of available oral iron have limited efficacy data available for analysis because of their being marketed for many years as nutritional supplements rather than therapeutic drug preparations.

Dosing

Dosing recommendations for oral iron therapy have been empiric for well over a century. However, recent research, including the discovery of hepcidin,[32] has greatly enhanced the understanding of iron dosing and subsequent absorption.[34] Studies of various iron-dosing regimens, serial measurements of hepcidin, and analysis of the fractional absorption of radiolabeled iron isotopes have been recently performed in iron-depleted, nonanemic healthy women.[48] An initial morning dose of oral iron ($\geq$60 mg) resulted in serum hepcidin being elevated for up to 24 hours, thereby limiting subsequent oral iron absorption. Therefore, to maximize the fractional absorption of iron (the percentage of the individual iron dose ingested), lower doses of iron (40–80 mg daily) should be given, and divided (ie, twice a day) dosing should be avoided.[48] A follow-up study involving a similar population administered 14 doses of iron on either consecutive days (14 doses in 14 days) or alternate days (14 doses in 28 days), with the alternate-day dosing regimen having 34% greater total iron absorption.[49] An analysis of split dosing (administering the same total amount of iron in 2 divided doses vs 1 large dose) found no benefit (ie, no increase in absorption) to divided dosing.[49]

Another study supporting the effectiveness of a low-dose regimen randomized 90 octogenarians with iron deficiency anemia to 15, 50, or 150 mg elemental iron daily.[50] All 3 groups had similar rates of improvement in anemia over 2 months despite the high-dose group having the most adverse effects.

Clinical trials comparing various dosing regimens in children with iron deficiency anemia are lacking. However, the BESTIRON study used a low-dose, once-daily regimen of 3 mg/kg elemental iron and demonstrated an excellent hematologic response.[25] Comparative studies of such "minimalist" dosing strategies are badly needed in children and adolescents. However, until such studies, based on the dosing in these available studies, for young children, the authors recommend 3 mg/kg elemental iron administered once daily, and in adolescents, they recommend 65 mg elemental iron (1 tablet) administered once daily.

Hematologic response

Children with mild iron deficiency anemia should have a normal Hgb within 1 month of initiating oral iron treatment assuming the cause of anemia has been identified and corrected. Those patients with moderate to severe anemia treated with oral iron should demonstrate reticulocytosis within 7 to 10 days and hemoglobin increment of ≥ 2 g/dL over the initial 4 weeks of therapy. Children with a suboptimal response should be assessed for poor adherence to the prescribed treatment regimen. Causes for persistent or refractory iron deficiency anemia are listed in **Table 5**. A minimum of 3 months of daily oral iron therapy is indicated in all patients. Many will require additional months of iron therapy to ensure adequate repletion of iron stores. Assessment of the serum ferritin level before therapy discontinuation may be prudent to ensure that the child's iron stores are adequate, thus reducing the risk of future recurrence of iron deficiency anemia even if the underlying cause has been corrected or eliminated.

Intravenous Iron Therapy

Indications

Several intravenous (IV) iron formulations are approved by the Food and Drug Administration (FDA) for use in children with the primary indication being chronic kidney disease. The next most common indication is children who fail oral iron therapy.[51–53] Reasons for oral iron treatment failure are broad but include nonadherence to oral iron,[54] continued low-iron diet, suboptimal iron absorption, and/or ongoing

Table 5
Reasons for "persistent" iron deficiency anemia or incomplete response to oral iron therapy in children

Reason	Examples
Incorrect diagnosis	Thalassemia trait Anemia of inflammation
Persistence of cause	Low-iron diet (ie, excessive milk intake) Ongoing blood loss
Insufficient oral iron intake	Nonadherence Insufficient dosing (ie, multivitamin) Poor administration or patient refusal
Malabsorption	Underlying gastrointestinal disorder Concomitant inflammatory condition Administration of oral iron with milk

uncontrolled blood loss experienced by some children with gastrointestinal disorders or adolescent girls with heavy menstrual bleeding.

Patients with concomitant iron deficiency anemia and anemia resulting from inflammation are unable to absorb oral iron effectively.[20] In such patients, IV iron should be used. Adolescent girls and young women with fatigue or restless legs syndrome have been shown to benefit from IV iron therapy, particularly when their serum ferritin is less than 15 mg/L.[55] Adults with heart failure have also demonstrated improved clinical outcomes as well as health-related quality of life following IV iron therapy.[56,57] Data on its use in children with heart failure are unavailable but warrant investigation.

Formulations

One distinguishing characteristic of the available IV iron preparations (**Table 6**) is the strength of the carbohydrate shell that binds the iron core. The strength of such binding determines the dose of iron that may be safely delivered in a single infusion. Excessive doses result in free iron release into the plasma, which can result in hypersensitivity or "pseudo-allergy" reactions that can mimic severe anaphylaxis.[58]

Immunogenicity is another distinguishing characteristic of these formulations. Current second-generation (iron sucrose, ferric gluconate, low-molecular-weight iron dextran) and third-generation (ferumoxytol, ferric carboxymaltose, iron isomaltoside) formulations have substantially lower rates of adverse effects than initial IV iron preparations introduced several decades ago. Nonetheless, low-molecular-weight iron dextran and ferumoxytol are 2 products that currently have a black box warning, with the former requiring a test dose before full-dose infusion.

Cost is variable among the more recently licensed preparations, with the newer drugs being more expensive. Third-generation formulations allow for larger doses to be administered, resulting in a reduction in the total number of infusions that are required. Therefore, their relatively higher cost may be offset by fewer iron infusion visits and ancillary costs. However, total charges for patients vary significantly based not only on the formulation chosen but also on their individual insurance coverage.

Dosing

The dosing of IV iron can be determined via package labeling of the individual formulations or alternatively calculated using the Ganzoni formula, which estimates a patient's total iron deficit (**Box 1**).[59] Several preparations use a weight-based dosing approach with a maximum amount per single infusion, whereas others provide dosing based on a patient's weight and current Hgb. The Ganzoni formula's first half incorporates the patient's weight and current and target Hgb to determine the amount of iron needed to restore the patient to a normal hemoglobin value. The second half of the formula estimates the amount of additional iron needed to fully replenish storage iron. After the iron deficit is calculated and the IV iron formulation to be given is selected, the total number of necessary infusions can be determined based on the maximum amount that may be delivered in a single infusion.

Safety

Localized adverse effects of IV iron include iron deposition and discoloration or staining of the skin, following local extravasation of iron. Extra care should therefore be taken to ensure that placement of a peripheral IV is within the vein and not the subcutaneous tissue. If a large amount of IV iron is deposited into the tissue, the subsequent iron staining can be quite significant. Case reports exist on the use of laser therapy for this complication, but the benefit of such an intervention is unclear. Over time (months), macrophages may engulf the deposited tissue iron leading to fading of the iron stain. More common reactions from IV iron include localized urticaria, nausea,

Table 6
Intravenous iron preparations available in the United States

Generic (Trade) Name	Iron Sucrose (Venofer)	Ferric Gluconate (Ferrlecit)	Low-Molecular-Weight Iron Dextran (INFeD)	Ferumoxytol (Feraheme)	Ferric Carboxymaltose (Injectafer)
Manufacturer	American Regent, Inc	Sanofi Aventis, Inc	Watson Pharmaceuticals	AMAG Pharmaceuticals	American Regent, Inc
FDA indication	CKD; iron deficiency anemia refractory to oral iron therapy	CKD on dialysis + erythropoiesis stimulating agents	CKD; oral iron administration unsatisfactory/impossible	CKD	Non-dialysis-dependent CKD; intolerance or unsatisfactory response to oral iron
FDA approved (pediatrics)	Yes ≥2 y	Yes ≥6 y	Yes ≥4 mo	No	No (>14 y, Europe)
Black box warning	No	No	Yes	Yes	No
Test dose required	No	No	Yes	No	No
Maximum FDA-approved single infusion dose	Initial: 100 mg Maintenance: 300 mg	125 mg	<5 kg: 25 mg 5–10 kg: 50 mg >10 kg: 100 mg	510 mg	750 mg
Total dose infusion possible	No	No	Yes (off-label)	Yes	Yes
Infusion time	Pediatrics: Diluted: 30–90 min Undiluted: 5 min	Diluted, 60 min	60 min	15–60 min	Diluted: ≥15 min Undiluted: slow IV push no faster than 100 mg/min
Iron concentration	12.5 mg/mL	20 mg/mL	50 mg/mL	30 mg/mL	50 mg/mL
Vial size	5 mL	5 mL	2 mL	17 mL	15 mL
Dilution	Diluted in NS at ≥1 mg/mL or undiluted	25 mL NS (Pediatrics)	250–1000 mL NS	50–200 mL NS or D5W (2–8 mg/mL iron)	>2 mg/mL or undiluted IV push

Abbreviations: CKD, chronic kidney disease; D5W, 5% dextrose in water; NS, normal saline.

Box 1
Ganzoni formula to estimate total iron deficit

Iron deficit (mg) = weight (kg) × (target − actual Hgb [g/dL]) × 2.4 + 15 × weight (kg)

From Mantadakis E. Advances in pediatric intravenous iron therapy. Pediatr Blood Cancer 2016;63(1):11–6; with permission.

---

abdominal pain, and flushing.[60] Most systemic reactions to IV iron administration may be related to mast cell activation resulting in a red man–type syndrome, similar to that seen with IV vancomycin. Such reactions can be prevented by using slower infusion times. More severe hypersensitivity reactions may cause diffuse urticaria. Many such reactions are nonimmunologically mediated with no demonstration of an elevation of serum tryptase or other evidence of drug-specific antibodies.[58] However, true anaphylaxis can rarely occur, so IV iron must always be administered in settings with appropriately trained staff and the availability of resuscitations medications and equipment.

Future potential uses of intravenous iron

Most data on use of IV iron in children are based on retrospective cohorts[51–53,61–63] rather than formal prospective clinical trials. However, the increased use of both on- and off-label use of IV iron therapy in children[64] warrants further investigation. Comparative effectiveness trials comparing oral and IV iron regimens and their effects on hematologic and patient-centered outcomes in a variety of settings are necessary in order to fully appreciate the potential benefits of such therapies in a variety of clinical settings.

SUMMARY

Iron is a tightly regulated element within the body: having too little or too much is detrimental. Iron deficiency anemia is the leading cause of anemia worldwide. Within the United States, 15% of young children are affected by nutritional iron deficiency and at least 11% of adolescent girls experience iron deficiency from acute or chronic excessive menstrual blood loss. Symptoms of iron deficiency may be subtle. Irritability, fatigue, pallor, or pica may be present in affected patients, but it is often identified on laboratory screening in the absence of significant signs or symptoms. A clinical diagnosis of iron deficiency anemia may be made on the basis of risk factors and microcytic anemia with the peripheral blood smear demonstrating hypochromic, microcytic cells. A hematologic response to a therapeutic trial of oral iron therapy is reassuring. In patients who require additional diagnostic confirmation, many iron laboratory measures are available with testing of the iron regulators hepcidin and ERFE now also possible, albeit not necessarily as a routine. Serum ferritin remains the best measure of total body iron status. Data on iron absorption in combination with clinical trial data support a "minimalist" treatment regimen of low-dose oral iron therapy at 3 mg/kg elemental iron administered just once daily (on an empty stomach) for young children and 65 mg of elemental iron once daily in adolescents. IV iron is indicated in children who have failed oral iron therapy or have complex medical conditions that complicate the diagnosis and tolerance of oral iron. Clinical trials that compare dosing regimens as well as benefits of oral versus IV iron in children are needed.

ACKNOWLEDGMENTS

Dr. Powers' research is supported by grant K23HL132001 from National Heart, Lung, and Blood Institute.

REFERENCES

1. Kassebaum NJ, Jasrasaria R, Naghavi M, et al. A systematic analysis of global anemia burden from 1990 to 2010. Blood 2014;123(5):615–24.
2. Gupta PM, Hamner HC, Suchdev PS, et al. Iron status of toddlers, nonpregnant females, and pregnant females in the United States. Am J Clin Nutr 2017; 106(Suppl 6):1640S–6S.
3. Gupta PM, Perrine CG, Mei Z, et al. Iron, anemia, and iron deficiency anemia among young children in the United States. Nutrients 2016;8(6) [pii:E330].
4. Sekhar DL, Murray-Kolb LE, Schaefer EW, et al. Risk-based questionnaires fail to detect adolescent iron deficiency and anemia. J Pediatr 2017;187:194–9.e1.
5. Cooke AG, McCavit TL, Buchanan GR, et al. Iron deficiency anemia in adolescents who present with heavy menstrual bleeding. J Pediatr Adolesc Gynecol 2017;30(2):247–50.
6. Powers JM, Stanek JR, Srivaths L, et al. Hematologic considerations and management of adolescent girls with heavy menstrual bleeding and anemia in U.S. Children's Hospitals. J Pediatr Adolesc Gynecol 2018;31(5):446–50.
7. Baker RD, Greer FR, Committee on Nutrition American Academy of Pediatrics. Diagnosis and prevention of iron deficiency and iron-deficiency anemia in infants and young children (0-3 years of age). Pediatrics 2010;126(5):1040–50.
8. Brotanek JM, Halterman JS, Auinger P, et al. Iron deficiency, prolonged bottle-feeding, and racial/ethnic disparities in young children. Arch Pediatr Adolesc Med 2005;159(11):1038–42.
9. Brotanek JM, Gosz J, Weitzman M, et al. Secular trends in the prevalence of iron deficiency among US toddlers, 1976-2002. Arch Pediatr Adolesc Med 2008; 162(4):374–81.
10. Ziegler EE. Consumption of cow's milk as a cause of iron deficiency in infants and toddlers. Nutr Rev 2011;69(Suppl 1):S37–42.
11. Salstrom JL, Kent M, Liang X, et al. Toddlers with anasarca and severe anemia: a lesson in preventive medicine. Curr Opin Pediatr 2012;24(1):129–33.
12. Nickerson HJ, Silberman T, Park RW, et al. Treatment of iron deficiency anemia and associated protein-losing enteropathy in children. J Pediatr hematology/oncology 2000;22(1):50–4.
13. Gasche C, Lomer MC, Cavill I, et al. Iron, anaemia, and inflammatory bowel diseases. Gut 2004;53(8):1190–7.
14. Haamid F, Sass AE, Dietrich JE. Heavy menstrual bleeding in adolescents. J Pediatr Adolesc Gynecol 2017;30(3):335–40.
15. Dang CV. Runner's anemia. JAMA 2001;286(6):714–6.
16. Fazal AA, Whittemore MS, DeGeorge KC. Foot-strike haemolysis in an ultramarathon runner. BMJ Case Rep 2017;2017 [pii:bcr-2017-220661].
17. McClung JP, Gaffney-Stomberg E, Lee JJ. Female athletes: a population at risk of vitamin and mineral deficiencies affecting health and performance. J Trace Elem Med Biol 2014;28(4):388–92.
18. Wiskin AE, Fleming BJ, Wootton SA, et al. Anaemia and iron deficiency in children with inflammatory bowel disease. J Crohns Colitis 2012;6(6):687–91.
19. Hershko C, Camaschella C. How I treat unexplained refractory iron deficiency anemia. Blood 2014;123(3):326–33.
20. Cappellini MD, Comin-Colet J, de Francisco A, et al. Iron deficiency across chronic inflammatory conditions: international expert opinion on definition, diagnosis, and management. Am J Hematol 2017;92(10):1068–78.

21. Buchanan GR, Sheehan RG. Malabsorption and defective utilization of iron in three siblings. J Pediatr 1981;98(5):723–8.
22. Heeney MM, Finberg KE. Iron-refractory iron deficiency anemia (IRIDA). Hematol Oncol Clin North Am 2014;28(4):637–52, ix.
23. Borgna-Pignatti C, Zanella S. Pica as a manifestation of iron deficiency. Expert Rev Hematol 2016;9(11):1075–80.
24. Moore DF Jr, Sears DA. Pica, iron deficiency, and the medical history. Am J Med 1994;97(4):390–3.
25. Powers JM, Buchanan GR, Adix L, et al. Effect of low-dose ferrous sulfate vs iron polysaccharide complex on hemoglobin concentration in young children with nutritional iron-deficiency anemia: a randomized clinical trial. JAMA 2017; 317(22):2297–304.
26. Canfield RL, Henderson CR Jr, Cory-Slechta DA, et al. Intellectual impairment in children with blood lead concentrations below 10 microg per deciliter. N Engl J Med 2003;348(16):1517–26.
27. Powers JM, Buchanan GR. Diagnosis and management of iron deficiency anemia. Hematol Oncol Clin North Am 2014;28(4):729–45, vi-vii.
28. Oski FA. Iron deficiency in infancy and childhood. N Engl J Med 1993;329(3): 190–3.
29. Infusino I, Braga F, Dolci A, et al. Soluble transferrin receptor (sTfR) and sTfR/log ferritin index for the diagnosis of iron-deficiency anemia. A meta-analysis. Am J Clin Pathol 2012;138(5):642–9.
30. Skikne BS, Punnonen K, Caldron PH, et al. Improved differential diagnosis of anemia of chronic disease and iron deficiency anemia: a prospective multicenter evaluation of soluble transferrin receptor and the sTfR/log ferritin index. Am J Hematol 2011;86(11):923–7.
31. Oustamanolakis P, Koutroubakis IE. Soluble transferrin receptor-ferritin index is the most efficient marker for the diagnosis of iron deficiency anemia in patients with IBD. Inflamm Bowel Dis 2011;17(12):E158–9.
32. Nemeth E, Ganz T. The role of hepcidin in iron metabolism. Acta Haematol 2009; 122(2–3):78–86.
33. Ganz T, Olbina G, Girelli D, et al. Immunoassay for human serum hepcidin. Blood 2008;112(10):4292–7.
34. Girelli D, Nemeth E, Swinkels DW. Hepcidin in the diagnosis of iron disorders. Blood 2016;127(23):2809–13.
35. Heeney MM, Guo D, De Falco L, et al. Normalizing hepcidin predicts TMPRSS6 mutation status in patients with chronic iron deficiency. Blood 2018;132(4): 448–52.
36. Pasricha SR. Is it time for hepcidin to join the diagnostic toolkit for iron deficiency? Expert Rev Hematol 2012;5(2):153–5.
37. Ganz T. Hepcidin and the global burden of iron deficiency. Clin Chem 2015;61(4): 577–8.
38. Pasricha SR, McQuilten Z, Westerman M, et al. Serum hepcidin as a diagnostic test of iron deficiency in premenopausal female blood donors. Haematologica 2011;96(8):1099–105.
39. Prentice AM, Doherty CP, Abrams SA, et al. Hepcidin is the major predictor of erythrocyte iron incorporation in anemic African children. Blood 2012;119(8): 1922–8.
40. Atkinson SH, Armitage AE, Khandwala S, et al. Combinatorial effects of malaria season, iron deficiency, and inflammation determine plasma hepcidin concentration in African children. Blood 2014;123(21):3221–9.

41. Kautz L, Jung G, Valore EV, et al. Identification of erythroferrone as an erythroid regulator of iron metabolism. Nat Genet 2014;46(7):678–84.

42. Kautz L, Jung G, Nemeth E, et al. Erythroferrone contributes to recovery from anemia of inflammation. Blood 2014;124(16):2569–74.

43. Kautz L, Jung G, Du X, et al. Erythroferrone contributes to hepcidin suppression and iron overload in a mouse model of beta-thalassemia. Blood 2015;126(17):2031–7.

44. Hanudel MR, Rappaport M, Chua K, et al. Levels of the erythropoietin-responsive hormone erythroferrone in mice and humans with chronic kidney disease. Haematologica 2018;103(4):e141–2.

45. El Gendy FM, El-Hawy MA, Shehata AMF, et al. Erythroferrone and iron status parameters levels in pediatric patients with iron deficiency anemia. Eur J Haematol 2018;100(4):356–60.

46. Ganz T, Jung G, Naeim A, et al. Immunoassay for human serum erythroferrone. Blood 2017;130(10):1243–6.

47. Powers JM, Buchanan GR, McCavit TL. Effect of different iron preparations for young children with iron-deficiency anemia-reply. JAMA 2017;318(13):1282–3.

48. Moretti D, Goede JS, Zeder C, et al. Oral iron supplements increase hepcidin and decrease iron absorption from daily or twice-daily doses in iron-depleted young women. Blood 2015;126(17):1981–9.

49. Stoffel NU, Cercamondi CI, Brittenham G, et al. Iron absorption from oral iron supplements given on consecutive versus alternate days and as single morning doses versus twice-daily split dosing in iron-depleted women: two open-label, randomised controlled trials. Lancet Haematol 2017;4(11):e524–33.

50. Rimon E, Kagansky N, Kagansky M, et al. Are we giving too much iron? Low-dose iron therapy is effective in octogenarians. Am J Med 2005;118(10):1142–7.

51. Crary SE, Hall K, Buchanan GR. Intravenous iron sucrose for children with iron deficiency failing to respond to oral iron therapy. Pediatr Blood Cancer 2011;56(4):615–9.

52. Plummer ES, Crary SE, McCavit TL, et al. Intravenous low molecular weight iron dextran in children with iron deficiency anemia unresponsive to oral iron. Pediatr Blood Cancer 2013;60(11):1747–52.

53. Powers JM, Shamoun M, McCavit TL, et al. Intravenous ferric carboxymaltose in children with iron deficiency anemia who respond poorly to oral iron. J Pediatr 2017;180:212–6.

54. Powers JM, Daniel CL, McCavit TL, et al. Deficiencies in the management of iron deficiency anemia during childhood. Pediatr Blood Cancer 2016;63(4):743–5.

55. Sharma R, Stanek JR, Koch TL, et al. Intravenous iron therapy in non-anemic iron-deficient menstruating adolescent females with fatigue. Am J Hematol 2016;91(10):973–7.

56. Anker SD, Comin Colet J, Filippatos G, et al. Ferric carboxymaltose in patients with heart failure and iron deficiency. N Engl J Med 2009;361(25):2436–48.

57. Ponikowski P, van Veldhuisen DJ, Comin-Colet J, et al. Beneficial effects of long-term intravenous iron therapy with ferric carboxymaltose in patients with symptomatic heart failure and iron deficiency dagger. Eur Heart J 2015;36(11):657–68.

58. Rampton D, Folkersen J, Fishbane S, et al. Hypersensitivity reactions to intravenous iron: guidance for risk minimization and management. Haematologica 2014;99(11):1671–6.

59. Mantadakis E. Advances in pediatric intravenous iron therapy. Pediatr Blood Cancer 2016;63(1):11–6.

60. Avni T, Bieber A, Grossman A, et al. The safety of intravenous iron preparations: systematic review and meta-analysis. Mayo Clin Proc 2015;90(1):12–23.
61. Mantadakis E, Roganovic J. Safety and efficacy of ferric carboxymaltose in children and adolescents with iron deficiency anemia. J Pediatr 2017;184:241.
62. Hassan N, Boville B, Reischmann D, et al. Intravenous ferumoxytol in pediatric patients with iron deficiency anemia. Ann Pharmacother 2017;51(7):548–54.
63. Laass MW, Straub S, Chainey S, et al. Effectiveness and safety of ferric carboxymaltose treatment in children and adolescents with inflammatory bowel disease and other gastrointestinal diseases. BMC Gastroenterol 2014;14:184.
64. Boucher AA, Pfeiffer A, Bedel A, et al. Utilization trends and safety of intravenous iron replacement in pediatric specialty care: a large retrospective cohort study. Pediatr Blood Cancer 2018;65(6):e26995.

Hemophilia in a Changing Treatment Landscape

Marie-Claude Pelland-Marcotte, MD[a],*, Manuel D. Carcao, MD, MSc[a,b]

KEYWORDS

- Hemophilia • Inhibitors • Extended half-life factors • Emicizumab • Fitusiran
- Concizumab • Gene therapy

KEY POINTS

- Prophylaxis with factor replacement has been the mainstay of treatment for persons with hemophilia but may be challenged by several novel treatment options in development.
- Emicizumab has been recently approved for persons with hemophilia A and inhibitors and may dramatically alter the care of patients with inhibitors.
- "Rebalanced hemostasis" by inhibition of natural anticoagulants is a potential strategy for managing hemophilia that is currently under intensive research.
- Gene therapy for hemophilia A and B seems very promising and is likely to change hemophilia management drastically in the future.

INTRODUCTION

Hemophilia A and B are X-linked inherited bleeding disorders caused by deficiency of factor VIII (FVIII) or factor IX (FIX), respectively. One out of 5000 men are born with hemophilia A, whereas 1 out of 30,000 men are born with hemophilia B. Hemophilia A and B vary as to their severity; persons with severe hemophilia essentially produce no active FVIII or FIX (ie, factor activity levels <1% of normal), whereas persons with moderate or mild hemophilia have factor activity levels of 1% to 5% and greater than 5% to 40%, respectively.[1] Bleeding is crudely proportional to baseline factor activity levels; accordingly, persons with severe hemophilia bleed considerably, whereas those with moderate hemophilia bleed less and those with mild hemophilia seldom bleed.

Disclosures: M-C. Pelland-Marcotte has no conflict of interest to disclose. M.D. Carcao reports having received research support from Bayer, Bioverativ/Sonofi, CSL Behring, Novo Nordisk, Octapharma, Pfizer, and Shire. He has also received honoraria for speaking/participating in advisory boards from Bayer, Bioverativ/Sonofi, Biotest, CSL Behring, Grifols, LFB, Novo Nordisk, Octapharma, Pfizer, Roche, and Shire.

[a] Division of Haematology/Oncology, Department of Paediatrics, The Hospital for Sick Children, University of Toronto, 555 University Avenue, Toronto M5G 1X8, Canada; [b] Child Health Evaluative Sciences, Research Institute, The Hospital for Sick Children, 555 University Avenue, Toronto M5G 1X8, Canada
* Corresponding author.
E-mail address: marie-claude.pelland-marcotte@sickkids.ca

Hematol Oncol Clin N Am 33 (2019) 409–423
https://doi.org/10.1016/j.hoc.2019.01.007
0889-8588/19/© 2019 Elsevier Inc. All rights reserved.

hemonc.theclinics.com

Historical Perspective

Until the early 1960s, very little could be offered to persons with hemophilia: consequently, severe hemophilia was a devastating disease resulting in repeated musculoskeletal bleeding, causing not only terrible acute pain but, over time, leading to hemophilic arthropathy, chronic pain, and disability. Furthermore, persons with severe hemophilia would experience life-threatening or fatal bleeding, such as intracranial hemorrhage.

The management of hemophilia has focused on the intravenous replacement of the missing/reduced factor. Beginning in the 1960s, the availability of fresh frozen plasma, cryoprecipitate, and, later, lyophilized (powdered) factor concentrates began transforming the lives of patients. Lyophilized factor concentrates allowed persons with hemophilia to maintain concentrates in their homes and use them as needed.

Initially treatment was given simply to stop bleeding when bleeds occurred (on-demand therapy). Many centers gradually started recognizing that instead of waiting for bleeds to occur, it was better to prevent bleeds by giving frequent regular infusions of factor (prophylaxis), providing persons with hemophilia at least some circulating factor to reduce the likelihood of bleeding. With home prophylaxis, persons with hemophilia could treat themselves and live relatively free of bleeds. Several clinical trials have shown clear superiority of prophylactic treatment with FVIII or FXI for severe hemophilia, compared with on-demand replacement.[2,3] Clearly the lives of persons with hemophilia were steadily improving throughout the 1970s. But some clinicians/researchers worried as to the safety of using factor concentrates that were not virally inactivated and were procured from thousands of mainly paid donors.

Tragedy struck in the late 1970s and early 1980s with the contamination of blood products with human immunodeficiency virus (HIV) and hepatitis B and C. Thousands of persons with hemophilia, along with their partners and children, were infected leading to shattered lives and tragic deaths. Researchers and pharmaceutical companies were driven to develop and implement effective viral inactivation technologies involving heat, solvent detergent, and/or nanofiltration. In addition, discovering the genes for FVIII and FIX became a priority, to create recombinant (synthetic) factor therapies. Over the next 20 years, factor concentrates became increasingly virally "safe" and prophylaxis continued to gain acceptance over on-demand therapy. However, there continues to be issues in the management of hemophilia, mainly due to the limitations of available plasma-derived and recombinant replacement therapies.

Limitations of Current Standard Replacement Therapies

Standard half-life (SHL) factor concentrates have many limitations, which the hemophilia community has traditionally tolerated in the absence of an adequate treatment alternative. With the advent of other therapies, these drawbacks are becoming increasingly unacceptable. Firstly, FVIII and FIX coagulation factors are only available intravenously and have had short half-lives of 8 to 12 hours and 16 to 24 hours, respectively. Thus, prophylactic therapy requires an intravenous infusion usually 3 to 4 times weekly for hemophilia A and 2 times weekly for hemophilia B, leading to a significant burden for persons with hemophilia and their families. The difficulties arising from the repeated intravenous treatments is such that adherence to therapy is far from ideal.

Secondly, even with such frequent intravenous infusions most people receiving SHL concentrates can only achieve factor trough levels of 1% to 3%. It has increasingly been recognized that these trough levels result in occasional clinical and subclinical bleeds, resulting in a slow, steady progression of joint disease over a lifetime.[4]

A third limitation of SHL factor concentrates has been their very high price, which has made them unaffordable and consequently unavailable in many parts of the world. This fortunately is improving, as prices of SHL factor concentrates are dropping.

Finally, 25% to 40% of persons with severe hemophilia A, 10% in those with mild/moderate hemophilia A, and 5% of those with severe hemophilia B develop inhibitory antibodies to factor, thereby making factor replacement therapy ineffective. In patients with inhibitors, bleeds are currently managed with high doses of factor concentrates (for low-titer inhibitors) or with bypassing agents, including recombinant factor VIIa (rFVIIa; NovoSeven) or activated prothrombin complex concentrates (FEIBA).

In this article, the authors focus on new therapies for hemophilia (**Tables 1** and **2**) and how they may influence principles of hemophilia care. Given the limitation of any paper to describe in depth all the new therapies in development, this article instead focuses on how we envision these therapies potentially fitting into hemophilia care.

NOVEL THERAPIES
Extended Half-Life Replacement Factors

To reduce treatment burden and increase compliance, several extended half-life (EHL) products have been developed, using technologies that involve attaching long-lasting molecules (Fc, albumin, or polyethylene glycol [PEG]) to recombinant FVIII or FIX.

Table 1
Extended half-life products available and/or in development

Product	Ref	Technology	Half-Life (h)	Cell Line	FDA Approval
FVIII					
rFVIII-Fc (Eloctate/Elocta)	44–47	Fusion protein of BDD rFVIII and the Fc fragment of IgG1	19	HEK	Jun 2014
BAX 855 (Adynovate/ Adynovi)	48–50	Random PEGylation to parent drug Advate (full length rFVIII)	14–16	CHO	Dec 2016
BAY94–9027 (Jivi)	51–54	Site-specific addition of PEG side chain to a BDD rFVIII	19	CHO	Aug 2018
N8-GP	55,56	Site-specific glycoPEGylation of BD-modified FVIII	19	CHO	NA
BIVV001	57	Fusion protein with addition of a region of VWF and XTEN polypeptides	37	HEK	NA
FIX					
rFIX-Fc (Alprolix)	11,58,59	Fusion protein with the Fc fragment of IgG1	82	HEK	Mar 2014
rFIX-FP (Idelvion)	10,60	Fusion protein with recombinant albumin	102	CHO	Mar 2016
N9-GP (Rebinyn/ Refixia)	9,61	Site-specific glycoPEGylation	93	CHO	May 2017

Abbreviations: BD, B-domain; BDD, B-domain deleted; CHO, Chinese Hamster Ovary; FDA, Food and Drug Administration; FIX, factor IX; FVIII, factor VIII; h, hours; HEK, human embryonic kidney; NA, not available; PEG, polyethylene glycol; rFVIII, recombinant factor VIII; VWF, von Willebrand factor.

Table 2
Nonfactor replacement therapies in hemophilia treatment

Product	Ref	Mechanism of Action	Administration Modalities	Clinical Stage
FVIII replacement products				
Emicizumab	[15–17]	mAB mimicking cofactor activity of FVIII	Weekly to monthly SQ injections	Licensed for clinical use
Inhibitors of anticoagulants				
Fitusiran	[23]	siRNA targeting antithrombin III	Weekly to monthly SQ injections	Clinical trials (phase 3)
Concizumab	[30]	Anti-TFPI (Kunitz-2 domain) mAB	Daily SQ injections	Clinical trials (phase 2)
PF-06741086	[29]	Anti-TFPI (Kunitz-1 and Kunitz-2 domains) mAB	SQ injections	Clinical trials (phase 2)
BAY1093884	[62]	Anti-TFPI (interface of Kunitz-1 and Kunitz-2 domains) mAB	SQ injections	Clinical trials (phase 1)
SerpinPC	[33]	Inhibition of activated protein C by modified α1-antitrypsin	NA	Preclinical
S77206	[34]	siRNA targeting protein S	NA	Preclinical
Gene therapy				
Hemophilia A[a]	[40]	Delivery of F8 gene by liver-specific viral vectors	Single IV infusion	Clinical trials (phase 1–2)
Hemophilia B[a]	[36–39]	Delivery of F9 gene (wild-type or Padua mutant) by liver-specific viral vectors	Single IV infusion	Clinical trials (phase 1–2)

Abbreviations: IV, intravenous; mAB, monoclonal antibody; NA, not available; siRNA, silencing microRNA; SQ, subcutaneous; TFPI, tissue factor pathway inhibitor.
[a] For a detailed review of ongoing gene therapy trials, the reader is referred to dedicated recent reviews.[63,64]

EXTENDED HALF-LIFE FACTOR VIII FOR HEMOPHILIA A

EHL FVIIIs currently available or in development are shown in **Table 1**. Adequate control of bleeding has been seen with all EHL factors currently available.[5] However, the half-life of the current EHL FVIIIs is only 1.4- to 1.6-fold higher compared with SHL FVIIIs; thus, most patients will need greater than 1 dose/week for effective prophylaxis. The modest extension of half-life is due to the binding of EHL FVIIIs to endogenous von Willebrand factor (VWF), which results in EHL FVIIIs still being subject to the clearance of VWF. This binding to VWF creates a "ceiling effect" for prolonging the half-life of FVIII. Despite the marginal improvement in half-life, there are increasing reports showing that EHL FVIIIs improve the quality of life (QOL) of persons with hemophilia and compliance to treatment by reducing the number of infusions.[6] Clinical trials have not raised substantial safety concern of EHL FVIIIs.[5]

A recombinant FVIII is in development, which avoids attachment to VWF by covering the FVIII binding site to VWF with a recombinant D′-D3 molecule. This D′-D3-FVIII is then attached to 2 Fc molecules and 2 XTEN polypeptides (protein polymers designed to increase the half-life of other proteins conjugated to them).[7] Preliminary results showed that this modified molecule exhibits a much longer half-life (37h), resulting in a median FVIII trough level of 5% with once weekly dosing.[8]

EXTENDED HALF-LIFE FACTOR IX FOR HEMOPHILIA B

Three EHL FIXs are currently commercially available (see **Table 1**). Unlike EHL FVIIIs, which all achieve similar half-life extension, EHL FIXs show significant variability in pharmacokinetic parameters. Both rFIXFP (Idelvion) and N9-GP (Rebinyn/Refixia) show substantially longer half-lives than rFIXFc (Alprolix), whereas N9-GP additionally shows a much higher recovery (ie, "peak" level following an infusion) than the others.

All 3 products allow for once weekly dosing in most patients with few or no bleeds reported; rFIXFP and N9-GP additionally allow for once every 2-week dosing while still maintaining protective FIX trough levels after 2 weeks. When given once per week, both rFIXFP and N9-GP (but not rFIXFc) can lead to FIX trough levels greater than 20% and in the case of N9-GP greater than 30% in many adults. All products have shown acceptable safety profiles in phase 3 clinical trials in previously treated patients.[9–11]

EHL factor concentrates, however, still carry some of the limitations of SHL concentrates; they are given intravenously, can lead to inhibitor development (the current literature does not allow to determine if the incidence of inhibitors with EHL factor concentrates will be more, less, or the same compared with SHL factor concentrates), and do not benefit persons with hemophilia and inhibitors. In addition, some of these products are more difficult to monitor using conventional laboratory assays such as the one-stage clotting assay.[12,13] Consequently, there is still room for improvement for hemophilia treatment.

FACTOR VIII REPLACEMENT PRODUCTS

Emicizumab (licenced as Hemlibra) is a humanized monoclonal antibody that mimics the cofactor activity of FVIII. Much like FVIII, emicizumab binds to both activated FIX and FX, leading to a significant acceleration of FIXa-mediated FX activation and ultimately to increased thrombin generation.[14] A series of clinical studies, the HAVEN trials, have been conducted in adults and children with or without inhibitors. These studies have shown substantial reductions in bleeding rates and improvement of health-related QOL.[15–17]

Obvious advantages of emicizumab are that it can be given subcutaneously and infrequently (weekly to potentially monthly). Moreover, emicizumab can be used in persons with inhibitors, offering such individuals for the first time a convenient and effective prophylactic option. Furthermore, emicizumab achieves steady state levels without the constant peak and troughs associated with factor replacement. It has been conjectured that at regular maintenance doses (1.5 mg/kg/wk), emicizumab provides similar hemostatic protection to a constant FVIII level of around 10% to 15%.[16] Such levels should be adequate to prevent most spontaneous bleeding and many minor trauma-induced bleeds, although they are likely insufficient to prevent bleeding in the setting of major trauma or surgery.

Concern has arisen when patients on emicizumab experience bleeds and require additional treatment with FVIII or bypassing agents (rFVIIa or FEIBA). As described by Lenting and colleagues,[18] emicizumab does not function exactly like FVIII and its activity is not subject to the same degree of self-regulation. Several cases of thrombotic microangiopathy, thrombosis, and death have occurred in patients on emicizumab receiving repeated, high doses of FEIBA ($\geq$100 U/kg/d for >1 day). The hypothesis is that FEIBA provides large doses of substrate (FIXa and FX) for emicizumab, leading to a massive synergistic effect on increasing thrombin generation. In vitro experiments showed that an analogue of emicizumab, combined with FEIBA, led to a 17-fold increase in thrombin generation, well above the normal physiologic range.[19] It is now recommended not to administer FEIBA to persons treated with emicizumab unless absolutely indicated and only in an inpatient setting. In contrast, rFVIIa or FVIII when given with emicizumab (in presence or absence of inhibitors, respectively), do not seem to create a huge synergistic burst in thrombin formation and thus seem safer.[19,20]

Inhibitors of Natural Anticoagulants

Coagulation represents a balance between procoagulants and anticoagulants. Factor concentrates and emicizumab aim to replace the missing/reduced procoagulant (FVIII or FIX). Of late, much research has gone toward improving clotting by instead reducing anticoagulants in an attempt to offset the procoagulant deficiency and rebalance coagulation (**Fig. 1**). There are analogies in nature in which persons with hemophilia

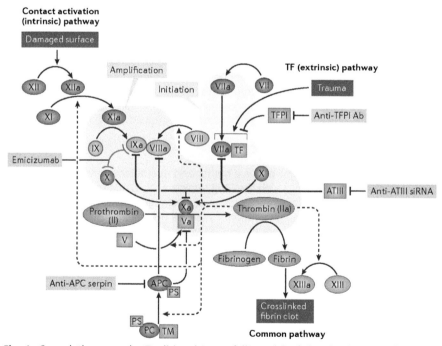

Fig. 1. Coagulation cascade. Traditional 'waterfall' model of the clotting cascade. Serine proteases (oval) and cofactors or other proteins (rectangles) of the intrinsic and extrinsic pathways converge at coagulation factor X (FX; coagulation factors are indicated using only the Roman numerals in the figure) in the common pathway and ultimately generate a stable fibrin clot. Amplification of the pathway occurs through the serial cleavage of clotting factors. The proteins that are absent in patients with hemophilia A or B, when activated, comprise the 'tenase' complex and are shown in pink. Selected non-factor therapies are shown in gray. Ab, antibody; APC, activated protein C; PC, protein C; PS, protein S; siRNA, small interfering RNA; TF, tissue factor; TFPI, tissue factor pathway inhibitor; TM, thrombomodulin. (*From* Peters R, Harris T. Advances and innovations in haemophilia treatment. Nat Rev Drug Discov 2018;17(7):494; with permission.)

and coinherited thrombophilic traits, such as Factor V Leiden, prothrombin gene mutation, or deficiencies in antithrombin, protein C, or S, have milder bleeding phenotypes.[21]

Downregulation of antithrombin

Antithrombin is an endogenous anticoagulant that inhibits thrombin, FX and, to a lesser degree, other procoagulant factors. Fitusiran is a small interfering RNA (siRNA) that silences posttranscriptional hepatic expression of the SERPINC1 gene, thereby reducing antithrombin levels in a dose-dependent manner.[22] Fitusiran, when given as a subcutaneous once-weekly or once-monthly infusion to either healthy volunteers or persons with hemophilia A or B, has been shown to reduce antithrombin levels to 70% to 80% of normal, which results in persons with hemophilia achieving thrombin generation values comparable to that observed in healthy individuals without hemophilia.[23] Early studies were very encouraging; however, studies were placed on hold when a fatal cerebral thrombosis occurred in a patient who, on fitusiran, had received therapeutic doses of FVIII concentrates for a musculoskeletal bleed.[24,25] Much like persons with hemophilia on emicizumab who are given FEIBA, when persons receiving fitusiran experience breakthrough bleeds and are given a prothrombotic agent such as FVIII, they may become excessively prothrombotic. The study was reopened after institution of a plan to use significantly lower doses of prothrombotic agents (FVIII and/or bypassing agents) to manage breakthrough bleeds.[26] Several phase 3 clinical trials are underway, in persons with severe hemophilia with and without inhibitors, to further assess the efficacy and safety of fitusiran.

Inhibition of tissue factor pathway inhibitor

Tissue factor pathway inhibitor (TFPI) inhibits the initiation pathway of coagulation through inhibition of FVIIa by its K (Kunitz) 1 domain and inhibition of FXa via its K2 domain.[27] Various companies have been developing different agents that inhibit TFPI.[28–30] Concizumab is a humanized monoclonal antibody targeting the TFPI binding site for FXa. In a phase 1 study in healthy volunteers and persons with hemophilia, Concizumab led to a concentration-dependent reduction in the residual level of TFPI and was generally well tolerated.[30] Phase 2 clinical trials are underway in persons with hemophilia with or without inhibitors. Other anti-TFPI monoclonal antibodies are currently under investigation.[28,29,31] As with emicizumab and fitusiran, TFPI inhibitors can be given subcutaneously. Like other rebalancing agents, the concern of potential thrombotic complications remains when persons with hemophilia on an anti-TFPI receive additional procoagulant therapy in the setting of a bleed or surgery.

Others (inhibition of activated protein C or protein S)

Activated protein C (APC) inhibits FVa and thus is an additional target to reduce endogenous anticoagulant activity. Several strategies are being investigated to block APC, including aptamers and mutated α-1-antitrypsin, thereby promoting thrombin generation.[32,33] Similarly, preliminary investigation is occurring in targeting protein S as a way of rebalancing coagulation.[34] These compounds are in early preclinical stages of development.

Gene Therapy

Nearly two decades after the first reports of gene therapy, several successful phase 1/2 gene therapy trials have recently been published. Most have used liver-specific tropic adenovirus-associated virus (AAV) as viral vectors to deliver the missing/faulty gene to liver hepatocytes. AAV viruses are thought to be nonpathogenic and do not integrate into the human genome (or if so, to a minimal degree), thus carrying a low theoretic risk of insertional mutagenesis compared with other viral vectors.

In hemophilia B, successful gene transfers have been reported with single infusions of both wild-type FIX and Padua FIX. The latter is a naturally occurring gain-of-function mutation (R338L), which increases the activity of FIX by 5 to 10 fold.[35] The Padua FIX gene allows for a reduced vector dose, which may translate into reduced immune cellular response to the viral capsid. Long-term steady state FIX levels of between 1% and 7% have been obtained with wild-type FIX,[36-38] whereas levels between 14% and 81% have been obtained using the Padua FIX.[39] Consequently, after gene therapy, these individuals have FIX levels in the normal or mild hemophilia range with significant reductions in annualized bleeding rates (ABRs) and factor consumption.

Before wide implementation of gene therapy, several questions remain. Firstly, all trials have enrolled persons with hemophilia without preexisting antibodies to AAV. However, it is estimated that approximately 30% of the population carry antibodies to AAV. These antibodies can also develop following gene therapy raising potential difficulties in children who may require additional future gene therapy due to the inability of AAV to integrate into the genome of dividing hepatocytes. Secondly, the efficacy and safety of gene therapy in persons with liver disease, including hepatitis C, who until now have been excluded from gene therapy trials, remains unknown. Thirdly, elevation of liver enzymes has been witnessed with infusion of high doses of AAV, usually within the first 12 weeks following infusion; this is probably related to dose-dependent cellular immunity to the viral capsid. Although not harmful to the individual, anticapsid cellular immunity has been associated with reduced FIX expression and thus mandates quick institution of immunomodulation, which may be associated with additional morbidity.[37,38]

Gene therapy in hemophilia A carries several specific challenges. First, FVIII (even in its B-domain deleted form) is a large molecule, making it difficult to be packaged within a viral genome. Also, for reasons that remain unclear, in vivo protein expression and secretion of FVIII is less efficient than FIX. Finally, FVIII is quite immunogenic and the risk of inhibitor development following gene therapy remains unknown. Nonetheless, early results of FVIII gene therapy trials are also promising: one trial has shown FVIII activity levels of 19% to 164% 52 weeks following a single gene therapy infusion.[40]

An alternate curative approach for hemophilia is gene editing to replace the mutant FVIII or FIX gene. This approach minimizes the risk of insertional mutagenesis. Preclinical trials with designer zinc finger nucleases, CRISP/Cas9, and nuclease-free targeting approach are underway.

PRINCIPLES OF HEMOPHILIA TREATMENT

Over the past 50 years, several key principles of care have been established: persons with hemophilia should be offered a treatment that is

1. Safe;
2. Timely;
3. Available at home;
4. Oriented toward prevention of bleeds;
5. Individualized; and
6. Focused on clinically relevant outcomes.

Finally, inhibitor development should be avoided, and inhibitors should be eradicated whenever possible. Although most of these principles will continue because new therapies are incorporated into practice, the paradigm may change for some of them.

Safety of Treatments

Since the hepatitis C and HIV tragedies, safety has become the main priority of persons with hemophilia and clinicians. Although contemporary products are considered safe for transmission of known viral pathogens, there remains a theoretic risk of transmission of unknown pathogens, in particular prions, such as variant Creutzfeldt-Jakob disease. Thus, there is a keen interest to avoid plasma-derived products. However, the consequences of manipulating recombinant products remain a concern, especially for inhibitor development. In addition, in altering the procoagulant-anticoagulant pendulum, many new therapies may lead to an increased risk of thrombosis. It is crucial for clinicians to remain vigilant of possible side effects (both expected and unexpected) of new therapies.

Rapid Treatment of Bleeds

A key principle of hemophilia management has been immediate treatment of a bleed to rapidly halt bleeding. This "treat first and fast" approach when there is any suspicion of a bleed has worked well until now. With factor replacement strategies, there is a significant margin of safety in that inadvertent factor overdose almost never results in harm. However, with future therapies there may be reason to alter this approach. This seems particularly true with inhibitors of natural anticoagulants, because the concurrent infusion of procoagulant agents (FVIII/FIX or bypassing agents) may transiently be associated with a prothrombotic state.

Home Care

In the 1960s, it was recognized that to accomplish immediate treatment of bleeds and, later, to allow persons with hemophilia to be on prophylaxis, treatment needed to be administered at home, ideally by the persons with hemophilia themselves or their families or, if that was not possible, through visiting nurses. Thus, a large part of any hemophilia management program has been to empower persons with hemophilia and their families, so that they can administer treatment at home.

Subcutaneous treatments are very appealing for prophylactic therapy. However, subcutaneous therapies do not lend themselves to rapid treatment of bleeds and consequently persons with hemophilia will still need occasional intravenous infusions. It is unclear if individuals will still be able to acquire and retain the ability to self-infuse intravenous therapies if they primarily use subcutaneous therapies.

Prevention of Bleeds

The current standard of care for severe hemophilia in most industrialized countries is regular prophylactic infusion of FVIII or FIX to prevent hemorrhage and hemophilic arthropathy. Yet because of the limitations of available treatments, prophylaxis has not been easy or as effective as desired and certainly has not been widely adopted in low- to middle-income countries. Newer therapies, both those administered subcutaneously as well as gene therapy, will substantially increase the bleed protection traditionally offered through FVIII or FIX trough levels of 1% to 3%.

Interindividual Heterogeneity of Hemophilia

Despite the generally accepted fact that bleeding is proportional to factor levels in hemophilia A and B, there is significant interindividual variability in bleeding phenotype and response to treatment, even between persons with comparable factor levels.

Box 1
Sources of interpatient variability in hemophilia phenotype

- Underlying hemophilia mutations, leading to slight differences in factor levels
- Levels of other prothrombotic (eg, fibrinogen, thrombin, FV, FVII, FXI, etc.) and anticoagulant (antithrombin, protein C, protein S, TFPI) factors
- Blood group and other variables that affect clearance of infused FVIII/FIX
- Joint structure
- Levels and patterns of activity

Abbreviations: FV, factor V; FVII, factor VII; FVIII, factor VIII; FIX, factor IX; FXI, factor XI; TFPI, tissue factor pathway inhibitor.

This variability is likely attributed to particular differences between persons with hemophilia (**Box 1**). Given these differences, individualization of prophylaxis has become a major focus of hemophilia care. Until now, individualization of hemophilia care has simply revolved around interpatient pharmacokinetic differences in how they use the same type of therapy—factor concentrates. In the future, individualization of therapy is likely to additionally involve interindividual differences in the type of therapy (eg, EHL factor replacement vs FVIII-mimetic agent vs rebalancing agent) from which an individual would most benefit. This is likely to increase the complexity of hemophilia care.

Focus on Outcomes

Currently, the efficacy of most hemostatic products is assessed using the ABR. This short-term outcome is fraught with limitations, in that it is very subjective and, as such, error prone. Furthermore, current therapies already achieve very low ABRs limiting the comparative value of the ABR to evaluate newer therapies. In addition, arthropathy can develop without clinically evident joint bleeds,[41] and consequently, low ABRs do not necessarily translate into the absence of hemophilic arthropathy, adequate functioning, and good QOL.

New indicators of treatment efficacy are therefore needed; these need to be clinically relevant, integrate patient-reported outcomes and economic evaluations. Moreover, long-term outcomes will be of utmost importance, especially with newer therapies that may be associated with long-term complications.

Inhibitor Management

Inhibitors are the most common complication of hemophilia and should be suspected in all patients who do not respond as expected to treatment. Several patient, disease, and treatment-related risk factors for the development of inhibitors have been reported (**Table 3**). Although research has led to a greater understanding of what triggers inhibitor development, there have been no effective strategies to reduce the incidence of inhibitors within clinical practice. Inhibitor development leads to two broad issues: (1) management and prevention of bleeds and (2) eradication of the inhibitor.

Although effective in treating bleeds, currently available bypassing agents (rFVIIa and FEIBA) are inconvenient, and neither is an ideal prophylactic agent. Given the high morbidity, significant cost, and inconvenience of having an inhibitor, eradication through immune tolerance induction (ITI) is currently the goal when persons with hemophilia develop an inhibitor. In ITI, frequent doses of factor are administered to

Table 3
Risk factors for the development of inhibitors in hemophilia A

Type of Risk Factors	Elements Associated with Higher Incidence of Inhibitors
Nonmodifiable risk factors	• Causative mutations, especially null mutations • Positive family history of inhibitors • Ethnicity—higher incidence in people of African-American or Hispanic descent • Polymorphisms in certain immune response genes
Treatment-related and environmental risk factors	• Type of factor concentrates • Context of factor exposure—on-demand vs prophylaxis • Intense exposure to factor concentrates at an early age

gradually render a person's immune system tolerant of factor. ITI usually requires several months of intensive treatment and is associated with high costs and burden of care for persons with hemophilia who tend to be very young children. Despite over 40 years of experience with ITI, the hemophilia community has still not resolved many important questions, including when to start ITI and whether ITI should be commenced immediately when a high titer inhibitor is detected or delayed until the inhibitor titer has fallen to a certain level. Other unresolved questions pertaining to ITI include when to discontinue when persons do not seem to respond; what is the ideal ITI regimen; and which is the type of factor to use.[42] Overall, ITI is effective in 60% to 80% of cases. Why ITI is ultimately successful or not is unknown, although certain predictors of success include younger patient age, lower historical inhibitor titer (<200 Bethesda Units [BU]) and lower inhibitor titer pre-ITI (<10 BU), lower inhibitor peak titers on ITI, and low-risk FVIII mutations.

Emicizumab will almost certainly have a valuable role in the management of persons with hemophilia and inhibitors. Emicizumab will likely replace traditional bypassing agents for prophylaxis, but bypassing agents will likely still be needed for episodic treatment of bleeding. However, many questions remain regarding the adoption of emicizumab. Should one or more courses of ITI still be attempted? If so, should immunosuppressive therapies still be attempted for those who fail a first course of ITI?[43] Will ITI regimens change with incorporation of emicizumab into inhibitor management? Can individuals stay on emicizumab exclusively following successful ITI or must they be maintained on some regular exposure to FVIII to maintain tolerance?

In addition to emicizumab, novel methods, several in the preclinical stage, are being studied to improve inhibitor eradication and care of persons with hemophilia and inhibitors. These methods have been recently reviewed elsewhere.[43]

SUMMARY

The future is promising for persons with hemophilia with the advent of so many new therapies. Clinicians caring for these individuals face a daunting future of how they will manage persons with hemophilia, with such an array of potential therapies. For now, it should be made clear to patients that treatment is changing, becoming more effective, and convenient. With gene therapy, many individuals with severe hemophilia will likely be cured of hemophilia or have factor levels in the mild hemophilia range. The authors envision a future in which joint disease from recurrent bleeds in persons with hemophilia will be incredibly rare. In anticipation of such a future, persons with hemophilia should be encouraged to prevent bleeds and their complication, recognizing that future therapies will be much more effective but are unlikely to reverse prior damage.

REFERENCES

1. Blanchette VS, Key NS, Ljung LR, et al. Definitions in hemophilia: communication from the SSC of the ISTH. J Thromb Haemost 2014;12(11):1935–9.
2. Manco-Johnson MJ, Abshire TC, Shapiro AD, et al. Prophylaxis versus episodic treatment to prevent joint disease in boys with severe hemophilia. N Engl J Med 2007;357(6):535–44.
3. Iorio A, Marchesini E, Marcucci M, et al. Clotting factor concentrates given to prevent bleeding and bleeding-related complications in people with hemophilia A or B. Cochrane Database Syst Rev 2011;(9):CD003429.
4. Oldenburg J. Optimal treatment strategies for hemophilia: achievements and limitations of current prophylactic regimens. Blood 2015;125(13):2038–44.
5. Mancuso ME, Santagostino E. Outcome of clinical trials with new extended half-life FVIII/IX concentrates. J Clin Med 2017;6(4):39–54.
6. Schwartz CE, Powell VE, Su J, et al. The impact of extended half-life versus conventional factor product on hemophilia caregiver burden. Qual Life Res 2018;27(5):1335–45.
7. Drager D, Patarroyo-White S, Chao H, et al. Recombinant FVIIIFC-VWF-XTEN demonstrates significant bioavailability following subcutaneous administration in hemophilia a mice. Blood 2015;126(23):3492.
8. Shapiro A, Quon D, Staber J, et al. BIVV001 - a novel, weekly dosing, VWF-independent, extended half-life FVIII therapy: First-in-human safety, tolerability, and pharmacokinetics. Haemophilia 2018;24(S5):209–18.
9. Collins PW, Young G, Knobe K, et al. Recombinant long-acting glycoPEGylated factor IX in hemophilia B: A multinational randomized phase 3 trial. Blood 2014;124(26):3880–6.
10. Santagostino E, Martinowitz U, Lissitchkov T, et al. Long-acting recombinant coagulation factor IX albumin fusion protein (rIX-FP) in hemophilia B: Results of a phase 3 trial. Blood 2016;127(14):1761–9.
11. Powell JS, Pasi KJ, Ragni MV, et al. Phase 3 study of recombinant factor IX Fc fusion protein in hemophilia B. N Engl J Med 2013;369(24):2313–23.
12. Kitchen S. Laboratory monitoring for long acting factor replacement therapy. Int J Lab Hematol 2016;38(Supplement 2):55.
13. Pruthi RK. Laboratory monitoring of new hemostatic agents for hemophilia. Semin Hematol 2016;53(1):28–34.
14. Uchida N, Sambe T, Yoneyama K, et al. A first-in-human phase 1 study of ACE910, a novel factor VIII-mimetic bispecific antibody, in healthy subjects. Blood 2016;127(13):1633–41.
15. Oldenburg J, Mahlangu JN, Kim B, et al. Emicizumab prophylaxis in hemophilia A with inhibitors. N Engl J Med 2017;377(9):809–18.
16. Shima M, Hanabusa H, Taki M, et al. Factor VIII-mimetic function of humanized bispecific antibody in hemophilia A. N Engl J Med 2016;374(21):2044–53.
17. Shima M, Hanabusa H, Taki M, et al. Long-term safety and efficacy of emicizumab in a phase 1/2 study in patients with hemophilia A with or without inhibitors. Blood Adv 2017;1(22):1891–9.
18. Lenting PJ, Denis CV, Christophe OD. Emicizumab, a bispecific antibody recognizing coagulation factors IX and X: how does it actually compare to factor VIII? Blood 2017;130(23):2463–8.
19. Hartmann R, Feenstra T, Valentino L, et al. In vitro studies show synergistic effects of a procoagulant bispecific antibody and bypassing agents. J Thromb Haemost 2018;16:1580–91.

20. Kruse-Jarres R, Callaghan MU, Croteau SE, et al. Surgical experience in two multicenter, open-label phase 3 studies of emicizumab in persons with hemophilia a with inhibitors (HAVEN 1 and HAVEN 2). Blood 2017;130(Supplement 1):S89.
21. Franchini M, Montagnana M, Targher G, et al. Interpatient phenotypic inconsistency in severe congenital hemophilia: a systematic review of the role of inherited thrombophilia. Semin Thromb Hemost 2009;35(3):307–12.
22. Sehgal A, Barros S, Ivanciu L, et al. An RNAi therapeutic targeting antithrombin to rebalance the coagulation system and promote hemostasis in hemophilia. Nat Med 2015;21(5):492–9.
23. Pasi KJ, Rangarajan S, Georgiev P, et al. Targeting of antithrombin in hemophilia A or B with RNAi therapy. N Engl J Med 2017;377(9):819–28.
24. World Federation of Hemophilia. Update: FDA lifts suspension of Fitusiran trial. 2017. Available at: https://news.wfh.org/update-fda-lifts-suspension-fitusiran-trial/. Accessed July 7, 2018.
25. World Federation of Hemophilia. Alnylam suspends fitusiran dosing due to thrombotic event in phase 2 open-label extension study 2017. Available at: https://news.wfh.org/alnylam-suspends-fitusiran-dosing-due-thrombotic-event-phase-2-open-label-extension-study/. Accessed July 7, 2018.
26. Callaghan MU, Sidonio R, Pipe SW. Novel therapeutics for hemophilia and other bleeding disorders. Blood 2018;132(1):23–30.
27. Wood JP, Bunce MW, Maroney SA, et al. Tissue factor pathway inhibitor-alpha inhibits prothrombinase during the initiation of blood coagulation. Proc Natl Acad Sci U S A 2013;110(44):17838–43.
28. Gu JM, Patel C, Kauser K. Plasma tissue factor pathway inhibitor (TFPI) levels in healthy subjects and patients with hemophilia a and B. Blood 2015;126(23):4672.
29. Cardinal M, Kantaridis C, Zhu T, et al. A first-in-human study of the safety, tolerability, pharmacokinetics and pharmacodynamics of PF-06741086, an anti-tissue factor pathway inhibitor mAb, in healthy volunteers. J Thromb Haemost 2018;16(9):1722–31.
30. Chowdary P, Lethagen S, Friedrich U, et al. Safety and pharmacokinetics of anti-TFPI antibody (concizumab) in healthy volunteers and patients with hemophilia: A randomized first human dose trial. J Thromb Haemost 2015;13(5):743–54.
31. Chowdary P. Inhibition of tissue factor pathway inhibitor (TFPI) as a treatment for haemophilia: rationale with focus on concizumab. Drugs 2018;78(9):881–90.
32. Hamedani NS, Ruhl H, Zimmermann JJ, et al. In vitro evaluation of aptamer-based reversible inhibition of anticoagulant activated protein C as a novel supportive hemostatic approach. Nucleic Acid Ther 2016;26(6):355–62.
33. Polderdijk SG, Adams TE, Ivanciu L, et al. Design and characterization of an APC-specific serpin for the treatment of hemophilia. Blood 2017;129(1):105–13.
34. Prince R, Bologna L, Manetti M, et al. Targeting anticoagulant protein S to improve hemostasis in hemophilia. Blood 2018;131(12):1360–71.
35. Simioni P, Tormene D, Tognin G, et al. X-linked thrombophilia with a mutant factor IX (factor IX Padua). N Engl J Med 2009;361(17):1671–5.
36. Miesbach W, Meijer K, Coppens M, et al. Gene therapy with adeno-associated virus vector 5-human factor IX in adults with hemophilia B. Blood 2018;131(9):1022–31.
37. Nathwani AC, Reiss UM, Tuddenham EGD, et al. Long-term safety and efficacy of factor IX gene therapy in hemophilia B. N Engl J Med 2014;371(21):1994–2004.
38. Nathwani AC, Tuddenham EG, Rangarajan S, et al. Adenovirus-associated virus vector–mediated gene transfer in hemophilia B. N Engl J Med 2011;365(25):2357–65.

39. George LA, Sullivan SK, Giermasz A, et al. Hemophilia B gene therapy with a high-specific-activity factor IX variant. N Engl J Med 2017;377(23):2215–27.
40. Rangarajan S, Walsh L, Lester W, et al. AAV5-factor VIII gene transfer in severe hemophilia a. N Engl J Med 2017;377(26):2519–30.
41. Manco-Johnson MJ, Soucie JM, Gill JC. Prophylaxis usage, bleeding rates, and joint outcomes of hemophilia, 1999 to 2010: a surveillance project. Blood 2017; 129(17):2368–74.
42. Hay CR, DiMichele DM. The principal results of the International Immune Tolerance Study: a randomized dose comparison. Blood 2012;119(6):1335–44.
43. Sherman A, Biswas M, Herzog RW. Tolerance induction in hemophilia: innovation and accomplishments. Curr Opin Hematol 2018;25(5):365–72.
44. Mahlangu J, Powell JS, Ragni MV, et al. Phase 3 study of recombinant factor VIII Fc fusion protein in severe hemophilia A. Blood 2014;123(3):317–25.
45. Young G, Mahlangu J, Kulkarni R, et al. Recombinant factor VIII Fc fusion protein for the prevention and treatment of bleeding in children with severe hemophilia A. J Thromb Haemost 2015;13(6):967–77.
46. Powell JS, Josephson NC, Quon D, et al. Safety and prolonged activity of recombinant factor VIII Fc fusion protein in hemophilia A patients. Blood 2012;119(13): 3031–7.
47. Nolan B, Mahlangu J, Perry D, et al. Long-term safety and efficacy of recombinant factor VIII Fc fusion protein (rFVIIIFc) in subjects with haemophilia A. Haemophilia 2016;22(1):72–80.
48. Konkle BA, Stasyshyn O, Chowdary P, et al. Pegylated, full-length, recombinant factor VIII for prophylactic and on-demand treatment of severe hemophilia A. Blood 2015;126(9):1078–85.
49. Mullins ES, Stasyshyn O, Alvarez-Roman MT, et al. Extended half-life pegylated, full-length recombinant factor VIII for prophylaxis in children with severe haemophilia A. Haemophilia 2017;23(2):238–46.
50. Brand B, Gruppo R, Wynn TT, et al. Efficacy and safety of pegylated full-length recombinant factor VIII with extended half-life for perioperative haemostasis in haemophilia A patients. Haemophilia 2016;22(4):e251–8.
51. Coyle TE, Reding MT, Lin JC, et al. Phase I study of BAY 94-9027, a PEGylated B-domain-deleted recombinant factor VIII with an extended half-life, in subjects with hemophilia A. J Thromb Haemost 2014;12(4):488–96.
52. Reding MT, Ng HJ, Poulsen LH, et al. Safety and efficacy of BAY 94-9027, a prolonged-half-life factor VIII. J Thromb Haemost 2017;15(3):411–9.
53. Reding MT, Ng HJ, Tseneklidou-Stoefer D, et al. Safety of long-term prophylaxis with BAY 94-9027: Interim results of >5 years of treatment in the PROTECT VIII extension trial. Haemophilia 2018;24(Supplement 5):17–8.
54. Santagostino E, Saxena K, Kenet G, et al. PROTECT VIII Kids trial results: BAY 94-9027 safety and efficacy in previously treated children with severe hemophilia A. Haemophilia 2016;22(Supplement 4):41.
55. Giangrande P, Andreeva T, Ehrenforth S, et al. Clinical evaluation of glycoPEGylated recombinant FVIII: efficacy and safety in severe haemophilia A. Thromb Haemost 2017;117(2):252–61.
56. Tiede A, Brand B, Fischer R, et al. Enhancing the pharmacokinetic properties of recombinant factor VIII: first-in-human trial of glyco PEG ylated recombinant factor VIII in patients with hemophilia A. J Thromb Haemost 2013;11(4):670–8.
57. Seth Chhabra E, Tie M, Dobrowsky T, et al. Pharmacokinetic profile of RFVIIIFC-VWF-XTEN (BIVV001) protein in cynomolgus monkey generated from a large-

scale manufacturing stable cell line. Blood Transfus 2017;15(Supplement 3): s484.

58. Fischer K, Kulkarni R, Nolan B, et al. Recombinant factor IX Fc fusion protein in children with haemophilia B (Kids B-LONG): results from a multicentre, non-randomised phase 3 study. Lancet Haematol 2017;4(2):e75–82.

59. Pasi KJ, Fischer K, Ragni M, et al. Long-term safety and efficacy of extended-interval prophylaxis with recombinant factor IX Fc fusion protein (rFIXFc) in subjects with haemophilia B. Thromb Haemost 2016;117(3):508–18.

60. Kenet G, Chambost H, Male C, et al. Long-acting recombinant fusion protein linking coagulation factor IX with albumin (rIX-FP) in children: Results of a phase 3 trial. Thromb Haemost 2016;116(4):659–68.

61. Carcao M, Zak M, Abdul Karim F, et al. Nonacog beta pegol in previously treated children with hemophilia B: results from an international open-label phase 3 trial. J Thromb Haemost 2016;14(8):1521–9.

62. Gu J-M, Zhao X-Y, Schwarz T, et al. Mechanistic modeling of the pharmacodynamic and pharmacokinetic relationship of tissue factor pathway inhibitor-neutralizing antibody (BAY 1093884) in cynomolgus monkeys. AAPS J 2017; 19(4):1186–95.

63. George LA. Hemophilia gene therapy comes of age. Hematology 2017;2017(1): 587–94.

64. Leebeek FW. Gene therapy for hemophilia: an update. Haemophilia 2018; 24(Supplement 1):20–1.

von Willebrand Disease in Pediatrics
Evaluation and Management

Sarah H. O'Brien, MD[a],*, Surbhi Saini, MD[b]

KEYWORDS

- von Willebrand disease • Pediatric • Diagnosis • Management

KEY POINTS

- von Willebrand disease (VWD) is a common inherited bleeding disorder with a variety of subtypes and bleeding phenotypes.
- Standardized bleeding assessment tools are predictive of both the diagnosis and severity of VWD.
- Major advances in laboratory evaluation, including improved von Willebrand (VW) functional assays and genetic testing, allow increasing accuracy in the diagnosis of VWD.
- Pharmacologic options for managing bleeding and perioperative care include desmopressin, antifibrinolytics, and plasma-derived or recombinant VW concentrates.

INTRODUCTION

Named after the Finnish internist who in 1926 first described a familial form of hemorrhagic diathesis in a 5-year-old girl from the Åland archipelago,[1] von Willebrand disease (VWD) is the most common inherited bleeding disorder. The reported prevalence of VWD varies between 0.1% and 1% in the general population, occurring across all races and ethnicities.[2,3] Inherited in an autosomal fashion, it affects men and women equally; however, symptomatic bleeding is more common in women of reproductive age because of the hemostatic challenges of menstruation and childbirth. This article reviews the pathophysiology of VWD, the use of bleeding assessment tools to

Disclosure: S.H. O'Brien has served on advisory boards for CSL Behring (manufacturer of Stimate) and Shire (manufacturer of Vonvendi).
[a] Division of Pediatric Hematology/Oncology, Nationwide Children's Hospital, The Ohio State University College of Medicine, Center for Innovation in Pediatric Practice, The Research Institute at Nationwide Children's Hospital, 700 Children's Drive, Office FB3444, Columbus, OH 43205, USA; [b] Division of Pediatric Hematology/Oncology, Penn State Hershey Children's Hospital, Penn State University College of Medicine, 500 University Drive, Hershey, PA 17036, USA
* Corresponding author.
E-mail address: sarah.obrien@nationwidechildrens.org

Hematol Oncol Clin N Am 33 (2019) 425–438
https://doi.org/10.1016/j.hoc.2019.01.010
0889-8588/19/© 2019 Elsevier Inc. All rights reserved.

hemonc.theclinics.com

identify patients at risk of VWD, laboratory evaluation with a focus on newly available testing, and pharmacologic treatment strategies.

Pathophysiology

von Willebrand factor (VWF) is a large, multimeric glycoprotein synthesized by endothelial cells and megakaryocytes, and stored within Weibel-Palade bodies and alpha granules, respectively. The VWF gene is located on the short arm of chromosome 12. VWF is essential for primary hemostasis as a result of binding to platelet surface glycoproteins and subendothelial collagen. In an intact blood vessel with normal, laminar blood flow, VWF multimers and platelets have minimal interactions. In a damaged blood vessel, the exposure of subendothelial collagen leads to binding of plasma VWF to several connective tissue collagens. Fast-flowing platelets are initially bound to VWF through the VWF binding site on the GPIbα of the platelet surface GPIb-IX-V complex. This initial tethering is strengthened by platelet binding to subendothelial collagen, and subsequently high-affinity binding of VWF to the GPIIb-IIIa complex of activated platelets. VWF also acts as a chaperone protein to plasma factor VIII. This interaction ensures that most circulating factor VIII is protected from proteolytic degradation and rapid clearance, thus prolonging its half-life.[4]

Nomenclature and Classification

VWD is characterized by disorders of concentration (quantitative) or structure/function (qualitative) of the VWF (**Table 1**). Broadly, VWD is classified as partial deficiency of VWF (type 1), severe deficiency of VWF (type 3), or impairment of VWF interactions with platelets or factor VIII (type 2). Approximately 75% of patients affected by VWD have the type 1 variant.[5] Most of the remaining patients have a type 2 variant, and type 3 disease is exceedingly rare ($\sim$1 in 1 million).

Clinical Presentation of von Willebrand Disease

Because most patients with VWD have milder subtypes of the disease, differentiating their bleeding symptoms from those seen in the general population can be a challenge. For example, in a study of 228 otherwise healthy children undergoing tonsillectomy, 39% reported epistaxis and 24% reported easy bruising.[6] The 2007 guidelines from the National Heart, Lung, and Blood Institute (NHLBI) regarding the diagnosis, evaluation, and management of VWD provide a list of recommended questions when screening a patient for a possible bleeding disorder[7] (**Box 1**).

However, bleeding history can be subjective and is influenced by patient-level and parent-level factors as well as the setting and format of the interview. A variety of objective bleeding assessment tools have been validated, most based on an instrument published by investigators in Vicenza, Italy, and have consistently shown high specificity and negative predictive value for VWD.[8] The Vicenza-based tools collect information on a variety of bleeding symptoms and score them from 0 (or −1) to 4 based on the frequency or severity of the symptom or the intensity of intervention required (**Fig. 1**).[9] A total score of greater than or equal to 3 in men and greater than or equal to 5 in women was found to be 98.6% specific and 69.1% sensitive for the identification of individuals with type 1 VWD.[10] The likelihood of VWD increases exponentially with each 1-point increase in the total bleeding score (**Fig. 2**), and correlates with VWF antigen (VWF:Ag) and activity levels in a seemingly linear relationship.[11,12]

A Pediatric Bleeding Questionnaire (PBQ) has also been validated, which is based on the Vicenza tools but includes an "other" category with pediatric-specific symptoms such as umbilical stump and postcircumcision bleeding.[13] Using a definition of greater than 2 as an abnormal PBQ score in children has a high negative predictive

Table 1
The pathobiology and genetics of the various subtypes of von Willebrand Disease

VWD Subtype	Pathobiology	Genetics
Type 1	Partial deficiency of VWF caused by impaired production, intracellular trafficking, storage, secretion, or enhanced clearance (type 1C or Vicenza subtype)	• Autosomal dominant with often incomplete penetrance and varied expressivity • Mutations throughout the VWF gene; ~75% missense mutations
Type 2A	Decreased VWF-dependent platelet adhesion caused by selective deficiency of HMWM as a result of defects in dimerization, multimer storage and secretion, or enhanced multimer cleavage by ADAMTS13	• Majority autosomal dominant; autosomal recessive forms rare • Mutations in the D2, D3, A1, A2, CK domains
Type 2B	Spontaneous affinity of VWF for platelet GP1bα; platelet-VWF aggregates cleared by ADAMTS13 with resultant thrombocytopenia and loss of HMWM	• Autosomal dominant • Gain-of-function missense variants affecting A1 domain
Type 2M	Decreased VWF-dependent platelet interaction not caused by selective deficiency of HMWM; reduced VWF binding to GPIbα or collagen	• Autosomal dominant • Missense variants affecting the A1 and A3 domains
Type 2N	Markedly decreased binding of VWF to factor VIII; reduced factor VIII half-life	• Autosomal recessive • Missense variants affecting D′–D3
Type 3	Complete or near-complete absence of VWF	• Autosomal recessive; rarely inheritance of 2 codominant mutant alleles • Large VWF gene deletions

Abbreviation: HMWM, high-molecular-weight multimer.

value (99%) for VWD. The median PBQ score in children with VWD is 7 (range, 0–29), compared with 0 (range, −1 to 2) in unaffected siblings. More recently, a self-administered PBQ has also been validated.[14]

LABORATORY EVALUATION
Screening Tests for von Willebrand Disease

The activated partial thromboplastin time (aPTT) and prothrombin time are the most commonly used tests to screen for coagulation defects. However, the aPTT is only prolonged in VWD if plasma levels of factor VIII are sufficiently reduced. Significant prolongation of aPTT rarely occurs outside of type 3 and type 2N VWD, in which it indicates factor VIII deficiency secondary to loss of factor VIII carrying capabilities of VWF.

Platelet function analyzers (PFA-100) are designed to assess primary platelet-plug formation after citrated whole blood is aspirated through cartridges coated with collagen/epinephrine and collagen/ADP at high shear stress, mimicking physiologic conditions. The PFA-100 has a high negative predictive value and excellent sensitivity to severe reductions in the VWF levels; however, its usability as a screening test is limited in the diagnosis of mild type 1 VWD, for which it is much less sensitive.[15] Definitive laboratory evaluation of VWF can be broadly classified into phenotypic

Box 1
Suggested questions when obtaining a bleeding history

1. Do you have a blood relative who has a bleeding disorder?
2. Have you ever had prolonged bleeding from trivial wounds, lasting more than 15 minutes or recurring spontaneously during the 7 days after the injury?
3. Have you ever had heavy, prolonged, or recurrent bleeding after surgical procedures, such as tonsillectomy?
4. Have you ever had bruising, with minimal or no apparent trauma, especially if you could feel a lump under the bruise?
5. Have you ever had a spontaneous nosebleed that required more than 10 minutes to stop or needed medical attention?
6. Have you ever had heavy, prolonged, or recurrent bleeding after dental extractions that required medical attention?
7. Have you ever had blood in your stool, unexplained by a specific anatomic lesion (such as an ulcer in the stomach) that required medical attention?
8. Have you ever had anemia requiring treatment or received a blood transfusion?
9. For women, have you ever had heavy menses, characterized by the presence of clots greater than 2.5 cm in diameter and/or changing a pad or tampon more than hourly, or resulting in anemia or low iron level?

Adapted from Nichols WL, Hultin MB, James AH, et al. von Willebrand disease (VWD): evidence-based diagnosis and management guidelines, the National Heart, Lung, and Blood Institute (NHLBI) Expert Panel report (USA). Haemophilia 2008;14(2):185; with permission.

Epistaxis	
0	No or trivial (less than 5)
1	> 5 or more than 10'
2	CONSULTATION ONLY
3	Packing or Cauterization or Antifibrinolytics
4	Blood transfusion or Replacement therapy or Desmopressin

Oral cavity	
0	No
1	Reported at least one
2	CONSULTATION ONLY
3	Surgical hemostasis or Antifibrinolytics
4	Blood transfusion or Replacement therapy or Desmopressin

Surgery	
−1	No bleeding in at least 2 surgeries
0	Not done or no bleeding in 1 surgery
1	Reported in <25% of all surgeries
2	Reported in >25% of all surgeries, no intervention
3	Surgical hemostasis or Antifibrinolytics
4	Blood transfusion or Replacement therapy or Desmopressin

Muscle hematoma	
0	Never
1	Post-trauma no therapy
2	Spontaneous no therapy
3	Spontaneous or traumatic requiring Desmopressin or Replacement therapy
4	Spontaneous or traumatic requiring Surgical intervention or Blood transf

Cutaneous	
0	No or trivial (<1 cm)
1	>1 cm and no trauma
2	CONSULTATION ONLY

GI bleeding	
0	No
1	Associated with ulcer, portal hypertension, hemorrhoids, angiodysplasia
2	Spontaneous
3	Surgical hemostasis or Blood transfusion or Replacement therapy or Desmopressin or Antifibrinolytics

Menorrhagia	
0	No
1	CONSULTATION ONLY
2	Antifibrinolytics or pill use
3	Curettage or Iron therapy
4	Blood transfusion or Replacement ther-apy or Desmopressin or Hysterectomy

Hemarthrosis	
0	Never
1	Post-trauma no therapy
2	Spontaneous no therapy
3	Spontaneous or traumatic requiring desmopressin or Replacement therapy
4	Spontaneous or traumatic requiring surgical intervention or blood transfusion

Bleeding from minor wounds	
0	No or trivial (less than 5)
1	> 5 or more than 5'
2	CONSULTATION ONLY
3	Surgical hemostasis
4	Blood transfusion or Replacement therapy or Desmopressin

Tooth extraction	
−1	No bleeding in at least 2 extractions
0	Not done or no bleeding in 1 extraction
1	Reported in <25% of all procedures
2	Reported in >25% of all procedures, no intervention
3	Resuturing or Packing
4	Blood transfusion or Replacement therapy or Desmopressin

Post-partum hemorrhage	
−1	No bleeding in at least 2 deliveries
0	No deliveries or no bleeding in 1 delivery
1	CONSULTATION ONLY
2	Curettage or Iron therapy or Antifibrinolytics
3	Blood transfusion or Replacement therapy or Desmopressin
4	Hysterectomy

CNS bleeding	
0	Never
1	-
2	-
3	Subdural, any intervention
4	Intracerebral, any intervention

Total assigned score:

Fig. 1. Condensed version of the bleeding assessment tool. CNS, central nervous system; GI, gastrointestinal. (*From* Tosetto A, Castaman G, Plug I, et al. Prospective evaluation of the clinical utility of quantitative bleeding severity assessment in patients referred for hemostatic evaluation. J Thromb Haemost 2011;9(6):1144; with permission.)

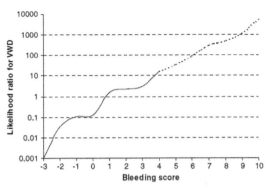

Fig. 2. Likelihood ratios for VWD based on the Vicenza bleeding assessment tool (−1 version). (*From* Tosetto A, Castaman G, Rodeghiero F. Assessing bleeding in von Willebrand disease with bleeding score. Blood Rev 2007;21(2):95; with permission.)

assessment of the quantity, structure, and function of VWF, and genetic investigation of VWD-causing mutations (**Fig. 3**).

Quantitative Assessment of von Willebrand Factor Antigen

The concentration of VWF in plasma can be measured by several immunoassay-based techniques. The traditional enzyme-linked immunosorbent assay (ELISA) for measuring VWF uses antibodies to human VWF. This technique is labor intensive with a high coefficient of variation, and is slowly being replaced by more precise automated latex immunoassays and chemiluminescent assays.

Functional Assessment of von Willebrand Factor

The activity of VWF can be assessed in the laboratory by the ex vivo estimation of its biologically important functions of binding to platelets, collagen, and factor VIII.

Ristocetin-based platelet binding
Ristocetin, a drug initially marketed as an antibiotic, mimics the physiologic shear stress that induces binding of VWF to platelets, and is used in the laboratory to measure the ability of the patient's plasma VWF to agglutinate platelets. Recently, automated immunoturbidimetric and chemiluminescent techniques have improved the reliability of ristocetin-based functional testing.[16] Nevertheless, all adaptations of ristocetin-based assays remain prone to intralaboratory and interlaboratory variability and are nonphysiologic because of the lack of conformational change to VWF induced by high shear stress.

Ristocetin-independent platelet binding
Ristocetin-based activity tests are currently being supplemented or replaced by assays based on the binding of VWF to a recombinant platelet glycoprotein (GP1bM).[17] Compared with methods that use ristocetin, the VWF:GP1bM assays show greater precision and higher sensitivity, especially in the diagnosis of type 2 VWD.[18] Automated and ELISA versions of the VWF:GP1bM assay are currently available at reference laboratories.

Collagen binding assays
In vivo, VWF binds collagens type I, III, IV, and VI. High-molecular-weight multimers of VWF increase its collagen binding capacity. Using ELISA methodology, this function of

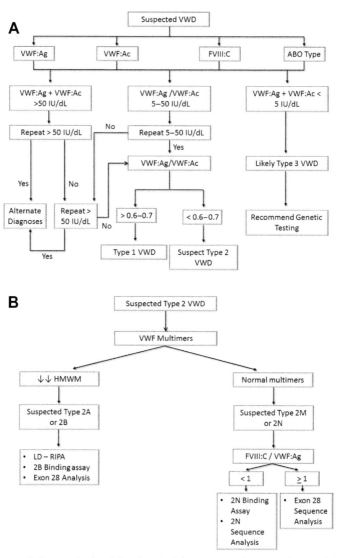

Fig. 3. Suggested diagnostic algorithm for the laboratory evaluation of VWD. (*A*) Owing to preanalytical, analytical, and biological variables that affect von Willebrand testing, the authors recommend that testing be repeated to confirm or rule out VWD. (*B*) Type 2 VWD is suspected when the VWF:Ac is substantially lower than the VWF:Ag, and further classified by multimeric and genetic analysis. FVIII:C, factor VIII activity; HMWM, high-molecular-weight multimers; LD-RIPA, low-dose ristocetin-induced platelet aggregation; VWF:Ac, VWF activity; VWF:Ag, VWF antigen.

VWF can be tested in the laboratory.[19] VWF collagen binding assays (VWF:CB) are more sensitive to the loss of high-molecular-weight VWF subunits than traditional functional tests but are limited by the lack of standardization of commercially available assays.[20]

2N binding assay
Type 2N VWD, often misdiagnosed as mild hemophilia A because of the characteristic prolongation of aPTT and low factor VIII levels, arises because of defective binding of

factor VIII to VWF. This interaction can be assessed in the laboratory by measuring ELISA-based binding of patient VWF to an excess of factor VIII. 2N binding assays aid in diagnosis when the patient's factor VIII:C/VWF:Ag ratio is less than 1.[21]

Platelet aggregometry

Platelet aggregation studies, in which increasing amounts of ristocetin are added to the patient plasma and platelets, are sensitive for the diagnosis of type 2B VWD, in which platelet agglutination is observed at low doses of ristocetin.

Structural Assessment of von Willebrand Factor (von Willebrand Factor Multimers)

Electrophoresis on 0.65% agarose gels in the presence of sodium dodecyl sulfate separates VWF multimers based on molecular weight. Historically, this has been considered the gold standard in diagnosing VWD subtypes with loss of high-molecular-weight subunits (type 2A, 2B). However, this test is technologically challenging and laborious, with considerable interlaboratory variation, which limits its value for VWD subtyping.

Genetic Analysis

Recent advancements in genetic testing have widened its availability and reduced the overall cost. Genetic testing in VWD is advantageous, circumventing the need for an array of tests, and precluding the influence of variables such as stress, infection, and inflammation. However, the clinical utility of VWF genetic testing is limited by various issues.

In type 1 VWD, the most prevalent type, mutations (predominantly missense) have been reported throughout the *VWF* gene.[22] However, almost 20% to 50% of patients with type 1 VWD lack causative mutations, particularly among those with VWF levels between 30 and 50 IU/dL.[22,23] More recently, variants in genes influencing VWF secretion and clearance have been shown to contribute to low VWF levels in patients with type 1 VWD.[24]

Genetic abnormalities are better characterized in patients with type 2 VWD, in which targeted variant analysis often helps confirm a phenotypic diagnosis of type 2A, 2B, 2M, or 2N VWD. Genetic mutations can be found in most patients with type 3 VWD. Null mutations are prevalent in patients with undetectable VWF levels, whereas missense mutations can be found in patients with less severe bleeding phenotypes.

DIAGNOSTIC CONSIDERATIONS IN THE LABORATORY EVALUATION OF VON WILLEBRAND DISEASE

Phenotypic characterization of VWD is a multistep process that involves several laboratory tests, each with its own limitations, as discussed earlier. Furthermore, laboratory diagnosis of VWD is rendered difficult by various preanalytical, analytical, and biological variables.

von Willebrand Factor Levels and ABO Blood Groups

Thirty years ago, Gill and colleagues[25] studied the VWF antigen levels of 1117 healthy blood donors and reported that persons with blood group O had the lowest mean VWF:Ag levels, followed by blood group A, B, and AB. VWF protein is the only nonerythrocytic protein that expresses terminal ABO blood group–related carbohydrate chains, with shortened survival of VWF protein carrying only the H antigen of blood group O.[26] The eventual bleeding tendency is most likely a result of plasma VWF levels, regardless of ABO blood type.[27]

von Willebrand Factor Levels and Estrogen

Although earlier studies reported VWF to be higher in women on estrogen, secondary to a heightened inflammatory response,[28,29] subsequent studies found little effect in healthy, nonsmoking women taking low-dose estrogens (<50 μg/d).[30] Although current literature supports that VWF levels can be appropriately investigated in healthy women taking low-dose estrogen without the need to withdraw treatment, it remains unclear whether the same strategy can be used for women with heavy menses and other bleeding symptoms, for whom the likelihood of VWD is higher. Our practice is to not withdraw treatment from adolescents undergoing a bleeding evaluation but to not definitively rule out VWD in patients found to have borderline VWF levels in the setting of estrogen therapy.

Benign Variants of von Willebrand Factor

Although persons of African American heritage tend to have higher VWF:Ag levels compared with white people, their mean VWF ristocetin cofactor (VWF:RCo) activity is similar. This finding can lead to a misdiagnosis of type 2 VWD, based on a decreased VWF:RCo/VWF:Ag ratio. African Americans also have an increased likelihood of carrying a polymorphism in the VWF gene, p.D1472H. This common variant has been shown to reduce ristocetin-dependent binding of VWF to platelet GP1bα, but this is a laboratory phenomenon rather than a true bleeding risk.[31]

Sample Collection, Processing, and Handling

As with every hemostasis test, laboratory testing for VWD is prone to several preanalytical issues. Ideally, free-flowing blood from a large-bore needle needs to be precisely collected in sodium citrate tubes. Atraumatic blood draws limit the activation of clotting factors in the sample. Struggling or crying in children or anxiety in adults, as well as inflammation or recent exercise, can falsely increase VWF and factor VIII levels. Furthermore, agitation of samples or extremes of temperature during transport and storage is likely to yield false abnormalities.[32]

CLASSIFICATION OF VON WILLEBRAND DISEASE

Laboratory criteria for VWD classification remain controversial. Laboratory cutoffs for type 1 VWD are most debated, but distinct issues still remain in the diagnosis of type 3 VWD as well as subtyping type 2 VWD.

Type 1 von Willebrand Disease

In 2005, the International Society on Thrombosis and Haemostasis defined the criteria for type 1 VWD as VWF:RCo and VWF:Ag greater than or equal to 2 standard deviations (SD) less than the population mean and ABO type adjusted mean on greater than or equal to 2 determinations, in addition to a personal and family history of bleeding.[33] However, since that time a variety of alternative definitions for type 1 VWD have been proposed (**Box 2**).[22,23,34,35] This disparity in laboratory criteria for type 1 VWD is challenging for practicing clinicians, exposing patients to the risk of overdiagnosis and overtreatment or underdiagnosis and undertreatment.

Type 2 von Willebrand Disease

The initial diagnosis of type 2 VWD often relies on the calculated ratio of the VWF activity to antigen levels. At most centers, VWF:RCo is the commonly used activity assay, and the inherent imprecision of this assay complicates ratio-dependent type 2 VWD diagnosis. In addition, up to a third of patients diagnosed as type 1 VWD

Box 2
Proposed definitions of type 1 von Willebrand disease

- Canadian Type 1 VWD Study: VWF:Ag and VWF:RCo between 5 and 50 IU/dL obtained on at least 2 occasions[22]

- NHLBI Expert Panel: VWF:Ag and/or VWF:RCo less than 30 IU/dL[7]

- European Group on von Willebrand disease: VWF:RCo or VWF:CB less than or equal to 40 IU/dL

- United Kingdom Hemophilia Centre Doctors Organization: VWF activity less than 30 IU/dL[34]

- Zimmerman Program and WiN (Willebrand in the Netherlands) Study: VWF:Ag, VWF:RCo, or VWF:CB less than 30 IU/dL[23,35]

- International Society on Thrombosis and Haemostasis: VWF:Ag and VWF:RCo greater than or equal to 2 SD less than the population mean and ABO type adjusted mean on greater than or equal to 2 determinations, in addition to a personal and family history of bleeding[33]

---

have abnormal multimer patterns. Type 2M VWD remains poorly understood and molecular studies of previously classified type 2M patients have shown considerable variability in clinical and laboratory phenotypes, as well as an overlap with type 2A VWD.[7,36,37]

Type 3 von Willebrand Disease

The distinction between severe type 1 and type 3 VWD is not always obvious. VWF propeptide (pp) levels can be used to characterize type 3 patients with virtually no synthesis of VWF (absent or very low VWFpp levels) from severe type 1 patients with rapid clearance of VWF (normal to high VWFpp levels).[38] Genetic analysis is important in making this distinction as well as in counseling patients about inheritance patterns.

Low von Willebrand Factor Levels

The diagnosis of type 1 VWD is complicated by a distinct cohort of patients with VWF levels between 30 and 50 IU/dL and bleeding symptoms. Patients with low VWF levels in the Zimmerman and Willebrand in the Netherlands (WiN) studies reported clinically significant bleeding history and bleeding scores that were similar to patients with VWF:Ag levels less than 30 IU/dL.[35] A later report on an Irish cohort of patients with low VWF levels found little correlation between bleeding tendency and plasma VWF levels within the range of 30 to 50 IU/dL.[39] Causative VWF genetic mutations are less common and blood group O is more common in patients with low VWF. Navigating the medical management of such patients remains difficult, and approaches vary widely between treating these patients as type 1 VWD and no treatment at all. It has been proposed that VWF levels in the population are a continuum and that the risk of bleeding increases as the VWF levels decrease, without a defining line between healthy and diseased states.[40]

PHARMACOLOGIC OPTIONS FOR PATIENTS WITH VON WILLEBRAND DISEASE

The mainstays of therapy to manage bleeding symptoms in patients with VWD include desmopressin, antifibrinolytics, and VWF products (human derived and recombinant). The mechanism and dosing for these agents, and strategies for common management scenarios encountered by treating hematologists, are reviewed here.

Desmopressin

Desmopressin (1-deamino-8-ᴅ-arginine vasopressin [DDAVP]) is a hormone that causes release of factor VIII and VWF from storage sites within endothelial cells, and can be given intranasally (high-dose version as opposed to the low-dose version for diuretic use), subcutaneously, or intravenously, although available formulations vary by geographic location. The intranasal dose is 1 spray (150 µg) for patients less than 50 kg, and 2 sprays for those greater than or equal to 50 kg. The intravenous and subcutaneous dose for DDAVP is 0.3 µg/kg (some institutions use a maximum dose of 20 µg). Patients typically undergo a so-called DDAVP challenge in the clinic setting, which assesses the magnitude and sustainability of their increase in VWF levels. In general, most patients with type 1 and some patients with type 2 have adequate responses to DDAVP, but it is not clinically useful for patients with type 3 disease.

The most common side effects of DDAVP include facial flushing, headache, hypotension (all caused by vasomotor side effects), and fluid retention. Fluid intake must be restricted to maintenance levels for 24 hours after each dose in order to prevent the complication of hyponatremia and, in rare cases, seizures. The NHLBI expert panel guidelines recommend that for management of minor bleeding (epistaxis, heavy menses, tooth extraction) with DDAVP and proper fluid restriction, laboratory monitoring is not necessary unless DDAVP is used more than 3 times in 72 hours. For major surgeries such as tonsillectomy and other inpatient procedures, our practice is to monitor sodium levels before administering the second dose of DDAVP, given that patients may have received more intravenous fluid than expected. We also avoid the use of DDAVP in patients less than 3 years of age, because younger patients are thought to be at greater risk of hyponatremia-related seizures.

Antifibrinolytics

Antifibrinolytic agents (aminocaproic acid and tranexamic acid) help prevent clot degradation by inhibiting the action of plasminogen. They are available in oral and

---

Box 3
Suggested durations of von Willebrand factor replacement for surgical procedures

Major surgery, 7 to 14 days
- Cardiothoracic
- Neurosurgery
- Open cholecystectomy
- Tonsillectomy

Minor surgery, 1 to 5 days
- Biopsy
- Complicated dental extractions
- Central line placement
- Laparoscopic procedures

Other procedures, if uncomplicated, single VWF treatment
- Cardiac catheterization
- Endoscopy (without biopsy)
- Lacerations
- Simple dental extractions

Adapted from Nichols WL, Hultin MB, James AH, et al. von Willebrand disease (VWD): evidence-based diagnosis and management guidelines, the National Heart, Lung, and Blood Institute (NHLBI) expert panel report (USA). Haemophilia 2008;14(2):205; with permission.

Table 2
Dosing recommendations for von Willebrand factor concentrate replacement for prevention or management of bleeding

	Major Surgery/Bleeding	Minor Surgery/Bleeding
Loading dose	40–60 VWF:RCo IU/kg	30–60 VWF:RCo IU/kg
Maintenance dose[a]	20–40 U/kg every 8–24 h	20–40 U/kg every 12–48 h
Therapeutic goal	Trough VWF:RCo and factor VIII >50 IU/dL for 7–14 d	Trough VWF:RCO and factor VIII >50 IU/dL for 3–5 d

[a] Can alternate maintenance factor replacement with DDAVP for later part of treatment.
Adapted from Nichols WL, Hultin MB, James AH, et al. von Willebrand disease (VWD): evidence-based diagnosis and management guidelines, the National Heart, Lung, and Blood Institute (NHLBI) Expert Panel report (USA). Haemophilia 2008;14(2):205; with permission.

intravenous formulations, and in general are better tolerated by patients than DDAVP. The most common side effects are gastrointestinal symptoms (nausea and/or diarrhea), but these typically resolve with dose reduction.[41] Dosing for aminocaproic acid is traditionally 50 to 60 mg/kg every 4 to 6 hours for aminocaproic acid and 10 to 15 mg/kg every 8 to 12 hours for tranexamic acid.[42]

In our practice, the authors use antifibrinolytics for patients undergoing procedures involving mucocutaneous membrane surfaces (tooth extractions, tonsillectomy), and those undergoing procedures who do not tolerate or adequately respond to DDAVP. Tranexamic acid at a dose of 1.3 g (2 tablets) 3 times daily during the first 5 days of menses is an effective primary treatment of heavy menstrual bleeding[43–45] and is also a helpful adjunct for adolescents with heavy menstrual bleeding not adequately responding to hormonal contraception therapy (and who do not have any risk factors for thrombosis).

von Willebrand Factor Replacement

Regular use of VWF concentrates is generally reserved for patients with type 3 disease. In those with milder forms of VWD, factor replacement is typically used during perioperative management of patients who do not respond to or tolerate DDAVP, or for lengthy surgeries (especially those expected to require a critical care stay afterward because of the anticipated difficulty in managing fluid restrictions). The NHLBI expert panel guidelines include recommendations for bolus and maintenance dosing of VWF concentrates for both major and minor bleeding (**Box 3**), as well as recommended durations of factor replacement (**Table 2**). Dosing is weight based using ristocetin cofactor units per kilogram. Most VWF concentrates are plasma derived, contain factor VIII as well as varying amounts of VWF, and are dual approved for VWD and factor VIII deficiency. The first recombinant VWF factor was approved by the US Food and Drug Administration in 2015.[46] Although this product does not contain factor VIII, early surgical studies suggest that patients can achieve hemostatic efficacy without coadministration of factor VIII.[47] Patients with severe VWD and chronic bleeding can benefit from regular prophylaxis with VWF concentrates.[48]

SUMMARY

Advances in the use of standardized bleeding assessment tools, VWF functional assays, and genetic testing have all improved the ability of hematologists to more accurately diagnose VWD in patients presenting with easy bruising or bleeding. A variety of treatment options exist, including desmopressin, antifibrinolytics, and both plasma-based and recombinant VWF products. The diagnosis of VWD remains complex and requires expertise in the appropriateness and interpretation of the many available tests. Questions still remain unanswered, in particular the appropriate classification and management of patients with low VWF levels.

REFERENCES

1. Lassila R, Lindberg O. Erik von Willebrand. Haemophilia 2013;19(5):643–7.
2. Rodeghiero F, Castaman G, Dini E. Epidemiological investigation of the prevalence of von Willebrand's disease. Blood 1987;69(2):454–9.
3. Werner EJ, Broxson EH, Tucker EL, et al. Prevalence of von Willebrand disease in children: a multiethnic study. J Pediatr 1993;123(6):893–8.
4. Swystun LL, Georgescu I, Mewburn J, et al. Abnormal von Willebrand factor secretion, factor VIII stabilization and thrombus dynamics in type 2N von Willebrand disease mice. J Thromb Haemost 2017;15(8):1607–19.
5. Castaman G, Federici AB, Rodeghiero F, et al. Von Willebrand's disease in the year 2003: towards the complete identification of gene defects for correct diagnosis and treatment. Haematologica 2003;88(1):94–108.
6. Nosek-Cenkowska B, Cheang MS, Pizzi NJ, et al. Bleeding/bruising symptomatology in children with and without bleeding disorders. Thromb Haemost 1991;65(3):237–41.
7. Nichols WL, Hultin MB, James AH, et al. von Willebrand disease (VWD): evidence-based diagnosis and management guidelines, the National Heart, Lung, and Blood Institute (NHLBI) Expert Panel report (USA). Haemophilia 2008;14:171–232.
8. Rydz N, James PD. The evolution and value of bleeding assessment tools. J Thromb Haemost 2012;10(11):2223–9.
9. Tosetto A, Castaman G, Plug I, et al. Prospective evaluation of the clinical utility of quantitative bleeding severity assessment in patients referred for hemostatic evaluation. J Thromb Haemost 2011;9(6):1143–8.
10. Rodeghiero F, Castaman G, Tosetto A, et al. The discriminant power of bleeding history for the diagnosis of type 1 von Willebrand disease: an international, multicenter study. J Thromb Haemost 2005;3(12):2619–26.
11. Tosetto A, Rodeghiero F, Castaman G, et al. A quantitative analysis of bleeding symptoms in type 1 von Willebrand disease: results from a multicenter European study (MCMDM-1 VWD). J Thromb Haemost 2006;4(4):766–73.
12. Tosetto A, Castaman G, Rodeghiero F. Assessing bleeding in von Willebrand disease with bleeding score. Blood Rev 2007;21(2):89–97.
13. Biss TT, Blanchette VS, Clark DS, et al. Quantitation of bleeding symptoms in children with von Willebrand disease: use of a standardized pediatric bleeding questionnaire. J Thromb Haemost 2010;8(5):950–6.
14. Casey LJ, Tuttle A, Grabell J, et al. Generation and optimization of the self-administered pediatric bleeding questionnaire and its validation as a screening tool for von Willebrand disease. Pediatr Blood Cancer 2017;64(10). https://doi.org/10.1002/pbc.26588.
15. Ardillon L, Ternisien C, Fouassier M, et al. Platelet function analyser (PFA-100) results and von Willebrand factor deficiency: a 16-year 'real-world' experience. Haemophilia 2015;21(5):646–52.
16. Stufano F, Lawrie AS, La Marca S, et al. A two-centre comparative evaluation of new automated assays for von Willebrand factor ristocetin cofactor activity and antigen. Haemophilia 2014;20(1):147–53.

17. Patzke J, Budde U, Huber A, et al. Performance evaluation and multicentre study of a von Willebrand factor activity assay based on GPIb binding in the absence of ristocetin. Blood Coagul Fibrinolysis 2014;25(8):860–70.
18. Vangenechten I, Mayger K, Smejkal P, et al. A comparative analysis of different automated von Willebrand factor glycoprotein Ib-binding activity assays in well typed von Willebrand disease patients. J Thromb Haemost 2018;16(7):1268–77.
19. Favaloro EJ. Von Willebrand factor collagen-binding (activity) assay in the diagnosis of von Willebrand disease: a 15-year journey. Semin Thromb Hemost 2002;28(2):191–202.
20. Favaloro EJ. Evaluation of commercial von Willebrand factor collagen binding assays to assist the discrimination of types 1 and 2 von Willebrand disease. Thromb Haemost 2010;104(5):1009–21.
21. Mohammed S, Favaloro EJ. Laboratory testing for von Willebrand factor: factor VIII binding (for 2N VWD). In: Favaloro EJ, Lippi G, editors. Hemostasis and Thrombosis: Methods and Protocols. Humana Press; 2017. p. 461–2.
22. James PD, Notley C, Hegadorn C, et al. The mutational spectrum of type 1 von Willebrand disease: results from a Canadian cohort study. Blood 2007;109(1): 145–54.
23. Flood VH, Christopherson PA, Gill JC, et al. Clinical and laboratory variability in a cohort of patients diagnosed with type 1 VWD in the United States. Blood 2016; 127(20):2481–8.
24. Sanders YV, van der Bom JG, Isaacs A, et al. CLEC4M and STXBP5 gene variations contribute to von Willebrand factor level variation in von Willebrand disease. J Thromb Haemost 2015;13(6):956–66.
25. Gill JC, Endres-Brooks J, Bauer PJ, et al. The effect of ABO blood group on the diagnosis of von Willebrand disease. Blood 1987;69(6):1691–5.
26. Gallinaro L, Cattini MG, Sztukowska M, et al. A shorter von Willebrand factor survival in O blood group subjects explains how ABO determinants influence plasma von Willebrand factor. Blood 2008;111(7):3540–5.
27. Nitu-Whalley IC, Lee CA, Griffioen A, et al. Type 1 von Willebrand disease - a clinical retrospective study of the diagnosis, the influence of the ABO blood group and the role of the bleeding history. Br J Haematol 2000;108(2):259–64.
28. Kluft C, Leuven JA, Helmerhorst FM, et al. Pro-inflammatory effects of oestrogens during use of oral contraceptives and hormone replacement treatment. Vascul Pharmacol 2002;39(3):149–54.
29. Oral Contraceptive and Hemostasis Study Group. The effects of seven monophasic oral contraceptive regimens on hemostatic variables: conclusions from a large randomized multicenter study. Contraception 2003;67(3):173–85.
30. Larsen JB, Bor MV, Hvas AM. Combined oral contraceptives do not influence von Willebrand factor related biomarkers despite an induced acute phase response. Thromb Res 2015;135(1):208–11.
31. Flood VH, Friedman KD, Gill JC, et al. No increase in bleeding identified in type 1 VWD subjects with D1472H sequence variation. Blood 2013;121(18):3742–4.
32. Favaloro EJ, Lippi G. Preanalytical issues that may cause misdiagnosis in haemophilia and von Willebrand disease. Haemophilia 2018;24(2):198–210.
33. Sadler JE, Rodeghiero F. Provisional criteria for the diagnosis of VWD type 1. J Thromb Haemost 2005;3(4):775–7.
34. Laffan MA, Lester W, O'Donnell JS, et al. The diagnosis and management of von Willebrand disease: a United Kingdom Haemophilia Centre Doctors Organization guideline approved by the British Committee for Standards in Haematology. Br J Haematol 2014;167(4):453–65.

35. Boender J, Eikenboom J, Fijnvandraat K, et al. No association between normalization of VWF levels and bleeding phenotype in patients with type 1 VWD - from the WiN study. Blood 2016;128(22):2577.

36. Larsen DM, Haberichter SL, Gill JC, et al. Variability in platelet- and collagen-binding defects in type 2M von Willebrand disease. Haemophilia 2013;19(4): 590–4.

37. Doruelo AL, Haberichter SL, Christopherson PA, et al. Clinical and laboratory phenotype variability in type 2M von Willebrand disease. J Thromb Haemost 2017;15(8):1559–66.

38. Sanders YV, Groeneveld D, Meijer K, et al. von Willebrand factor propeptide and the phenotypic classification of von Willebrand disease. Blood 2015;125(19): 3006–13.

39. Lavin M, Aguila S, Schneppenheim S, et al. Novel insights into the clinical phenotype and pathophysiology underlying low VWF levels. Blood 2017;130(21): 2344–53.

40. Sadler JE. Low von Willebrand factor: sometimes a risk factor and sometimes a disease. Hematol Am Soc Hematol Educ Program 2009;106–12. https://doi.org/10.1182/asheducation-2009.1.106.

41. Mikhail S, Kouides P. von Willebrand disease in the pediatric and adolescent population. J Pediatr Adolesc Gynecol 2010;23(6 Suppl):S3–10.

42. Mannucci PM. Treatment of von Willebrand's disease. N Engl J Med 2004;351(7): 683–94.

43. Chi C, Pollard D, Tuddenham EG, et al. Menorrhagia in adolescents with inherited bleeding disorders. Pediatr Adolesc Gynecol 2010;23(4):215–22.

44. Srivaths LV, Dietrich JE, Yee DL, et al. Oral tranexamic acid versus combined oral contraceptives for adolescent heavy menstrual bleeding: a pilot study. Pediatr Adolesc Gynecol 2015;28(4):254–7.

45. O'Brien SH, Saini S, Ziegler H, et al. An open-label, single-arm, efficacy study of tranexamic acid in adolescents with heavy menstrual bleeding. J Pediatr Adolesc Gynecol 2019. [Epub ahead of print].

46. Peyvandi F, Mamaev A, Wang JD, et al. Phase 3 study of recombinant von Willebrand factor in patients with severe von Willebrand disease who are undergoing elective surgery. J Thromb Haemost 2018;17(1):52–62.

47. Abshire T, Cox-Gill J, Kempton CL, et al. Prophylaxis escalation in severe von Willebrand disease: a prospective study from the von Willebrand Disease Prophylaxis Network. J Thromb Haemost 2015;13(9):1585–9.

48. Castaman G, Goodeve A, Eikenboom J. Principles of care for the diagnosis and treatment of von Willebrand disease. Haematologica 2013;98(5):667–74.

Thrombosis in Children
Approach to Anatomic Risks, Thrombophilia, Prevention, and Treatment

Arash Mahajerin, MD, MSCr[a],*, Marisol Betensky, MD, MPH[b,c],
Neil A. Goldenberg, MD, PhD[b,d,e,f,1]

KEYWORDS

- Venous thromboembolism • Pediatrics • Thrombophilia • Prevention • Treatment

KEY POINTS

- The incidence of pediatric venous thromboembolism is increasing.
- Risk-assessment models are limited in clinical utility, but the multi-institutional Children's Hospital-Acquired Thrombosis Registry may provide a novel model.
- Best practices for treatment are lacking, but the Multicenter Evaluation of the Duration of Therapy for Thrombosis in Children and Young Adults trial will provide novel and direct evidence in treatment of provoked venous thromboembolism.

INTRODUCTION

Incidence of pediatric venous thromboembolism (VTE), including deep vein thrombosis (DVT) and pulmonary embolism (PE), has significantly increased over the last 2 decades. An analysis of the Pediatric Health Information System database noted a 70% increase from 2001 to 2007.[1] This increase is attributed to improved survival of children with chronic conditions, increased use of central venous catheters, and other lifesaving technology, among other factors. Estimated incidence of pediatric VTE has ranged from 0.07 to 0.49 per 10,000 children.[2,3] Hospitalized children have significantly higher rates of 4.9 to 21.9 per 10,000 hospital admissions.[2–4]

Disclosure: The authors report no conflicts of interest.
[a] Division of Hematology, 1201 West La Veta Avenue, Orange, CA 92868, USA; [b] Department of Pediatrics, Johns Hopkins University School of Medicine, Baltimore, MD, USA; [c] Pediatric Thrombosis Program, Johns Hopkins All Children's Cancer and Blood Disorder Institute, Johns Hopkins Medicine, 600 5th Street South, 4th Floor, St Petersburg, FL 33701, USA; [d] Department of Medicine, Division of Hematology, Johns Hopkins University School of Medicine, Baltimore, MD, USA; [e] Pediatric Thrombosis Program, Johns Hopkins All Children's Hospital, Johns Hopkins All Children's Cancer and Blood Disorder Institute, Johns Hopkins Medicine, 600 5th Street South, 3rd Floor, St Petersburg, FL 33701, USA; [f] Johns Hopkins Children's Center, Baltimore, MD, USA
[1] Senior author.
* Corresponding author.
E-mail address: amahajerin@choc.org

Hematol Oncol Clin N Am 33 (2019) 439–453
https://doi.org/10.1016/j.hoc.2019.01.009
0889-8588/19/© 2019 Elsevier Inc. All rights reserved.

hemonc.theclinics.com

Besides the associated increase in morbidity, pediatric VTE has significant cost implications, with an estimated increased mean hospital cost of $27,686 and mean length of stay extension of 8.1 days in children with hospital-acquired VTE.[5] This article describes the classification of VTE, thrombophilia, risk assessment, and treatment in children.

CLASSIFICATION

There are several VTE classifications. When used in combination, these classifications inform decisions regarding length of therapy and outcomes predictions.

Anatomic

The primary means of classification is based on anatomic site with further dissection into specific veins.(**Table 1**) Most pediatric data on anatomic distribution are from in-hospital VTE. Data from the Children's Hospital-Acquired Thrombosis (CHAT) Registry, a multi-institutional registry of pediatric in-hospital VTE, have shown that 79% of pediatric VTE occur in the extremities.[6] The Multicenter Evaluation of the Duration of Therapy for Thrombosis in Children and Young Adults (Kids-DOTT) trial found in the pilot/feasibility (P/F) phase that 63.7% of pediatric VTEs occur in the extremities.[7]

Presence of Symptoms

VTE is often classified as symptomatic (ie, associated with signs or symptoms) or asymptomatic. Extremity or caval VTE presents with painful limb swelling and edema; PE can present with pleuritic chest pain, dyspnea, and hemoptysis, whereas cerebral sinovenous thrombosis can induce headache with or without cranial nerve findings.

Table 1 Anatomic classification of venous thromboembolism	
Lower Extremity	**Nonextremity Sites**
Distal	Cerebral sinovenous system
Popliteal vein	Superior sagittal sinus
Calf veins	Sigmoid sinus
Tibial veins (anterior and posterior)	Transverse sinus
Peroneal, soleal, and gastrocnemius vein	Straight sinus
Foot veins	
Proximal	Pulmonary arteries
Iliac system	Main and lobar arteries
External iliac and internal iliac veins	Segmental arteries
Common iliac vein	Subsegmental arteries
Femoral system	Isolated internal jugular vein
Deep femoral and superficial femoral	Renal vein
Common femoral vein	
Upper Extremity	
Distal	Caval system
Ulnar and radial vein	Superior vena cava
Interosseous veins	Inferior vena cava
Proximal	Splanchnic vein
Brachial vein	Portal vein
Axillary vein	Hepatic vein
Subclavian vein	Mesenteric vein
Brachiocephalic/innominate vein	

Intra-abdominal thromboses have variable presentation but abdominal pain is a common symptom. Hepatic vein thrombosis can be associated with nausea, emesis, diarrhea, ascites, and splenomegaly.[8] Mesenteric vein thrombosis presents with fecal occult blood positivity in 50% of cases, whereas melena, hematochezia, and hematemesis are seen in 15% of adult cases.[9] Other common manifestations of portal vein thrombosis include fever, ascites, and splenomegaly.[10]

Renal vein thrombosis has a specific constellation of symptoms including flank pain/tenderness, hypertension, hematuria, and thrombocytopenia. Depending on severity, hydronephrosis and subsequent acute kidney failure can develop.[11]

Provoked/Unprovoked

Provoked VTE is associated with an overt clinical risk factor and occurs in greater than 90% of pediatric VTE.[12] The International Society on Thrombosis and Haemostasis (ISTH) Scientific and Standardization Committee (SSC) refined this definition further to recommend identifying the risk factor as transient (ie, resolved after triggering VTE event; eg, surgery) or persistent (eg, metastatic cancer).[13] Although there are many known risks factors in pediatric VTE, central venous catheters (CVCs) represent the most common provoking factor for children, present in 80% of cases of hospital-associated VTE in the CHAT Registry and 46.4% in the Kids-DOTT P/F phase.[6,7]

Idiopathic/Nonidiopathic

VTE is idiopathic when there is a lack of an overt clinical risk factor and a clinically significant thrombophilia. This situation differs from an unprovoked VTE because of the additional absence of thrombophilia.

THROMBOPHILIA

Thrombophilia refers to the predisposition to develop VTE in the presence of acquired and/or inherited traits that result in hypercoagulability. The available evidence on the risks associated with the presence of thrombophilia have yielded inconclusive or contradictory findings.[14] Thrombophilia plays a role in the development of pediatric VTE; however, the extent of this role is likely influenced by the specific pediatric subgroups (eg, provoked vs unprovoked VTE, first episode vs recurrent VTE) in whom other risks factors, such as the presence of CVCs or underlying medical conditions, may play a more important role.

At present, there is no evidence to support testing for primary prevention in the general population, although there may be a role for testing of first-degree relatives of individuals who have a personal history of early-onset VTE. Inherited thrombotic traits are listed in **Table 2**. Acquired thrombotic traits include antiphospholipid antibodies (APAs) and increased factor VIII level.

Antiphospholipid Antibodies

The diagnosis of APA syndrome is established when a patient develops a thrombosis and is noted to have positivity of the lupus anticoagulant (LA) and/or immunoglobulin (Ig) G or IgM anticardiolipin antibodies (aCLs) present in medium or high titer (>99th percentile) or IgG or IgM anti–beta-2-glycoprotein antibodies (>99th percentile). Testing should show positivity on 2 or more consecutive occasions separated by a minimum of 12 weeks.[15] Prevalence estimates in healthy children are 3.3% to 25%. However, only 10% of children with APAs develop thrombosis.[16,17] Children are more likely to have LA positivity of the 3 antibodies.[18] In addition to VTE, APAs are implicated in arterial events, particularly neonatal arterial ischemic stroke.[16]

Table 2
Inherited thrombophilia traits

Inherited Thrombophilia Trait	Mechanism	Gene/Classification	Prevalence	VTE Risk[66] OR (95% CI)
Antithrombin deficiency	Serine protease inhibitor Irreversible inhibition of factors IIa and Xa (primary targets), and IXa, XIa, XIIa, and VIIa (secondary targets)[14]	SERPINC1 gene, chromosome 1 Type 1: quantitative (detectable levels) Type 2: qualitative; 2a defect in reactive domain; 2b defect in heparin binding site Type 3: quantitative (undetectable); most likely incompatible with life[15]	VTE population: 1 in 20–1 in 200[16] Pediatric-specific prevalence poorly defined: none in The Canadian Registry (n = 171)[16] and 1.1% on a single-institution Indiana cohort[17]	First VTE Fixed model: 9.44 (3.34–26.66) Random model: 8.73 (3.12–24.42) Recurrent VTE Fixed model: 3.01 (1.43–6.33) Random model: 3.37 (1.57–7.2)
PC	Vitamin K–dependent protein Activated by thrombin-thrombomodulin Inactivates factors Va and VIIIa[14]	PROC gene, chromosome 2 Homozygous or compound heterozygous present with life-threatening disorders on first days of life Type 1: quantitative; both functional and antigenic levels reduced Type 2: reduction of functional activity greater than antigenic activity[14,18]	Unclear estimates: 1 in 20,000 clinically significant PC deficiency[18] 1 in 400,000 to 1 in 1 million homozygous PC deficiency[14] The Canadian Registry: 0.6%[16] Indiana cohort: 2.1%[17]	First VTE Fixed model: 7.72 (4.44–13.42) Random model: 7.75 (4.48–3.38) Recurrent VTE Fixed model: 2.39 (1.21–4.36) Random model: 2.53 (1.3–4.92)
Protein S deficiency	Vitamin K–dependent protein cofactor for PC accelerating PC's activity 10-fold Cofactor for tissue factor pathway inhibitor[19]	PROS gene, chromosome 3 Homozygous or compound heterozygous present with life-threatening disorders on first days of life	The Canadian Registry: 1.2%[16] Indiana cohort: 1%[17]	First VTE Fixed model: 5.77 (3.03–10.97) Random model: 5.77 (3.07–10.85) Recurrent VTE Fixed model: 3.12 (1.5–6.45) Random model: 3.76 (1.76–8.04)

FVL	Point mutation with single amino acid substitution (arginine 506 to glutamine) at the APC cleavage site This Va variant is resistant to cleavage by APC, leading to excess of activated FVL[14]	*FV* gene, chromosome 1 Heterozygous or homozygous	Heterozygous: 3%–8% of general population in the United States (higher prevalence in Europe) VTE population: 20%–25%[20]	First VTE Fixed model: 3.77 (2.98–4.77) Random model: 3.56 (2.57–4.93) Recurrent VTE Fixed model: 0.64 (0.35–1.18) Random model: 0.77 (0.4–1.45)
Factor II G20210A mutation	Single guanine to adenine substitution at position 20,210. Associated with increased production of plasma prothrombin, which protects factor Va from APC's cleavage[22]	*Prothrombin* gene, chromosome 11 Heterozygous or homozygous	White people: 2%–3% VTE population: 4%–8%[23]	First VTE Fixed model: 2.64 (1.6–4.41) Random model: 2.63 (1.61–4.29) Recurrent VTE Fixed model: 1.88 (1.01–3.49) Random model: 2.15 (1.12–4.10)
Lp(a) increase	Similar structure to plasminogen Lp(a) competes with plasminogen for the binding domain in endothelial cells leading to decreased plasminogen activity on the endothelial cell surface[14]	Level>300 mg/L has been shown to increase risk of cardiovascular disease and AIS in pediatrics, role in VTE remains unclear[29,30]	General population: 7%–10.3%	First VTE Fixed model: 4.49 (3.26–6.18) Random model: 4.5 (3.19–6.35) Recurrent VTE Fixed model: 0.81 (0.49–1.36) Random model: 0.84 (0.5–1.4)
Hyperhomocysteinemia	Increased levels are thought to induce endothelial damage and reduce thrombomodulin activity Further research is needed to determine specific role in VTE	Increased levels (>11 μmol/L) can be seen in patients homozygous for the *MTHFR* C677T polymorphism or in compound heterozygous (C677T/A1298C genotype)	General population (homozygous C677T genotype): 10% Prevalence in pediatric VTE population similar to that of the general population	Pediatric VTE risk not accurately determined Adequate vitamin B₁₂/folate intake can lower homocysteine levels to normal range but do not decrease thrombotic risk[28]

Abbreviations: AIS, arterial ischemic stroke; APC, activated protein C; CI, confidence interval; FVL, factor V Leiden mutation; Lp(a), lipoprotein a; OR, odds ratio; PC, protein C deficiency.

Factor VIII Increase

Increase in factor VIII level greater than 150 IU/dL increases risk of initial and recurrent VTE. Persistently increased levels correlate with poor outcomes (ie, lack of resolution, recurrence, and postthrombotic syndrome).[19] It remains unclear whether factor VIII represents congenital thrombophilia, acquired prothrombotic tendency, or an acute phase reactant.[20]

ANATOMIC PREDISPOSITION SYNDROMES
Atretic Inferior Vena Cava

Anomalies of the inferior vena cava occur secondary to embryologic disorders during the fifth to seventh weeks of gestation. These abnormalities lead to inadequate blood return, increased lower extremity pressure, venous stasis, and subsequent predisposition to thromboses.[21] Prevalence is estimated at 0.4% to 1% in the general population, and at 5% in unprovoked lower extremity VTE cases.[22,23] VTE is bilateral in more than 50% of cases.[24] Standard treatment guidelines do not exist but acute management often consists of parenteral anticoagulation and catheter-directed thrombolysis followed by chronic anticoagulation.

May-Thurner Anomaly

The May-Thurner anomaly (iliac vein compression syndrome) results when the left common iliac vein is chronically compressed between an overlying right common iliac artery and an underlying vertebral body. The resultant compression and endothelial damage induces venous congestion and stasis predisposing to VTE.[25,26] Clinically, it is characterized by left lower extremity swelling; pain; claudication and, in chronic cases, ulceration; skin hyperpigmentation; and the development of varicose veins. True prevalence is unknown but one series of 50 patients evaluated in an emergency room for abdominal pain found that 24% of the cohort had greater than 50% compression and 66% had at least 25% compression.[27] Prevalence in patients with left lower extremity venous insufficiency is estimated at 2% to 5%.[25] Acute management consists of parenteral anticoagulation with catheter-directed thrombolysis followed by conventional anticoagulation. Stenting has been shown to improve patency rates and is recommended by both the Society of Interventional Radiology[28] and Society for Vascular Surgery.[29]

Paget-Schroetter Syndrome

Paget-Schroetter syndrome (venous thoracic outlet syndrome or so-called effort thrombosis) occurs when VTE develops in the axillary and/or subclavian veins at the costoclavicular junction. The subclavian vein is highly susceptible to injury where it passes by the junction of the first rib and clavicle. Repetitive motions can lead to recurrent injury, endothelial damage, and extrinsic compression resulting in VTE.[30,31] True incidence is unknown but estimated as 1 to 2 cases per 100,000 people per year.[30] It typically affects male adolescents and young adults.

Management is a multimodal approach that includes the use of anticoagulation, thrombolysis, and surgical thoracic outlet decompression. Acute management consists of parenteral anticoagulation with catheter-directed thrombolysis and transition to outpatient anticoagulation, which is followed by thoracic outlet decompression via first rib resection. There is debate about surgical timing but it is often done shortly after acute management to avoid the risk of rethrombosis, which remains while the compression persists.[30,32]

RISK-ASSESSMENT AND RISK MODELING FOR INCIDENT VENOUS THROMBOEMBOLISM

Several risk-assessment models have been published for pediatric health care–associated (HA) VTE (**Table 3**).[33–38] Branchford and colleagues[35] showed independent risk with mechanical ventilation, systemic infection, and hospital stay greater than or equal to 5 days. Sharathkumar and colleagues[39] derived 6 independent risk factors with various point values, and a cumulative score of greater than or equal to 3 yielded a positive predictive value of 2.45% for HA-VTE at a prevalence of 0.71%.

Two separate risk-assessment models, for critically ill and non–critically ill children, respectively, were created from a single institution by retrospective, case-control study designs.[33,34] In non–critically ill children, scores of 8, 7, and less than or equal to 6 correlated to risk of HA-VTE of 12.5%, 1.1%, and 0.1%, respectively.[34] In critically ill children, scores of 15, 7 to 14, and less than or equal to 6 correlated to risk of HA-VTE of 8.8%, 1.3%, and 0.03%, respectively.[33]

Kerlin and colleagues[40] used a retrospective derivation and retrospective validation method to determine an equation that uses 0 or 1 for absence or presence of certain factors.

Reiter and colleagues[38] created an intensive care unit (ICU)–specific (cardiac ICU excluded) model for prehospital and in-hospital thromboses but included venous and arterial events. They derived 12 risk factors via literature review and assigned 1 point per factor. Each 1 point increased the risk of symptomatic thrombosis 1.57-fold (95% confidence interval, 0.132–5.49) to 2.12-fold (95% confidence interval, 0.175–18.34) for prehospital and in-hospital thrombi, respectively ($P<.05$).[38]

The model by Prentiss[37] describes levels of risk, risk score 1 to 3, but does not detail which risk factors comprise the scoring system. Additional models have been derived for children with acute lymphoblastic leukemia,[41] patients admitted to the cardiovascular ICU,[42] pediatric oncology patients with a CVC-related VTE,[43] and pediatric trauma.[44]

VENOUS THROMBOEMBOLISM TREATMENT

Determining treatment of pediatric VTE entails many considerations, including differing epidemiology from adults, developmental hemostasis, differing pharmacokinetic and pharmacodynamic considerations in children, issues with vascular access, parenteral administration, and limited oral treatment options.

Treatment Goals

The initial goal of therapy is to halt thrombus progression and prevent further propagation and/or embolization. With clot stability and reduction in local inflammation, endogenous fibrinolytic systems break down existing clot material, whereas anticoagulation prevents further clot formation. Longer term goals include prevention of recurrence and chronic complications.

Treatment Options

Acute VTE treatment is typically with a heparin product, either unfractionated heparin (UFH) or low-molecular-weight heparin (LMWH). Direct thrombin inhibitors, argatroban and bivalirudin, can be used in pediatrics but are typically reserved for scenarios in which UFH is contraindicated; for example, heparin-induced thrombocytopenia.[45]

Agents used for subacute and chronic therapy are LMWH, fondaparinux, and warfarin. LMWH has advantages of being widely used, predictable bioavailability, and any dose strength can be administered (which is a key advantage in infants) given

Table 3
Pediatric venous thromboembolism risk-assessment models

	Branchford	Sharathkumar	Arlikar	Atchison	Reiter[a]	Kerlin
Pediatric Population	All	All	ICU	Non-ICU	ICU	All
Study Design for Score Derivation	Retrospective case control (1:2)	Retrospective case control (1:2)	Retrospective case control (1:3)	Retrospective case control (1:7)	Literature review	Retrospective cohort
N	78:160	173:346	57:171	50:350	—	389
Validation Method	—	Retrospective case control (1:1)	—	—	Prospective, observational cohort study	Retrospective cohort
N	—	100:100	—	—	742	149
Risk Factors Comprising Score	MV Infection LOS ≥ 5 d	Immobilization LOS ≥ 7 d OCP CVC Bacteremia Direct ICU admission	CVC LOS ≥ 4 d Infection	CVC Infection LOS ≥ 4 d	CVC Immobility>72 h Infection Orthopedic surgery Major trauma (ISS>15) Malignancy OCP Burns>30% BSA Thrombophilia Age<1 y or >14 y Obesity Hypercoagulable state	Male gender Asymmetric extremity CVC Active cancer Alternative diagnosis[b]

Abbreviations: BSA, body surface area; ICU, intensive care unit; ISS, injury severity score; LOS, length of stay; MV, mechanical ventilation; OCP, oral contraceptive pill.
[a] Included VTE and arterial thromboembolism in their study.
[b] Presence of this factor results in point reduction from score.

the availability of multiuse vials. The key disadvantage is twice-daily subcutaneous injections. Fondaparinux is a once-daily injection but is difficult to use in small children because of fixed-dose preparations. Warfarin, a vitamin K antagonist, has the advantage of oral dosing but can be challenging in children given frequent dose monitoring with venipuncture and changing dietary patterns affecting dose titration.

At the time of this writing, none of the direct oral anticoagulants (DOACs) are approved for use in pediatrics and experience is limited to clinical trials and off-label use. However, current trials are evaluating the use of both IIa and Xa inhibitors in all pediatric ages, including neonates and infants, with evaluation of liquid formulations as well as concomitant evaluation of health-related quality of life compared with standard of care. Furthermore, there are trials evaluating certain DOACs in specific clinical scenarios; for example, rivaroxaban as thromboprophylaxis after the Fontan cardiac surgical procedure and apixaban as thromboprophylaxis in children with leukemia who have a CVC and have received pegylated L-asparaginase.

Thrombolysis

Thrombolysis can be administered systemically or site directed via an endovascular approach. Systemic thrombolysis is typically indicated in the setting of life-threatening or limb-threatening thrombosis but more recently has been investigated in completely occlusive proximal limb DVT and found to reduce postthrombotic syndrome (PTS; discussed later) versus no reduction in unselected cases.[46] Success (complete and partial) and major bleeding (per ISTH criteria[47]) rates have been reported as 79% and 15%, respectively.[48] Endovascular therapy is typically performed for extremity and/or pelvic VTE with full occlusion. Full resolution has been noted in 76% of cases, partial resolution in 17%, and no resolution in 7%.[48]

Duration of Anticoagulation

The duration of therapy often depends on patient-specific and thrombus-specific characteristics. The American College of Chest Physicians guidelines recommend anticoagulation therapy for 3 months in children presenting with a provoked VTE, and longer, at prophylactic or therapeutic dosing, if the provoking factor is still present.[49] For a recurrent provoked VTE, therapy is continued for 3 months from the event. For a first idiopathic VTE, therapy is for 6 to 12 months and, if recurrent, chronic anticoagulation is recommended.[49]

Kids-DOTT is a National Institutes of Health–sponsored multinational ongoing randomized controlled trial investigating noninferiority of a 6-week (shortened) versus 3-month (conventional) duration of anticoagulation in patients aged less than 21 years with provoked venous thrombosis. The primary efficacy and safety end points are symptomatic recurrent VTE and anticoagulant-related, clinically relevant bleeding, respectively, within 1 year.

Complications of Treatment

The primary safety concern of antithrombotic therapy is bleeding. Bleeding risk has been reported as 1.5% to 24% with UFH, and 2.9% and 23.4% for major and minor bleeding respectively, with LMWH. Bleeding rates with warfarin depend on the target International Normalized Ratio (INR) and have been reported as high as 12.2% for major bleeding with INRs of 2 to 3.[49] Clinically relevant bleeding risk at 1 year post-diagnosis in the Kids-DOTT pilot phase, including mostly patients treated with LMWH and approximately half with a shortened duration of anticoagulation, was approximately 1%.[7]

Heparin-induced thrombocytopenia has been reported in up to 2.3% of pediatric patients receiving UFH but data are vexed by differences in patient population and laboratory techniques. Osteoporosis is a rare but worrisome complication of chronic anticoagulation. In pediatrics, most data have come from case reports in which there may be other factors that affect bone density.[49]

LONG-TERM OUTCOMES
Recurrent Venous Thromboembolism

Risk of VTE recurrence has been variably reported but is estimated at around 6% to 10% in children and 3% in neonates.[1,19,50] The risk of symptomatic recurrent VTE at 1 year postdiagnosis in the Kids-DOTT pilot phase was approximately 2% in a study population that consisted of patients less than 21 years old with provoked VTE.[7] The likelihood of recurrence is influenced by a host of variables including comorbidities and thrombophilia status. Longitudinal assessment of D-dimer and/or factor VIII level may be helpful in identifying patients at higher risk for recurrence when there is persistent increase (>500 ng/mL and >150 IU/dL, respectively).[19]

Postthrombotic Syndrome

PTS is the most common long-term complication in pediatric patients with an extremity DVT. Impaired venous return, caused by valvular reflux or thrombotic veno-occlusion, leads to venous hypertension and chronic venous insufficiency.[51] It is characterized by presence of edema; pain; changes to skin pigmentation; varicosities; and, in severe cases, stasis dermatitis and ulceration.[52]

PTS incidence varies significantly, from 0% to 70%, which reflects heterogeneity of study designs, patient population, duration of follow-up, and assessment methods. A systematic review identified a weighted mean frequency of 26%.[53] Proposed risks factors include older age, higher body mass index, extent of initial DVT, number of vessels involved, lack of resolution, presence of the LA, and CVC.[33]

PTS is typically diagnosed with a validated assessment tool. In pediatrics, 2 key tools exist: the Manco-Johnson Instrument[54] and the modified Villalta Scale (**Table 4**).[55] Although the ISTH SSC has stated that there is insufficient evidence to endorse one tool rather than the other,[56] the Manco-Johnson Instrument has undergone reliability and validity testing as well as validation for both upper and lower extremity DVT.[54,57]

Basic treatment involves regular activity, periodic elevation of the affected extremity, and maintenance of a healthy weight. The use of elastic compression stockings has minimal evidence in children and is hampered by difficulty with sizing (particularly as the child grows) and poor compliance in adolescents and young adults.[58] There are insufficient data to make recommendations for use of pharmacologic agents in pediatrics but adult trials of vasoactive drugs have been inconsistent and do not support routine use.[59]

Chronic Thromboembolic Pulmonary Hypertension

An emerging complication of PE in pediatrics is chronic thromboembolic pulmonary hypertension (CTEPH). This condition is thought to occur because of incomplete thrombus resolution in pulmonary arteries leading to chronic thrombosis and fibrosis. The resultant obstruction reduces the cross-sectional area of pulmonary arteries, leading to vasoconstriction and further vascular remodeling. These processes result in pulmonary hypertension and right ventricular pressure overload.[60]

Table 4
Comparison of postthrombotic syndrome instruments

	Manco-Johnson Instrument		Modified Villalta Scale	
	Components	Scoring	Components	Scoring
Signs	Edema[a] Dilated superficial collateral veins Venous stasis dermatitis Venous stasis ulcers	Each scored 0 or 1 (absent/present)	Change in skin color Increased limb circumference[b] Pitting edema Venous collaterals on skin Pigmentation Tenderness on palpation Head swelling Varicosities Venous ulcer	Each scored 0 or 1 (absent/present) 1 moderate; 2 severe 1 moderate; 2 severe 9 (present)
Symptoms	Chronic lower extremity pain • Limiting aerobic activities • Limiting activities of daily living • At rest	Each scored 0–5 (Wong-Baker FACES scale)	Pain or abnormal use[c] Swelling[c]	Each scored 0 or 1 (absent/present)
PTS Classification	PTS absent Any PTS present Physically and functionally significant PTS	0 points 1 or more points ≥1 sign and ≥1 symptoms	No PTS Mild PTS Moderate PTS Severe PTS	0 points 1–3 points 4–8 points >8 points

[a] More than 1-cm increase in circumference in the affected extremity compared with the contralateral extremity.
[b] More than 3% compared with contralateral side.
[c] Reported by patient, parent, caregiver or proxy.

Most data, from adult studies, have noted an incidence of 2% to 4%.[61,62] Incidence rates in pediatrics are not clearly defined but it is suspected to be underdiagnosed.[63]

The diagnosis of CTEPH is made when patients with history of VTE present with symptoms of exercise intolerance, fatigue, dyspnea, and/or chest pain, associated with an echocardiogram showing pulmonary hypertension. A ventilation/perfusion (V/Q) lung scan and/or computed tomography angiography should be performed. If confirmed, patients are often assessed by right heart catheterization and the final diagnosis of CTEPH is made when precapillary pulmonary hypertension (mean pulmonary arterial pressure ≥25 mm Hg, pulmonary capillary wedge pressure <15 mm Hg) is identified after at least 3 months of anticoagulation.[64] Pediatric-specific catheterization values to diagnose CTEPH have not been determined. However, if the clinical suspicion is present and pulmonary hypertension has been diagnosed, the next step is to continue anticoagulation[64] and explore possible pulmonary thromboendarterectomy (PTE).[65] One pediatric case series (n = 17) of patients who underwent PTE noted significantly improved cardiopulmonary hemodynamics and functional status.[63] This case series noted a markedly higher risk of rethrombosis (n = 6, 35%) compared with rates from adult studies (1%–4%). The investigators noted that their population had a high rate of thrombophilia (67%), were more likely to have unilateral main pulmonary artery disease, and 2 out of the 6 patients with rethrombosis discontinued anticoagulation prematurely.[63]

SUMMARY

The incidence of pediatric VTE is increasing but there are emerging data on best practices for risk prediction, management, and use of thrombophilia testing. Ongoing research such as the CHAT Registry and Kids-DOTT trial highlights the complexity, but also now the feasibility, of investigator-initiated cooperative studies in pediatric VTE. In addition, ongoing pediatric trials of DOACs hold potential to expand the options for treatment in children.

REFERENCES

1. Raffini L, Huang YS, Witmer C, et al. Dramatic increase in venous thromboembolism in children's hospitals in the United States from 2001 to 2007. Pediatrics 2009;124(4):1001–8.
2. Andrew M, David M, Adams M, et al. Venous thromboembolic complications (VTE) in children: first analyses of the Canadian Registry of VTE. Blood 1994; 83(5):1251–7.
3. Stein PD, Kayali F, Olson RE. Incidence of venous thromboembolism in infants and children: data from the National Hospital Discharge Survey. J Pediatr 2004;145(4):563–5.
4. Kim SJ, Sabharwal S. Risk factors for venous thromboembolism in hospitalized children and adolescents: a systemic review and pooled analysis. J Pediatr Orthop B 2014;23(4):389–93.
5. Goudie A, Dynan L, Brady PW, et al. Costs of venous thromboembolism, catheter-associated urinary tract infection, and pressure ulcer. Pediatrics 2015;136(3): 432–9.
6. Jaffray J, Mahajerin A, Young G, et al. A multi-institutional registry of pediatric hospital-acquired thrombosis cases: The Children's Hospital-Acquired Thrombosis (CHAT) project. Thromb Res 2018;161:67–72.
7. Goldenberg NA, Abshire T, Blatchford PJ, et al. Multicenter randomized controlled trial on Duration of Therapy for Thrombosis in Children and Young Adults (the Kids-DOTT trial): pilot/feasibility phase findings. J Thromb Haemost 2015;13(9):1597–605.
8. Sabol TP, Molina M, Wu GY. Thrombotic venous diseases of the liver. J Clin Transl Hepatol 2015;3(3):189–94.
9. Hmoud B, Singal AK, Kamath PS. Mesenteric venous thrombosis. J Clin Exp Hepatol 2014;4(3):257–63.
10. Chawla YK, Bodh V. Portal vein thrombosis. J Clin Exp Hepatol 2015;5(1):22–40.
11. Asghar M, Ahmed K, Shah SS, et al. Renal vein thrombosis. Eur J Vasc Endovasc Surg 2007;34(2):217–23.
12. Parasuraman S, Goldhaber SZ. Venous thromboembolism in children. Circulation 2006;113(2):e12–6.
13. Kearon C, Ageno W, Cannegieter SC, et al. Categorization of patients as having provoked or unprovoked venous thromboembolism: guidance from the SSC of ISTH. J Thromb Haemost 2016;14(7):1480–3.
14. Nowak-Göttl U, van Ommen H, Kenet G. Thrombophilia testing in children: what and when should be tested? Thromb Res 2018;164:75–8.
15. Miyakis S, Lockshin MD, Atsumi T, et al. International consensus statement on an update of the classification criteria for definite antiphospholipid syndrome (APS). J Thromb Haemost 2006;4(2):295–306.
16. Aguiar CL, Soybilgic A, Avcin T, et al. Pediatric antiphospholipid syndrome. Curr Rheumatol Rep 2015;17(4):27.

17. Avcin T, Ambrozic A, Kuhar M, et al. Anticardiolipin and anti-beta(2) glycoprotein I antibodies in sera of 61 apparently healthy children at regular preventive visits. Rheumatology (Oxford) 2001;40(5):565–73.

18. Keeling D, Mackie I, Moore GW, et al, British Committee for Standards in Haematology. Guidelines on the investigation and management of antiphospholipid syndrome. Br J Haematol 2012;157(1):47–58.

19. Goldenberg NA, Knapp-Clevenger R, Manco-Johnson MJ, Mountain States Regional Thrombophilia Group. Elevated plasma factor VIII and D-dimer levels as predictors of poor outcomes of thrombosis in children. N Engl J Med 2004; 351(11):1081–8.

20. Jenkins PV, Rawley O, Smith OP, et al. Elevated factor VIII levels and risk of venous thrombosis. Br J Haematol 2012;157(6):653–63.

21. Sarlon G, Bartoli MA, Muller C, et al. Congenital anomalies of inferior vena cava in young patients with iliac deep venous thrombosis. Ann Vasc Surg 2011;25(2): 265.e5-8.

22. Bianchi M, Giannini D, Balbarini A, et al. Congenital hypoplasia of the inferior vena cava and inherited thrombophilia: rare associated risk factors for idiopathic deep vein thrombosis. A case report. J Cardiovasc Med (Hagerstown) 2008;9(1): 101–4.

23. Eifert S, Villavicencio JL, Kao TC, et al. Prevalence of deep venous anomalies in congenital vascular malformations of venous predominance. J Vasc Surg 2000; 31(3):462–71.

24. Gayer G, Luboshitz J, Hertz M, et al. Congenital anomalies of the inferior vena cava revealed on CT in patients with deep vein thrombosis. AJR Am J Roentgenol 2003;180(3):729–32.

25. Kaltenmeier CT, Erben Y, Indes J, et al. Systematic review of May-Thurner syndrome with emphasis on gender differences. J Vasc Surg Venous Lymphat Disord 2018;6(3):399–407.e4.

26. Knuttinen MG, Naidu S, Oklu R, et al. May-Thurner: diagnosis and endovascular management. Cardiovasc Diagn Ther 2017;7(Suppl 3):S159–64.

27. Kibbe MR, Ujiki M, Goodwin AL, et al. Iliac vein compression in an asymptomatic patient population. J Vasc Surg 2004;39(5):937–43.

28. Vedantham S, Millward SF, Cardella JF, et al. Society of Interventional Radiology position statement: treatment of acute iliofemoral deep vein thrombosis with use of adjunctive catheter-directed intrathrombus thrombolysis. J Vasc Interv Radiol 2006;17(4):613–6.

29. Meissner MH, Gloviczki P, Comerota AJ, et al. Early thrombus removal strategies for acute deep venous thrombosis: clinical practice guidelines of the Society for Vascular Surgery and the American Venous Forum. J Vasc Surg 2012;55(5): 1449–62.

30. Illig KA, Doyle AJ. A comprehensive review of Paget-Schroetter syndrome. J Vasc Surg 2010;51(6):1538–47.

31. Naeem M, Soares G, Ahn S, et al. Paget-Schroetter syndrome: a review and algorithm (WASPS-IR). Phlebology 2015;30(10):675–86.

32. Alla VM, Natarajan N, Kaushik M, et al. Paget-Schroetter syndrome: review of pathogenesis and treatment of effort thrombosis. West J Emerg Med 2010; 11(4):358–62.

33. Arlikar SJ, Atchison CM, Amankwah EK, et al. Development of a new risk score for hospital-associated venous thromboembolism in critically-ill children not undergoing cardiothoracic surgery. Thromb Res 2015;136(4):717–22.

34. Atchison CM, Arlikar S, Amankwah E, et al. Development of a new risk score for hospital-associated venous thromboembolism in noncritically ill children: findings from a large single-institutional case-control study. J Pediatr 2014;165(4):793–8.

35. Branchford BR, Mourani P, Bajaj L, et al. Risk factors for in-hospital venous thromboembolism in children: a case-control study employing diagnostic validation. Haematologica 2012;97(4):509–15.

36. Kerlin BA, Stephens JA, Hogan MJ, et al. Development of a pediatric-specific clinical probability tool for diagnosis of venous thromboembolism: a feasibility study. Pediatr Res 2015;77(3):463–71.

37. Prentiss AS. Early recognition of pediatric venous thromboembolism: a risk-assessment tool. Am J Crit Care 2012;21(3):178–83 [quiz: 184].

38. Reiter PD, Wathen B, Valuck RJ, et al. Thrombosis risk factor assessment and implications for prevention in critically ill children. Pediatr Crit Care Med 2012;13(4):381–6.

39. Sharathkumar AA, Mahajerin A, Heidt L, et al. Risk-prediction tool for identifying hospitalized children with a predisposition for development of venous thromboembolism: Peds-Clot clinical Decision Rule. J Thromb Haemost 2012;10(7):1326–34.

40. Kerlin BA, Smoyer WE, Tsai J, et al. Healthcare burden of venous thromboembolism in childhood chronic renal diseases. Pediatr Nephrol 2015;30(5):829–37.

41. Mitchell L, Lambers M, Flege S, et al. Validation of a predictive model for identifying an increased risk for thromboembolism in children with acute lymphoblastic leukemia: results of a multicenter cohort study. Blood 2010;115(24):4999–5004.

42. Atchison CM, Amankwah E, Wilhelm J, et al. Risk factors for hospital-associated venous thromboembolism in critically ill children following cardiothoracic surgery or therapeutic cardiac catheterisation. Cardiol Young 2018;28(2):234–42.

43. Revel-Vilk S, Yacobovich J, Tamary H, et al. Risk factors for central venous catheter thrombotic complications in children and adolescents with cancer. Cancer 2010;116(17):4197–205.

44. Connelly CR, Laird A, Barton JS, et al. A clinical tool for the prediction of venous thromboembolism in pediatric trauma patients. JAMA Surg 2016;151(1):50–7.

45. Moffett BS, Teruya J. Trends in parenteral direct thrombin inhibitor use in pediatric patients: analysis of a large administrative database. Arch Pathol Lab Med 2014;138(9):1229–32.

46. Vedantham S, Goldhaber SZ, Julian JA, et al. Pharmacomechanical catheter-directed thrombolysis for deep-vein thrombosis. N Engl J Med 2017;377(23):2240–52.

47. Schulman S, Kearon C, Subcommittee on Control of Anticoagulation of the Scientific and Standardization Committee of the International Society on Thrombosis and Haemostasis. Definition of major bleeding in clinical investigations of antihemostatic medicinal products in non-surgical patients. J Thromb Haemost 2005;3(4):692–4.

48. Albisetti M. Thrombolytic therapy in children. Thromb Res 2006;118(1):95–105.

49. Monagle P, Chan AKC, Goldenberg NA, et al. Antithrombotic therapy in neonates and children: Antithrombotic Therapy and Prevention of Thrombosis, 9th ed: American College of Chest Physicians Evidence-Based Clinical Practice Guidelines. Chest 2012;141(2 Suppl):e737S–801S.

50. Spentzouris G, Scriven RJ, Lee TK, et al. Pediatric venous thromboembolism in relation to adults. J Vasc Surg 2012;55(6):1785–93.

51. Prandoni P, Frulla M, Sartor D, et al. Vein abnormalities and the post-thrombotic syndrome. J Thromb Haemost 2005;3(2):401–2.

52. Kuhle S, Koloshuk B, Marzinotto V, et al. A cross-sectional study evaluating post-thrombotic syndrome in children. Thromb Res 2003;111(4–5):227–33.

53. Goldenberg NA, Donadini MP, Kahn SR, et al. Post-thrombotic syndrome in children: a systematic review of frequency of occurrence, validity of outcome measures, and prognostic factors. Haematologica 2010;95(11):1952–9.

54. Goldenberg NA, Pounder E, Knapp-Clevenger R, et al. Validation of upper extremity post-thrombotic syndrome outcome measurement in children. J Pediatr 2010;157(5):852–5.

55. Raffini L, Davenport J, Bevilacqua L, et al. Comparison of 3 postthrombotic syndrome assessment scales demonstrates significant variability in children and adolescents with deep vein thrombosis. J Pediatr Hematol Oncol 2015;37(8):611–5.

56. Goldenberg NA, Brandao L, Journeycake J, et al. Definition of post-thrombotic syndrome following lower extremity deep venous thrombosis and standardization of outcome measurement in pediatric clinical investigations. J Thromb Haemost 2012;10(3):477–80.

57. Goldenberg NA, Durham JD, Knapp-Clevenger R, et al. A thrombolytic regimen for high-risk deep venous thrombosis may substantially reduce the risk of post-thrombotic syndrome in children. Blood 2007;110(1):45–53.

58. Biss TT, Kahr WH, Brandão LR, et al. The use of elastic compression stockings for post-thrombotic syndrome in a child. Pediatr Blood Cancer 2009;53(3):462–3.

59. Betensky M, Goldenberg NA. Post-thrombotic syndrome in children. Thromb Res 2018;164:129–35.

60. Piazza G, Goldhaber SZ. Chronic thromboembolic pulmonary hypertension. N Engl J Med 2011;364(4):351–60.

61. Pengo V, Lensing AW, Prins MH, et al. Incidence of chronic thromboembolic pulmonary hypertension after pulmonary embolism. N Engl J Med 2004;350(22):2257–64.

62. Becattini C, Agnelli G, Pesavento R, et al. Incidence of chronic thromboembolic pulmonary hypertension after a first episode of pulmonary embolism. Chest 2006;130(1):172–5.

63. Madani MM, Wittine LM, Auger WR, et al. Chronic thromboembolic pulmonary hypertension in pediatric patients. J Thorac Cardiovasc Surg 2011;141(3):624–30.

64. Wilkens H, Lang I, Behr J, et al. Chronic thromboembolic pulmonary hypertension (CTEPH): updated Recommendations of the Cologne Consensus Conference 2011. Int J Cardiol 2011;154(Suppl 1):S54–60.

65. Ivy DD, Abman SH, Barst RJ, et al. Pediatric pulmonary hypertension. J Am Coll Cardiol 2013;62(25 Suppl):D117–26.

66. Young G, Albisetti M, Bonduel M, et al. Impact of inherited thrombophilia on venous thromboembolism in children: a systematic review and meta-analysis of observational studies. Circulation 2008;118(13):1373–82.

Vascular Anomalies
Diagnosis of Complicated Anomalies and New Medical Treatment Options

Denise M. Adams, MD[a],*, Kiersten W. Ricci, MD[b]

KEYWORDS

- Vascular anomaly • Vascular malformation • Vascular tumor
- Kaposiform hemangioendothelioma • Lymphatic anomalies
- Kaposiform lymphangiomatosis • Sirolimus • PIK3CA

KEY POINTS

- Vascular anomalies are classified as tumors and malformations.
- Vascular anomalies are best cared for by an interdisciplinary team.
- Some of the most aggressive vascular anomalies have a lymphatic component.
- The mammalian target of Rapamycin inhibitor sirolimus has proved to be safe and efficacious for many vascular anomalies when standard protocols are used.
- Correlation of phenotype and genotype in vascular anomalies is important for classification and treatment.

INTRODUCTION

Vascular anomalies, characterized by the abnormal development or growth of blood and/or lymphatic vessels, comprise a spectrum of diseases that have a wide range of complications and varying severity. Diagnosis can be challenging because of phenotype heterogeneity and overlapping symptoms among these conditions. In addition, affected individuals commonly present across various medical and surgical subspecialties, further necessitating accurate diagnosis and common terminology in order to provide appropriate evaluation and optimal management of these conditions.

Recognizing the need for uniformity, Mulliken and Glowacki[1] first proposed a classification system in 1982 that characterized nonmalignant vascular lesions as

[a] Division of Hematology and Oncology, Vascular Anomalies Center, Boston Children's Hospital, Harvard Medical School, 300 Longwood Avenue, Fegan 3, Boston, MA 02115, USA;
[b] Division of Hematology, Hemangioma and Vascular Malformation Center, Cincinnati Children's Hospital Medical Center, University of Cincinnati College of Medicine, 3333 Burnet Avenue, MLC 7015, Cincinnati, OH 45229, USA
* Corresponding author.
E-mail address: Denise.Adams@childrens.harvard.edu

Hematol Oncol Clin N Am 33 (2019) 455–470
https://doi.org/10.1016/j.hoc.2019.01.011
0889-8588/19/© 2019 Elsevier Inc. All rights reserved.

hemonc.theclinics.com

hemangiomas and malformations. With the intent of creating a universal system, the International Society for the Study of Vascular Anomalies (ISSVA) adopted and modified this classification in 1996 to divide vascular anomalies as tumors or malformations based on clinical and histologic characteristics. Since that time, ISSVA has revised this classification system multiple times to incorporate new clinical entities and genetic discoveries. The ISSVA classification system was most recently updated in 2018 and can be accessed at www.issva.org/classification.[2,3]

Vascular anomalies may cause clinical problems such as disfigurement, acute and chronic pain, coagulopathy, bleeding, thrombosis, organ and musculoskeletal dysfunction, and death. These disorders, especially the most severe, are progressive and have lifelong complications.[4] A multidisciplinary team that includes medical, surgical, and radiology experts is frequently essential in the long-term management of these complex patients. Pediatric hematologists/oncologists are key members of these teams, providing clinical acumen in diagnostics, guiding medical management, and coordinating long-term follow-up. Furthermore, hematologists/oncologists have been and will continue to be at the forefront of clinical trial development. The focus of this article is on the diagnosis and management of complicated vascular anomalies with an emphasis on current treatments and new rational and targeted medical therapies (**Table 1**).

COMPLICATED VASCULAR TUMORS
Kaposiform Hemangioendothelioma with Kasabach-Merritt Phenomenon

Kaposiform hemangioendothelioma (KHE) is a rare, locally aggressive vascular tumor that typically presents in infancy and early childhood, although initial symptoms have been reported in adulthood.[5,6] KHE tumors are rapidly growing vascular lesions that are usually unifocal and most commonly involve the extremities, trunk, retroperitoneum, or head and neck regions. Most commonly occurring in infants with KHE, Kasabach-Merritt phenomenon (KMP) is a potentially life-threatening coagulopathy, characterized by profound thrombocytopenia, hypofibrinogenemia, and microangiopathic hemolytic anemia.[7–10] In patients with KHE and KMP, the skin is tense, warm, and indurated and appears purpuric with deep red-purple discoloration that frequently is surrounded by petechiae. Risk factors for the development of KMP include young age of presentation, lesions greater than 8 cm, and retroperitoneal and mediastinal primary sites.[5] Although these tumors do not metastasize, regional perinodal soft tissue involvement and multifocal bone KHE have been reported.[11–15]

On histology, KHE is composed of infiltrating nodules and sheets of spindled endothelial cells and slitlike vascular channels. Platelet microthrombi, hemosiderin, and extravasated red blood cells can also be seen. KHE endothelial cells stain negatively for the hemangioma marker, GLUT-1, and positively for the lymphatic markers, D2-40 (podoplanin) and PROX-1.[16] On T1-weighted MRI, KHE appears as an infiltrative lesion that lacks well-demarcated margins and traverses different tissue planes (from skin to muscle/bone). Stranding in the subcutaneous fat, caused by lymphatic obstruction and invasion, can be seen on T2-weighted imaging.[17]

Treatments have included steroids, single or multiple chemotherapy agents, interferon, antifibrinolytics, aspirin, propranolol, and recently sirolimus.[18–22] A multidisciplinary consensus statement in 2013 concluded that initial therapy for KHE with KMP should include a combination of steroids and vincristine (0.05–0.065 mg/kg/dose or 1–1.5 mg/m^2/dose).[23] However, this statement was released before the publication of the results of the phase 2 prospective clinical trial of sirolimus use in complicated vascular anomalies. In this prospective trial, all 12 patients with KHE complicated by

Table 1
Clinicopathologic features and medical treatment of complicated vascular anomalies

Complicated Vascular Anomaly	Clinical Manifestations	Histopathology/ Molecular Genetics	Drug Treatments

Tumors
  KHE with Kasabach-Merritt phenomenon
	• Unifocal, rapidly growing, tense, warm, red-purple mass
	• Coagulopathy: severe thrombocytopenia, hypofibrinogenemia, and microangiopathic hemolytic anemia
	• May progress to multiorgan failure
		Infiltrating nodules of spindled endothelial cells and slitlike vascular channels, platelet microthrombi, hemosiderin, and extravasated RBCs
		Mutation: GNA14 (somatic)[57]
			First line:
			  Corticosteroids
			  Sirolimus
			  Vincristine

Malformations GSD	• Vanishing bone disease → pathologic fractures, functional issues, CSF leaks, meningitis, spinal instability, deformity • Effusions • Chronic pain	PROX-1, D2-40-positive abnormal lymphatics with increased osteoclast activity and destruction of bone cortex Mutation: unknown	Sirolimus Bisphosphonates NSAIDs
GLA	• Multisite lymphatic malformation of soft tissue, viscera (spleen and liver common) and bones; bone lesions are multiple and noncontiguous • Effusions • Chronic pain	Increased number of dilated anastomosing lymphatic channels, lined by endothelial cells, stains PROX-1 and D2-40 positive Mutation: PIK3CA (somatic)	Sirolimus Bisphosphonates NSAIDs *PIK3CA inhibitor is a consideration in uncontrolled disease
PIK3CA-related overgrowth syndromes (including Klippel-Trenaunay and CLOVES syndrome)	• Capillary lymphatic venous malformation • Benign and malignant tumors • Bone and/or soft tissue overgrowth → deformity, functional issues • Venous thromboembolism associated with ectatic veins • Spinal/neurologic issues • Venous and lymphatic stasis • Recurrent soft tissue infection • Chronic pain	Histology dependent on area of affected tissue and malformation sampled: dilated capillaries, tortuous and dilated veins, embryonal avalvular veins, abnormal lymphatic channels and cysts, fatty or lipomatous masses Mutation: PIK3CA (somatic)	Sirolimus Anticoagulation (heparins, DOACs) NSAIDs *PIK3CA inhibitor is a consideration in uncontrolled disease and/or overgrowth

(continued on next page)

458

Complicated Vascular Anomaly	Clinical Manifestations	Histopathology/ Molecular Genetics	Drug Treatments
Vascular malformations with low-grade intravascular coagulopathy	• Venous or mixed venous malformations-usually extensive or multifocal • Superficial and deep venous thrombosis • Coagulopathy: high D-dimer, low fibrinogen and/or low platelet count • Risk of progression to DIC with surgery, trauma, and severe illness • Chronic pain	Enlarged venous channels, flattened layer of endothelial cells, sparse smooth muscle cells; thrombi may be present; PROX-1, D2-40 positive only with lymphatic component Mutations: TIE2 (germline and somatic), PIK3CA (somatic)	Perioperative or long-term anticoagulation (heparins, DOACs) Sirolimus NSAIDs (consider celecoxib with anticoagulation)
KLA[a]	• Multifocal lymphatic anomaly that often involves thorax, bones, viscera • Progressive involvement, severe morbidity, high mortality • Coagulopathy: severe hypofibrinogenemia, thrombocytopenia, and high rate of bleeding complications • Effusions • Hemorrhage • Respiratory and multiorgan failure	Focal areas of spindled lymphatic endothelial cells with abnormal lymphatics; similar to KHE but the spindle cell component is more dispersed and arranged in poorly defined clusters or anastomosing strands/sheets Mutation: NRAS (somatic)	First line, a combination of: Sirolimus Corticosteroids Vincristine *MEK inhibitor is a consideration in uncontrolled disease Bisphosphonates
CCLA[b]	• Enlarged lymphatic channels/cysts in abdomen and/or thorax • Reflux of lymphatic fluid → pleural and pericardial effusions, ascites, massive edema • Protein loss • Recurrent infections • Organ dysfunction	Dilated lymphatic channels-vessels are not malformed but are dysfunctional or distally obstructed Mutation: EPHB4 (germline, unknown if also somatic)	Surgical intervention is recommended, if possible Consider sirolimus *Consider MEK inhibitor

Abbreviations: CCLA, central conducting lymphatic anomalies; CLOVES, congenital lipomatous overgrowth, vascular malformations, epidermal nevi, scoliosis/skeletal/spinal anomalies; CSF, cerebrospinal fluid; DIC, disseminated intravascular coagulopathy; DOACs, direct-acting oral anticoagulants; GLA, generalized lymphatic anomaly; GSD, Gorham-Stout disease; KHE, kaposiform hemangioendothelioma; KLA, kaposiform lymphangiomatosis; NSAIDs, nonsteroidal anti-inflammatory drugs; RBCs, red blood cells; PIK3CA, phosphoinositide-3-kinase.

[a] KLA was recently classified by ISSVA as a vascular malformation but this remains controversial given its tumorlike features.

[b] CCLA is considered a channel-type lymphatic anomaly caused by lymphatic vessel dysfunction rather than congenital deformation/malformation.

* There are no clinical trials in vascular anomalies presently available using these medications.

KMP experienced partial response to sirolimus.[24] Other treatment options include resection of isolated small lesions, embolization of feeding vessels, and compression therapy when lymphedema is present.[17] Radiation therapy has also been reported to be effective to control KHE in refractory cases.

Consultation with a hematologist/oncologist is essential for KMP management. Platelet transfusions should only be given for active bleeding or immediately before or during surgery. Because of platelet trapping within the tumor, platelet transfusions have minimal effect on the platelet count and cause tumor engorgement, pain, and worsening of the underlying coagulopathy. The consensus panel recommends that patients with plasma fibrinogen levels <100 mg/dL receive fresh frozen plasma or cryoprecipitate; a higher threshold should be considered in the presence of bleeding.[23]

Even with successful therapy, KHE does not fully regress and continues to be visible on imaging and/or physical examination. Biopsy of residual lesions continues to show viable tumor.[25] Long-term issues with chronic pain, lymphedema, and/or orthopedic problems may persist despite tumor control.[26] Case series, predating recent therapeutic regimens, approximated a mortality of 10% to 37% for patients with KHE and KMP.[5,27]

COMPLICATED LYMPHATIC ANOMALIES

Comprising several diagnoses with overlapping symptoms, imaging features, and complications, complex lymphatic anomalies are associated with significant morbidity and include Gorham-Stout disease (GSD), generalized lymphatic anomaly, central collecting lymphatic anomaly, and kaposiform lymphangiomatosis. These malformations are caused by embryologic errors in lymphangiogenesis, resulting in malformed and dysfunctional lymphatic channels that most commonly occur in soft tissue but may involve bone and viscera. Impaired flow of lymphatic fluid can lead to lymphatic hypertension and reflux and cause significant complications, such as effusions and organ damage.[28]

Gorham-Stout Disease

GSD or vanishing bone disease was originally described in 1838 and was first characterized in 1955.[29,30] Documentation of progressive osteolysis with destruction of bone cortex is critical for diagnosis. MRI shows lytic lesions of the spine and axial skeleton, often in a contiguous pattern, with a T2-bright enhancing soft tissue component (if present). Histology reveals abnormal lymphatic channels of the bone with increased osteoclast activity and bone loss, presumably caused by increased osteoclast activity. Orthopedic stabilization of the spine may be indicated but consideration of active disease is also necessary, because lesion progression may result in destruction of adjacent bones and lead to instability of the hardware. Stabilization of disease has been reported with interferon and/or bisphosphonates.[31–33] The use of sirolimus with and without bisphosphonate therapy in GSD is currently being studied with early promising results.[34] A recently published retrospective study demonstrated radiographic stabilization or improvement of disease in all 5 patients with GSD. The majority of these individuals (80%) also experienced increased quality of life.[35]

Generalized Lymphatic Anomaly

Generalized lymphatic anomaly (GLA), although similar to GSD, is a distinctly different condition that also involves the bones, viscera, retroperitoneum, and mediastinum and is associated with effusions and organ compromise. In contrast with GSD, GLA favors the appendicular skeleton and typically involves multiple body sites in a noncontiguous or "skip lesion" pattern. Importantly, GLA bone lesions do not cause destruction of bone cortex.[29] Diagnosis of GLA can often be made with adequate radiographic imaging and a comprehensive physical examination. If biopsy is needed, histology shows bony changes along with the presence of abnormal lymphatic channels that stain positively for PROX-1 and D2-40. Notably, biopsy of rib lesions should not be performed in individuals with suspected or confirmed GLA because this may lead to refractory pleural effusions.[28] Management of GLA is supportive and guided by anatomic involvement and complications. Symptomatic pleural and pericardial effusions have historically been treated with surgical options such as drainage and pleurodesis, but recent advances in drug therapies are changing this treatment paradigm. Responses to sirolimus, as a single agent or in combination with bisphosphonates, have also been reported in individuals with GLA.[24,33] Five pathologic phosphoinositide-3-kinase (PIK3CA) mutations were recently reported in small case series of patients with GLA.[36] Recently, a retrospective study of 13 patients with GLA reported that 92% of the individuals treated with sirolimus experienced improvement in one aspect of disease including clinical/functional status, quality of life, and radiologic imaging. The affected patients also had improvement of pleural and pericardial effusions, 83% and 67% respectively.[35]

Central Conducting Lymphatic Anomaly

Central conducting lymphatic anomalies (CCLAs) are progressive disorders caused by dysfunction of the thoracic duct and/or cisterna chyli, a dilated sac of the lower thoracic duct that receives lymph from the intestinal and lumbar lymphatic trunks, with subsequent reflux and leakage of lymphatic fluid into the lungs, pleura, pericardium, peritoneum, bone, soft tissue, and other organs.[28] Pleural and pericardial effusions, ascites, and massive edema can lead to organ dysfunction, protein loss, and infections. Diagnosis requires lymphangiography, which shows enlargement of lymphatic channels (lymphangiectasia), lymphatic fluid reflux, and/or failure to empty into the thoracic duct or the subclavian vein at the thoracic duct outlet. Advanced radiologic techniques such as intranodal MRI and intranodal lymphangiography are available at certain centers for use in diagnostic imaging and treatment.[37] Treatment is largely supportive, although interventional and surgical procedures, such as ligation of refluxing channels or reimplantation of the thoracic duct or other structures, should be considered if appropriate expertise is available.[38] Medical therapies such as sirolimus have been used, but response remains unclear. Recently, Li and colleagues[39] identified a pathogenic EPHB4 variant in CCLA, which suggests that mammalian target of Rapamycin (mTOR) and mitogen-activated protein kinase (MAPK)/MEK inhibitors may be beneficial.

Kaposiform Lymphangiomatosis

Kaposiform lymphangiomatosis (KLA), a newly described entity, is an aggressive lymphatic anomaly that has features of both tumors and malformations. KLA most commonly involves the thoracic cavity, bone, and spleen and is associated with a life-threatening coagulopathy characterized by severe hypofibrinogenemia, thrombocytopenia, and bleeding complications. Disease progression is common, with hemorrhage and effusions causing the most significant morbidity. Imaging features and initial presentation are similar to GLA, and lymphatic channel dysfunction comparable with CCLA may also be present.[30,40] Histologic evaluation reveals focal areas of spindle cells with lymphatic disease similar to KHE but the spindle cell component is more dispersed and arranged in poorly defined clusters or anastomosing strands/sheets. Outcomes are poor, with a reported 5-year survival of 51%.[40] Current therapy is supportive with sirolimus, frequently in combination with steroids and/or vincristine.[17]

COMBINED HIGH-RISK VASCULAR MALFORMATIONS
Congenital Lipomatous Overgrowth, Vascular Malformations, Epidermal Nevi, Scoliosis/Skeletal/Spinal Anomalies Syndrome

CLOVES (congenital lipomatous overgrowth, vascular malformations, epidermal nevi, scoliosis/skeletal/spinal anomalies) syndrome[41–43] is a noninherited rare disorder, which was recently found to be associated with a somatic mutation of PIK3CA. Affected individuals may experience a wide array of complications, including recurrent infections, benign and malignant tumors, venous thromboembolism associated with ectatic veins, and limb and spinal abnormalities. Treatment with sirolimus has been beneficial in some patients, particularly in those with a lymphatic component.[24]

Klippel-Trénaunay Syndrome

Klippel-Trénaunay syndrome (KTS) is characterized by a capillary lymphatic venous malformation and variable overgrowth of soft tissue and bone. Somatic mutations of PIK3CA have also been identified in patient with KTS. Patients with this syndrome can have chronic debilitating pain, a coagulopathy with risk for bleeding and thrombosis, orthopedic issues, pulmonary hypertension, disfigurement, recurrent infections, and progressive disease. Sirolimus therapy has been reported to improve pain, function, coagulopathy, and quality of life[24,44,45]; benefits seem to be greatest in individuals with a significant lymphatic component.

Vascular Malformations with Low-Grade Intravascular Coagulopathy

Venous malformations or mixed venous malformations (slow-flow malformations) are associated with a low-grade intravascular coagulopathy (LIC). Individuals with extensive or multiple venous or combined venous malformations are at highest risk for LIC. The pathophysiology of this coagulopathy is poorly understood, but it is hypothesized that blood stagnation within the venous channels of the lesion induces activation of the coagulation cascade with subsequent consumption of circulating coagulation factors.[46,47] Patients with LIC have an increased risk of hematologic complications (ie, bleeding or thrombosis), particularly during or after major surgical or interventional procedures.[48] This coagulopathy can be aggravated secondary to trauma, puberty, infection, severe systemic illnesses, or vessel manipulation or aggravation with surgical or interventional procedures. Pain is also common secondary to superficial thrombosis and calcified phleboliths.

The basic laboratory tests for the evaluation of patients at risk include a complete blood count, blood smear, prothrombin time, activated partial thromboplastin time, fibrinogen, and D-dimer level. Patients with venous malformations associated with coagulopathy or venous ectasia and those undergoing major debulking surgery should be referred for hematology consultation. No established protocols are currently available to guide hematologic management of these patients. Depending on the location and morbidity caused by the lesions, sclerotherapy and/or surgical interventions may be considered. Medical treatment options include compression garments, anticoagulation, and sirolimus.

MEDICAL TREATMENT AND NEW DISCOVERIES

Over the past several years, both germline and somatic mutations have been discovered leading to correlation of phenotype and genotype in vascular anomalies (**Fig. 1**). Although the pathophysiology of these lesions is not well understood, these genetic discoveries have led to new therapeutic options for these patients and improved disease outcomes. The currently available disease-modifying medical treatment of

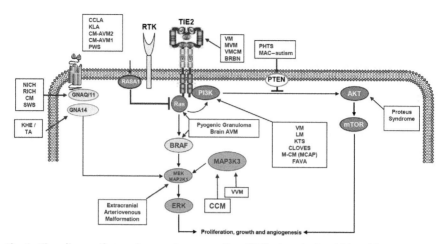

Fig. 1. Signaling pathways in vascular anomalies. PI3K, phosphoinositide-3-kinase.

complicated vascular anomalies as well as possible new therapeutic agents are discussed here.

Mammalian Target of Rapamycin Inhibitors: Sirolimus/Everolimus

Sirolimus (Rapamune) is a specific and potent inhibitor of mTOR, a serine/threonine kinase in the PI3K/AKT pathway that regulates numerous cellular processes, including cellular catabolism and anabolism, cell motility, angiogenesis, and cell growth.[49] Components of the PIK3CA/AKT/mTOR and RAS/MAPK/MEK pathways interact and regulate each other via cross-inhibition and cross-activation. Overactivation of the PI3K/AKT/mTOR or the RAS/MAPK/MEK pathway leads to dysregulation of normal cellular functions, resulting in cellular proliferation, survival advantage, and angiogenesis and is thought to be the driver for the development and/or progression of vascular anomalies.

Before its use in vascular anomalies, sirolimus was used to treat patients with tuberous sclerosis and lymphangioleiomyomatosis, both of which involve the PI3K/AKT pathway. Given its effectiveness in these conditions and the knowledge mutations in phophatase and tensin homolog gene (PTEN) and the angiopoeitin receptor, TIE-2, in certain vascular anomalies, sirolimus was first trialed for compassionate use in an infant with KHE/KMP in whom all traditional medical treatments had been exhausted. The patient had complete resolution of coagulopathy within 2 months of sirolimus treatment and the tumor decreased in size by 4 months.[50] This initial success prompted the prospective phase 2 clinical trial assessing the safety and efficacy of sirolimus in the treatment of complicated vascular anomalies, which showed efficacy and safety for 85% of all patients treated. Many of these patients experienced improvement in clinical symptoms and quality of life regardless of whether improvement was noted radiologically.[24] These encouraging results, along with identification of somatic PIK3CA mutations further supporting mTOR inhibition, have rapidly expanded the use of sirolimus in complicated vascular anomalies.[44,51-53]

Sirolimus has emerged as one of the first-line treatments for KHE with KMP. Several retrospective studies have reinforced the efficacy of sirolimus therapy, often initially in combination with steroids. Decreased pain, resolution of KMP and organ dysfunction, reduced tumor size, and improved quality of life and physical functioning have all been reported.[54-57] In the prospective phase 2 clinical trial, Adams and colleagues[24] reported 10 patients with KHE and KMP with 100% partial response. More specifically, hematologic parameters improved substantially with sirolimus. Three patients with KHE without KMP were also treated: 2 had partial response and 1 patient with multiple bone disease had progressive disease. A randomized phase 2 clinical trial for high-risk KHE comparing efficacy of vincristine-based with sirolimus-based treatment, both used in conjunction with corticosteroids in the initial treatment period, is currently open to enrollment (NCT02110069). Despite the apparent benefits of sirolimus, its therapeutic mechanism of action remains unknown in KHE. Everolimus, a derivative of sirolimus that more selectively inhibits mTORC1 with little impact on the mTORC2 complex, seems to be advantageous in treating KHE with KMP, but clinical studies are lacking.[58,59]

Sirolimus also seems to have some benefit in other benign vascular tumors, including hemangiomas, PTEN hamartomas, and fibroadipose vascular anomaly (FAVA). Multiple case studies and small series have reported that oral sirolimus is effective for infantile hemangiomas that are refractory to conventional therapies such as oral propranolol and systemic steroids.[60–62] A few case reports have published that individuals with PTEN hamartomas experience improved functioning and less pain with sirolimus therapy.[24,63–65] Rapid improvement of pain and quality of life with use of sirolimus has also been reported in 2 patients with FAVA.[66]

Although prospective clinical trials have been limited, numerous reports have been published on the efficacy of sirolimus treatment of macrocystic and microcystic lymphatic malformations as well as combined malformations with a lymphatic component.[44,51,67] Decreased size or volume of the malformation, reduced number of lymphatic blebs and malformation-associated infections, complete or partial alleviation of pain, and improvement in quality of life have all been reported with sirolimus use in individuals with lymphatic malformations. A recent systematic review, analyzing 20 published studies, reported that 60 of 71 patients with pure or combined lymphatic malformations receiving sirolimus therapy experienced partial remission of disease.[45] In complex lymphatic malformations, including GLA and GSD, sirolimus has been shown to stabilize or improve associated pleural/pericardial effusions, bony disease, pain, and mobility.[24,33,34,68]

Topical sirolimus is also showing promise as a useful treatment of the cutaneous manifestations of lymphatic malformations and seems to have minimal systemic absorption and side effects.[69–71] Based on the experience of several institutions, many patients experience decreased lymphatic leakage, bleeding, and number and size of blebs with the use of topical 1% sirolimus applied once or twice daily.

Somatic activating PIK3CA mutations within the affected tissue have been identified in pure lymphatic malformations as well as in combined malformations with a lymphatic component associated with overgrowth syndromes, including CLOVES syndrome, KTS, congenital infiltrating facial lipomatosis, and CLAPO (capillary malformation of the lower lip, lymphatic malformation of the face and neck, asymmetry of face and limbs, and partial or generalized overgrowth) syndrome.[72–75] Although sirolimus and everolimus are known to inhibit overactive PIK3CA signaling, the exact cellular mechanisms in which mTOR inhibitors are beneficial in treating lymphatic malformations have not been completely elucidated.

Sirolimus has also shown efficacy in the management of KLA as a single agent and as a combined regimen with steroids and/or vincristine. mTOR inhibition has been shown to stabilize or improve pleural/pericardial effusions, consumptive coagulopathy, and life-threatening hemorrhage in patients with KLA, although long-term follow-up is needed.[24,76,77]

Sirolimus seems to have an emerging role in the treatment of some complicated venous malformations, including blue rubber bleb nevus syndrome and pure venous malformations. Germline and somatic TIE2 mutations and somatic PIK3CA mutations are found in venous malformations, both of which are gain-of-function mutations that result in constitutive activation of the PIK3KA/AKT/mTOR pathway.[78–80] A recent study using targeted exome sequencing of cancer-associated genes in pure venous malformations also identified mutations in GNAQ, NF1, MAP2K1, MAP3K1, AKT2, AKT3, and IRS2 alone or in combination with TIE2 or PIK3CA mutations, all of which likely overactivate the PIK3CA/mTOR pathway.[79] In a pilot study of 10 patients with venous malformations refractory to standard treatments, patients treated with oral sirolimus experienced pain relief, functional improvement of the affected body part, improved self-perceived quality of life, improved coagulopathy, and reduction in size of the malformation.[80] In addition to stabilizing or reducing lesion size, sirolimus has also been reported to decrease anemia, coagulopathy, transfusion requirements, and pain in individuals with complex venous malformations.[81] Verrucous venous malformations (previously called verrucous hemangiomas), which harbor MAP3K3 mutations upstream of mTOR, were also shown to decrease in volume when treated with systemic sirolimus.[82] A prospective multicenter phase 3 trial (NCT02638389) is currently underway in Europe evaluating the efficacy of sirolimus in pediatric and adult patients with venous, lymphatic, or combined vascular malformations that are refractory to standard treatment.

The role of sirolimus in the treatment of capillary malformations is unclear at this time. Some small studies report that topical and oral sirolimus may enhance the efficacy of laser treatment of capillary malformations.[83] The benefit of systemic sirolimus is also unknown in the treatment of hereditary hemorrhagic telangiectasia (HHT), an inherited disease characterized by bleeding from mucocutaneous telangiectasia and/or visceral arteriovenous malformations (AVMs). Only 1 case report documents the resolution of telangiectasia of the skin, buccal mucosa, and upper gastrointestinal tract in a patient with HHT while on sirolimus therapy.[84]

Benefit of sirolimus in the treatment of extracranial AVMs has also not yet been determined. The phase 2 clinical trial assessing the safety and efficacy of sirolimus restricted inclusion of fast-flow lesions to those associated with PTEN.[24] In Europe, there currently is an open study investigating the efficacy of sirolimus in the treatment of extracranial AVMs in children and adults (NCT02042326).

Sirolimus is administered orally as a tablet or liquid suspension once or twice daily. In the phase 2 clinical trial, sirolimus was given at an initial dose of 0.8 mg/m^2 per dose every 12 hours and titrated to maintain a goal serum trough level of 10 to 15 ng/mL. This goal drug level was based on the use of sirolimus in pediatric renal transplant patients.[24] However, lower levels of sirolimus have been efficacious in patients with vascular anomalies so many providers now titrate the dose to desired effect with consideration of side effects. In general, low-dose/intermediate-dose sirolimus (levels <8 ng/mL) are used for symptomatic relief, whereas high-dose sirolimus (levels $\geq$ 8 ng/mL) are reserved for patients with severe coagulopathy, multiorgan failure, and/or life-threatening or aggressive lesions. Compared with older children and adults, clearance of sirolimus differs in neonates and young children; recommended starting sirolimus doses for infants and young children have recently been reported based on pharmacokinetics in this special population.[85] Side effects tend to be dose dependent and most commonly include mouth sores, gastrointestinal upset, headaches, bone marrow suppression, and metabolic/laboratory disturbances. Although data are limited, everolimus also seems to be efficacious in treating patients with vascular malformations and is a treatment option in those with intolerable side effects from sirolimus. Frequent physical examinations and laboratory bloodwork are necessary while on sirolimus therapy to ensure adequate drug levels and to monitor for toxicities. Because of immunosuppression, *Pneumocystis jiroveci* pneumonia prophylaxis is also recommended.[24] Sirolimus is contraindicated in pregnancy and should be discontinued at least 12 weeks before attempted conception.[86] There is also some evidence that sirolimus is associated with impaired spermatogenesis and thus men of child-bearing age should be informed of the risks associated with exposure to sirolimus.[87] Time to response varies among patients but maximal effect generally does not occur until months after achieving adequate doses. Length of treatment is not defined and must be determined on an individual basis.

RATIONALE FOR OTHER THERAPEUTIC AGENTS

Complicated vascular anomalies often cause disfigurement, chronic pain, and organ dysfunction with significant morbidity and mortality. Sirolimus has improved the outcomes for many of these patients but preliminary long-term follow-up data from the phase 2 sirolimus trial indicate the need for continuous use of medication in most patients. Furthermore, 12% and 15% of patients had progressive disease at 6 and 12 months respectively, and others have needed additional medical therapies after the end of the study.[24] It is imperative that other medical therapies are investigated or developed, based on phenotype/genotype correlation, for sirolimus nonresponders and for those diagnoses with highest morbidity or poor survival rates.

PIK3CA Inhibitors

In a recent article by Venot and colleagues[88] the PIK3CA inhibitor BYL719 was used for compassionate use to treat 19 patients with PIK3CA-related overgrowth syndrome (PROS)/CLOVES. The drug improved symptoms in all patients. Although these results are encouraging, this study was not prospective, and this drug is presently only available for compassionate use in complicated patients with PROS/CLOVES. This group also developed a mouse model with a similar phenotype to PROS/CLOVES. The mice treated with BYL719 not only had an overtly normal appearance but also had improved survival compared with those treated with placebo. BYL719 was also more efficacious at reducing tumor burden in the mice compared with sirolimus.

MEK Inhibitors

The RAS/MAPK/MEK signaling pathway has also been identified in patients with complicated vascular anomalies. Mutations in EPHB4, KRAS, HRAS, NRAS, BRAF, RAF1, PTPN11, and SOS1 have recently been reported in vascular anomalies, resulting in dysregulation of the RAS pathway. These mutations have been found in lymphedema syndromes, KHE, KLA, CCLA, and capillary malformation/AVM2.[38,89–91] A single somatic activating NRAS variant (c.182A>G, p.Q61R) was recently identified at low levels within affected tissue of individuals with KLA.[90] This NRAS mutation has also been identified in melanoma and other cancers and results in the constitutive activation of the RAS/MAPK/MEK signaling pathway, conferring a selective growth advantage. Somatic MAP2K1 mutations have also been reported in extracranial AVMs.[92] Protocols with MEK inhibitors, already in use in pediatric oncology, are currently in development to treat these complicated vascular anomalies with dysregulation of the RAS/MAPK signaling pathway.

SUMMARY

Patients with complicated vascular anomalies require an interdisciplinary treatment approach and hematologists/oncologists play a major role in their care. Clinical and scientific research, along with genomic discovery, has improved understanding of the clinical behavior, pathology, and molecular biology of vascular anomalies. Additional therapeutic options, based on genotype/phenotype correlation, are needed.

REFERENCES

1. Mulliken JB, Glowacki J. Hemangiomas and vascular malformations in infants and children: a classification base on endothelial characteristics. Plast Reconstr Surg 1982;69(3):412–22.
2. Wassef M, Blei F, Adams D, et al. Vascular anomalies classification: recommendations from the International Society for the Study of Vascular Anomalies. Pediatrics 2015;136(1):e203–14.
3. ISSVA Classification of vascular Anomalies © 2018 International Society for the Study of Vascular Anomalies. Available at: issva.org/classification. Accessed September 2, 2018.
4. Killion E, Mohan K, Lee EI. A review of vascular anomalies: genetics and common syndromes. Semin Plast Surg 2014;28(2):64–8.
5. Croteau SE, Liang MG, Kozakewich HP, et al. Kaposiform hemangioendothelioma: atypical features and risks of Kasabach-Merritt phenomenon in 107 referrals. J Pediatr 2013;162:142.
6. Lee B, Chiu M, Soriano T, et al. Adult-onset tufted angioma: a case report and review of the literature. Cutis 2006;78:341.
7. Kasabach H, Merritt K. Capillary hemangioma with extensive purpura: report of a case. Am J Dis Child 1940;59:1063–70.
8. Zukerberg LR, Nickoloff BJ, Weiss SW. Kaposiform hemangioendothelioma of infancy and childhood. An aggressive neoplasm associated with Kasabach-Merritt syndrome and lymphangiomatosis. Am J Surg Pathol 1993;17:321.
9. Sarkar M, Mulliken JB, Kozakewich HP, et al. Thrombocytopenic coagulopathy (Kasabach-Merritt phenomenon) is associated with Kaposiform hemangioendothelioma and not with common infantile hemangioma. Plast Reconstr Surg 1997;100(6):1377–86.
10. Enjolras O, Wassef M, Mazoyer E, et al. Infants with Kasabach-Merritt syndrome do not have "true" hemangiomas. J Pediatr 1997;130(4):631–40.
11. San Miguel FL, Spurbeck W, Budding C, et al. Kaposiform hemangioendothelioma: a rare cause of spontaneous hemothorax in infancy. Review of the literature. J Pediatr Surg 2008;43:e37–41.
12. Deraedt K, Vander Poorten V, Van Geet C, et al. Multifocal kaposiform haemangioendothelioma. Virchows Arch 2006;448:843–6.
13. Gianotti R, Gelmetti C, Alessi E. Congenital cutaneous multifocal kaposiform hemangioendothelioma. Am J Dermatopathol 1999;21:557–61.
14. Zhang HZ, Jiang ZM, Zhou J, et al. Primary intermediate hemangioendothelioma of bone: a study of 5 cases. Zhonghua Bing Li Xue Za Zhi 2012;41:39–43.
15. Veening MA, Verbeke JI, Witbreuk MM, et al. Kaposiform (spindle cell) hemangioendotelioma in a child with an unusual presentation. J Pediatr Hematol Oncol 2010;32:240–2.
16. Arai E, Kuramochi A, Tsuchida T, et al. Usefulness of D2-40 immunohistochemistry for differentiation between kaposiform hemangioendothelioma and tufted angioma. J Cutan Pathol 2006;33:492.
17. Adams DM, Brandão LR, Peterman CM, et al. Vascular anomaly cases for the pediatric hematologist oncologists-An interdisciplinary review. Pediatr Blood Cancer 2018;65(1). https://doi.org/10.1002/pbc.26716.
18. Jiang RS, Hu R. Successful treatment of Kasabach-Merritt syndrome arising from kaposiform hemangioendothelioma by systemic corticosteroid therapy and surgery. Int J Clin Oncol 2012;17:512.

19. Blei F, Karp N, Rofsky N, et al. Successful multimodal therapy for kaposiform he-mangioendothelioma complicated by Kasabach-Merritt phenomenon: case report and review of the literature. Pediatr Hematol Oncol 1998;15:295.
20. Michaud AP, Bauman NM, Burke DK, et al. Spastic diplegia and other motor dis-turbances in infants receiving interferon-alpha. Laryngoscope 2004;114:1231.
21. Chiu YE, Drolet BA, Blei F, et al. Variable response to propranolol treatment of ka-posiform hemangioendothelioma, tufted angioma, and Kasabach-Merritt phe-nomenon. Pediatr Blood Cancer 2012;59:934.
22. Blatt J, Stavas J, Moats-Staats B, et al. Treatment of childhood kaposiform he-mangioendothelioma with sirolimus. Pediatr Blood Cancer 2010;55:1396.
23. Drolet BA, Trenor CC 3rd, Brandão LR, et al. Consensus-derived practice stan-dards plan for complicated Kaposiform hemangioendothelioma. J Pediatr 2013;163:285.
24. Adams DM, Trenor CC 3rd, Hammill AM, et al. Efficacy and safety of sirolimus in the treatment of complicated vascular anomalies. Pediatrics 2016;137(2): e20153257.
25. Enjolras O, Mulliken JB, Wassef M, et al. Residual lesions after Kasabach-Merritt phenomenon in 41 patients. J Am Acad Dermatol 2000;42:225.
26. Schaefer BA, Wang D, Merrow AC, et al. Long-term outcome for kaposiform heman-gioendothelioma: a report of two cases. Pediatr Blood Cancer 2017;64(2):284–6.
27. Kelly M. Kasabach-Merritt phenomenon. Pediatr Clin North Am 2010;57(5): 1085–9.
28. Trenor CC 3rd, Chaudry G. Complex lymphatic anomalies. Semin Pediatr Surg 2014;23(4):186–90.
29. Lala D, Mulliken JB, Alomari AI, et al. Gorham-Stout disease and generalized lymphatic anomaly - clinical, radiologic, and histologic differentiation. Skeletal Radiol 2013;42(7):917–24.
30. Ozeki M, Fujino A, Matsuoka K, et al. Clinical features and prognosis of general-ized lymphatic anomaly, kaposiform lymphangiomatosis, and Gorham-Stout dis-ease. Pediatr Blood Cancer 2016;63(5):832–8.
31. Kose M, Pekcan S, Dogru D, et al. Gorham-Stout Syndrome with chylothorax: successful remission by interferon alpha-2b. Pediatr Pulmonol 2009;44(6):613–5.
32. Kuriyama DK, McElligott SC, Glaser DW, et al. Treatment of Gorham-Stout dis-ease with zoledronic acid and interferon-alpha: a case report and literature re-view. J Pediatr Hematol Oncol 2010;32(8):579–84.
33. Venkatramani R, Ma NS, Pitukcheewanont P, et al. Gorham's disease and diffuse lymphangiomatosis in children and adolescents. Pediatr Blood Cancer 2011; 56(4):667–70.
34. Cramer SL, Wei S, Merrow AC, et al. Gorham-Stout disease successfully treated with sirolimus and zoledronic acid therapy. J Pediatr Hematol Oncol 2016;38(3): e129–32.
35. Ricci KW, Hammill AM, Mobberley-Schuman P, et al. Efficacy of syndtemic siro-limus in the treatment of generalized lymphatic anomaly and Gorham-Stout dis-ease. Pediatr Blood Cancer 2019;66(5):e27614.
36. Laguna LR, Agra N, Trujillo G, et al. Generalized lymphatic anomaly is caused by somatic activating PIK3CA mutations. Abstract presented at: Biannual Meeting of International Society for the Study of Vascular Anomalies. Amsterdam, Netherlands, May 29 – June 1, 2018.
37. Krishnamurthy R, Hernandez A, Kavuk S, et al. Imaging the central conducting lymphatics: initial experience with dynamic MR lymphangiography. Radiology 2015;274(3):871–8.

38. Taghinia AH, Upton J, Trenor CC 3rd, et al. Lymphaticovenous bypass of the thoracic duct for the treatment of chylous leak in central conducting lymphatic anomalies. J Pediatr Surg 2019;54(3):562–8.
39. Li D, Wenger TL, Seiler C, et al. Pathogenic variant in EPHB4 results in central conducting lymphatic anomaly. Hum Mol Genet 2018;27(18):3233–45.
40. Croteau SE, Kozakewich HP, Perez-Atayde AR, et al. Kaposiform lymphangiomatosis: a distinct aggressive lymphatic anomaly. J Pediatr 2014;164(2):383–8.
41. Peterman CM, Fevurly RD, Alomari AI, et al. Sonographic screening for Wilms tumor in children with CLOVES syndrome. Pediatr Blood Cancer 2017;64(12). https://doi.org/10.1002/pbc.26684.
42. Reis J 3rd, Alomari AI, Trenor CC 3rd, et al. Pulmonary thromboembolic events in patients with congenital lipomatous overgrowth, vascular malformations, epidermal nevi, and spinal/skeletal abnormalities and Klippel-Trénaunay syndrome. J Vasc Surg Venous Lymphat Disord 2018;6(4):511–6.
43. Uller W, Fishman SJ, Alomari AI. Overgrowth syndromes with complex vascular anomalies. Semin Pediatr Surg 2014;23(4):208–15.
44. Vlahovic AM, Vlahovic NS, Haxhija EQ. Sirolimus for the treatment of a massive capillary-lymphatico-venous malformation: a case report. Pediatrics 2015; 136(2):e513–6.
45. Wiegand S, Wichmann G, Dietz A. Treatment of lymphatic malformations with the mTOR inhibitor sirolimus: a systematic review. Lymphat Res Biol 2018;16(4): 330–9.
46. Enjolras O, Ciabrini D, Mazoyer E, et al. Extensive pure venous malformations in the upper or lower limb: a review of 27 cases. J Am Acad Dermatol 1997;36: 219–25.
47. Mazoyer E, Enjolras O, Laurian C, et al. Coagulation abnormalities associated with extensive venous malformations of the limbs: differentiation from Kasabach-Merritt syndrome. Clin Lab Haematol 2002;24(4):243–51.
48. Mason KP, Neufeld EJ, Karian VE, et al. Coagulation abnormalities in pediatric and adult patients after sclerotherapy or embolization of vascular anomalies. Am J Roentgenol 2001;177:1359–63.
49. Huber S, Bruns CJ, Schmid G, et al. Inhibition of the mammalian target of rapamycin impedes lymphangiogenesis. Kidney Int 2007;71(8):771–7.
50. Hammill AM, Wentzel M, Gupta A, et al. Sirolimus for the treatment of complicated vascular anomalies in children. Pediatr Blood Cancer 2011;57(6):1018–24.
51. Akyuz C, Atas E, Varan A. Treatment of a tongue lymphangioma with sirolimus after failure of surgical resection and propranolol. Pediatr Blood Cancer 2014;61: 931–2.
52. Triana P, Dore M, Cerezo VN, et al. Sirolimus in the treatment of vascular anomalies. Eur J Pediatr Surg 2017;27(1):86–90.
53. Iacobas I, Simon ML, Amir T, et al. Decreased vascularization of retroperitoneal kaposiform hemangioendothelioma induced by treatment with sirolimus explains relief of symptoms. Clin Imaging 2015;39(3):529–32.
54. Wang Z, Li K, Dong K, et al. Successful treatment of Kasabach-Merritt phenomenon arising from kaposiform hemangioendothelioma by sirolimus. J Pediatr Hematol Oncol 2015;37(1):72–3.
55. Lackner H, Karastaneva A, Schwinger W, et al. Sirolimus for the treatment of children with various complicated vascular anomalies. Eur J Pediatr 2015;174(12): 1579–84.
56. Oza VS, Mamlouk MD, Hess CP, et al. Role of sirolimus in advanced kaposiform hemangioendothelioma. Pediatr Dermatol 2016;33(2):e88–92.

57. Lim YH, Bacchiocchi A, Qiu J, et al. GNA14 somatic mutation causes congenital and sporadic vascular tumors by MAPK activation. Am J Hum Genet 2016;99(2): 443–50.
58. Uno T, Ito S, Nakazawa A, et al. Successful treatment of kaposiform hemangioendothelioma with everolimus. Pediatr Blood Cancer 2015;62(3):536–8.
59. Matsumoto H, Ozeki M, Hori T, et al. Successful everolimus treatment of kaposiform hemangioendothelioma with Kasabach-Merritt phenomenon: clinical efficacy and adverse effects of mTOR inhibitor therapy. J Pediatr Hematol Oncol 2016;38(8):e322–5.
60. Hutchins KK, Ross RD, Kobayashi D, et al. Treatment of refractory infantile hemangiomas and pulmonary hypertension with sirolimus in a pediatric patient. J Pediatr Hematol Oncol 2017;39(7):e391–3.
61. Warren D, Diaz L, Levy M. Diffuse hepatic hemangiomas successfully treated using sirolimus and high-dose propranolol. Pediatr Dermatol 2017;34(5):e286–7.
62. Kaylani S, Theos AJ, Pressey JG. Treatment of infantile hemangiomas with sirolimus in a patient with PHACE syndrome. Pediatr Dermatol 2013;30(6):e194–7.
63. Marsh DJ, Trahair TN, Martin JL, et al. Rapamycin treatment for a child with germline PTEN mutation. Nat Clin Pract Oncol 2008;5:357–61.
64. Schmid GL, Kässner F, Uhlig HH, et al. Sirolimus treatment of severe PTEN hamartoma tumor syndrome: case report and in vitro studies. Pediatr Res 2014; 75(4):527–34.
65. Iacobas I, Burrows PE, Adams DM, et al. Oral rapamycin in the treatment of patients with hamartoma syndromes and PTEN mutation. Pediatr Blood Cancer 2011;57(2):321–3.
66. Erickson J, McAuliffe W, Blennerhassett L, et al. Fibroadipose vascular anomaly treated with sirolimus: successful outcome in two patients. Pediatr Dermatol 2017;34(6):e317–20.
67. Kim D, Benjamin L, Wysong A, et al. Treatment of complex periorbital venolymphatic malformation in a neonate with a combination therapy of sirolimus and prednisolone. Dermatol Ther 2015;28(4):218–22.
68. Dvorakova V, Rea D, O'Regan GM, et al. Generalized lymphatic anomaly successfully treated with long-term, low-dose sirolimus. Pediatr Dermatol 2018; 35(4):533–4.
69. Ivars M, Redondo P. Efficacy of topical sirolimus (rapamycin) for the treatment of microcystic lymphatic malformations. JAMA Dermatol 2017;153(1):103–5.
70. García-Montero P, Del Boz J, Sanchez-Martínez M, et al. Microcystic lymphatic malformation successfully treated with topical rapamycin. Pediatrics 2017; 139(5) [pii:e20162105].
71. Le Sage S, David M, Dubois J, et al. Efficacy and absorption of topical sirolimus for the treatment of vascular anomalies in children: a case series. Pediatr Dermatol 2018;35(4):472–7.
72. Nathan N, Keppler-Noreuil KM, Biesecker LG, et al. Mosaic disorders of the PI3K/PTEN/AKT/TSC/mTORC1 signaling pathway. Dermatol Clin 2017;35(1):51–60.
73. Kurek KC, Luks VL, Ayturk UM, et al. Somatic mosaic activating mutations in PIK3CA cause CLOVES syndrome. Am J Hum Genet 2012;90:1108–15.
74. Downey C, López-Gutiérrez JC, Roé-Crespo E, et al. Lower lip capillary malformation associated with lymphatic malformation without overgrowth: part of the spectrum of CLAPO syndrome. Pediatr Dermatol 2018;35(4):e243–4.
75. Keppler-Noreuil KM, Parker VE, Darling TN, et al. Somatic overgrowth disorders of the PI3K/AKT/mTOR pathway & therapeutic strategies. Am J Med Genet C Semin Med Genet 2016;172(4):402–21.

76. Fernandes VM, Fargo JH, Saini S, et al. Kaposiform lymphangiomatosis: unifying features of a heterogeneous disorder. Pediatr Blood Cancer 2015;62(5):901–4.
77. Safi F, Gupta A, Adams D, et al. Kaposiform lymphangiomatosis, a newly characterized vascular anomaly presenting with hemoptysis in an adult woman. Ann Am Thorac Soc 2014;11(1):92–5.
78. Vikkula M, Boon LM, Carraway KL, et al. Vascular dysmorphogenesis caused by an activating mutation in the receptor tyrosine kinase TIE2. Cell 1996;87:1181–90.
79. Nätynki M, Kangas J, Miinalainen I, et al. Common and specific effects of TIE2 mutations causing venous malformations. Hum Mol Genet 2015;24:6374–89.
80. Boscolo E, Limaye N, Huang L, et al. Rapamycin improves TIE2-mutated venous malformation in murine model and human subjects. J Clin Invest 2015;125: 3491–504.
81. Salloum R, Fox CE, Alvarez-Allende CR, et al. Response of blue rubber bleb nevus syndrome to sirolimus treatment. Pediatr Blood Cancer 2016;63(11): 1911–4.
82. Zhang G, Chen H, Zhen Z, et al. Sirolimus for treatment of verrucous venous malformation: a retrospective cohort study. J Am Acad Dermatol 2019;80(2):556–8.
83. Marqués L, Núñez-Córdoba JM, Aguado L, et al. Topical rapamycin combined with pulsed dye laser in the treatment of capillary vascular malformations in Sturge-Weber syndrome: phase II, randomized, double-blind, intraindividual placebo-controlled clinical trial. J Am Acad Dermatol 2015;72(1):151–8.
84. Skaro AI, Marotta PJ, McAlister VC. Regression of cutaneous and gastrointestinal telangiectasia with sirolimus and aspirin in a patient with hereditary hemorrhagic telangiectasia. Ann Intern Med 2006;144:226.
85. Mizuno T, Fukuda T, Emoto C, et al. Developmental pharmacokinetics of sirolimus: implications for precision dosing in neonates and infants with complicated vascular anomalies. Pediatr Blood Cancer 2017;64:e26470.
86. EBPG Expert Group on Renal Transplantation. European best practice guidelines for renal transplantation. Section IV: long-term management of the transplant recipient. IV.10. Pregnancy in renal transplant recipients. Nephrol Dial Transplant 2002;17(Suppl 4):50.
87. Zuber J, Anglicheau D, Elie C, et al. Sirolimus may reduce fertility in male renal transplant recipients. Am J Transplant 2008;8(7):1471–9.
88. Venot Q, Blanc T, Rabia SH, et al. Targeted therapy in patients with PIK3CA-related overgrowth syndrome. Nature 2018;558(7711):540–6.
89. Manevitz-Mendelson E, Leichner GS, Barel O, et al. Somatic NRAS mutation in patient with generalized lymphatic anomaly. Angiogenesis 2018;21(2):287–98.
90. Amyere M, Revencu N, Helaers R, et al. Germline loss-of-function mutations in EPHB4 cause a second form of capillary malformation-arteriovenous malformation (CM-AVM) deregulating RAS-MAPK signaling. Circulation 2017;136(11): 1037–48.
91. Barclay SF, Inman KW, Luks VL, et al. A somatic activating NRAS variant associated with kaposiform lymphangiomatosis. Genet Med 2018. [Epub ahead of print].
92. Couto JA, Huang AY, Konczyk DJ, et al. Somatic MAP2K1 Mutations are associated with extracranial arteriovenous malformation. Am J Hum Genet 2017;100(3): 546–54.

Inherited Platelet Disorders

A Modern Approach to Evaluation and Treatment

Michele P. Lambert, MD, MSTR[a,b,c],*

KEYWORDS

- Inherited platelet disorders • Inherited thrombocytopenia • Macrothrombocytopenia
- Familial platelet disorders • Storage pool deficiency • Platelet function disorders

KEY POINTS

- Inherited platelet disorders, although individually rare, together account for a significant proportion of inherited mild bleeding disorders.
- Inherited platelet disorders are associated with variable bleeding ranging from mild or no bleeding to severe, life-threatening hemorrhage.
- Inherited platelet disorders may have variable thrombocytopenia, but if most platelets on the peripheral blood smear are macrothrombocytes, the diagnosis is likely to be an inherited platelet disorder.
- Next-generation sequencing has significantly expanded the spectrum of the phenotypes associated with many platelet disorders.

INTRODUCTION

Epistaxis and bruising are common complaints in pediatrics. Up to 9% of children have epistaxis[1] and 12% of infants in the general pediatric population (age 6–12 months) demonstrate bruising on examination.[2] Although epistaxis in children with bleeding disorders is difficult to differentiate from epistaxis in the healthy pediatric population based on history,[1] bruising is increased in children with bleeding disorders and occurs in even premobile infants.[3] Petechiae, the canonical platelet disorder

Disclosure Statement: Consultancy: Amgen, Kedrion, Bayer, CSL Behring, Novartis, Shionogi, and Sysmex. Research Funding: AstraZeneca. Off-Label use: TPO-receptor agonists for congenital thrombocytopenia.

[a] Department of Pediatrics, Perelman School of Medicine at the University of Pennsylvania, Philadelphia, PA, USA; [b] Special Coagulation Laboratory, The Children's Hospital of Philadelphia, Philadelphia, PA, USA; [c] Frontier Program in Immune Dysregulation, Division of Hematology, The Children's Hospital of Philadelphia, Philadelphia, PA, USA
* Division of Hematology, The Children's Hospital of Philadelphia, 3615 Civic Center Boulevard, Abramson Research Building, Room 316G, Philadelphia, PA 19104.
E-mail address: lambertm@email.chop.edu

cutaneous manifestation, can occur in healthy children, especially in infancy (10%–27% of infants <12 month old can have a few petechiae[4,5]) but may also be a symptom of a platelet-based bleeding disorder. Differentiating the children who have normal symptoms from those with a true bleeding diathesis is not always easy because many children have not had any significant hemostatic challenges. Additional mucosal bleeding symptoms of oral bleeding, bleeding with tooth extraction or exfoliation, gastrointestinal bleeding, dysfunctional uterine bleeding (either heavy or prolonged) or hematuria, all suggest a more significant bleeding disorder.[6] Intracranial hemorrhage and hemarthrosis can occur rarely with platelet-type bleeding as a result of platelet dysfunction or thrombocytopenia.

In addition, isolated thrombocytopenia is also a common hematologic problem, although in this case, a patient at any age is far more likely to have an acquired form of thrombocytopenia as a result of autoimmune disease[7,8], increased platelet consumption, bone marrow suppression, or bone marrow failure. Previous studies suggested that less than 5% of patients presenting with a chief complaint of thrombocytopenia have an inherited disorder; however, this has recently been challenged by several groups, and a recent French study looking at adult patients with chronic thrombocytopenia suggested that up to 40% of patients may have inherited thrombocytopenia.[9] Important clues to inherited thrombocytopenia are its chronicity/duration of symptoms and a positive family history of thrombocytopenia.[10,11] In children with suspected immune thrombocytopenia (ITP), failure to respond to typical ITP therapy is associated with increased probability of diagnosis of an inherited platelet disorder (IPD).

The diagnostic tools available to identify and categorize the IPDs have improved over the past few years with additional modalities offering more information to clinicians about patients with suspected IPDs. More importantly, with the advent of next-generation sequencing (NGS), the phenotypes of some of the characteristic disorders have been expanded, and molecular understanding of the causes of IPDs has significantly improved allowing better anticipatory guidance to families and better characterization of diseases. This article covers the current guidelines on the diagnostic approach to IPD and suggests ways in which novel testing in development may be able to streamline diagnosis and provide better information to families, potentially decreasing costs overall in terms of time and diagnostics.

THE CLASSICAL DIAGNOSTIC APPROACH

In 2015, the scientific subcommittee on platelet physiology of the International Society of Thrombosis and Haemostasis released guidelines for the diagnosis of IPD.[12] Using this approach, history and physical examination are the key features of the evaluation, followed by evaluation of platelet count and morphology, followed by evaluation of platelet function by light transmission aggregometry (LTA), and then evaluation by a panel of tests to assess granule contents and platelet surface markers (**Fig. 1**). With this methodology, patients with a history of abnormal bleeding have a normal or nondiagnostic platelet evaluation in 60% to 70% of evaluations.[13,14] In addition, prior studies have suggested that the degree of in vitro platelet dysfunction correlates poorly with severity of bleeding[13,14] and guidelines vary on recommendations for next steps after LTA in suspected platelet disorders regardless of whether that testing is normal or abnormal. For example, several studies have suggested that patients with dense granule deficiencies can have normal LTA.[15,16]

Since the publication of the International Society of Thrombosis and Haemostasis guidelines, NGS has greatly expanded the molecular repertoire of the IPD in terms

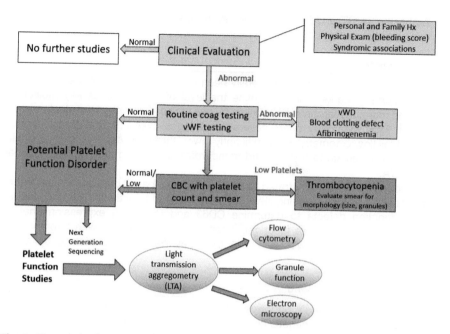

Fig. 1. Diagnostic algorithm flowchart. CBC, complete blood count; vWD, von Willebrand disease; vWF, von Willebrand factor. (*Modified from* Gresele P, Subcommittee on Platelet Physiology of the International Society on Thrombosis and Hemostasis. Diagnosis of inherited platelet function disorders: guidance from the SSC of the ISTH. J Thromb Haemost 2015;13(2):315; with permission.)

of the number of defined disorders (there are now approximately 51 recognized platelet disorder genes.[17] In addition to the discovery of novel platelet disorders, NGS has expanded phenotypes for many of the better known platelet disorders and allowed for deeper characterization of some of the IPDs, and for recognition of the association of thrombocytopenia or platelet dysfunction with other disorders not previously known to have these issues. As NGS has become more common, especially in some more developed countries, it has moved earlier in the diagnostic algorithm.

UPDATED DIAGNOSTIC TOOLS

Classically, platelet dysfunction has been evaluated by the use of LTA. This testing, initially described by Born in 1962,[18] is the current gold standard for the diagnosis of platelet dysfunction in vitro. By measuring the amount of light that is transmitted through platelet-rich plasma, LTA captures platelet ability to aggregate in response to various agonists at multiple concentrations. This testing is, however, time consuming; user dependent; and, despite considerable efforts by international committees, poorly standardized.[19–21] In addition, the volume of blood required makes testing difficult in small patients and is limited in patients with thrombocytopenia.[22] Whole blood impedance aggregometry, an alternative method of measuring platelet aggregation, requires significantly lower blood volumes, but is still limited by thrombocytopenia.[23] Both of these tools, however, are generally sufficient to diagnose significant platelet dysfunction and the characteristic platelet disorders of Glanzmann thrombasthenia (GT) and Bernard-Soulier syndrome (BSS), which present with distinctive aggregation patterns.

Flow Cytometry

Previously, flow cytometry has generally been used to demonstrate the presence of platelet surface markers and to define the level of expression of key molecules. More and more, researchers are refining the use of flow cytometry to evaluate platelet function. Flow cytometry offers several advantages over LTA: the blood volumes required for flow cytometry are significantly lower, thrombocytopenia is not a significant barrier to accurate testing, and standardization is no more complicated than that of LTA.

Studies have now demonstrated that flow cytometry–based platelet function testing corresponds well with bleeding severity,[24] can be used in patients with documented platelet function defects to determine CD63 and P-selectin expression (thereby measuring δ and α granule function),[25] can be used in patients with thrombocytopenia,[24] and correlates well with LTA (but may be better at picking up subtle abnormalities).[24]

Next-Generation Sequencing

Genetic testing was rarely performed in the IPDs when only individual tests were available because of the genetic heterogeneity of this group of disorders, which often preclude the selection of individual genes for testing based on laboratory and clinical phenotype alone. However, since the advent of NGS, the scale and cost-effectiveness of available genetic testing has vastly improved and has resulted in significant advances in the understanding of these disorders.[26] These advances allow for molecular diagnosis in approximately 40% to 50% of patients with IPDs. Difficulties now center not only on understanding which genes are important in platelet disorders (although most clinical tests only report variants in genes that are clearly associated with the platelet disorders), but on the interpretation of pathologic variants. **Table 1** lists some of the most common platelet disorders and their associated genes.

Multiplex and Automated or Semiautomated Platelet Function Testing

Several assays aimed at developing a high throughput, automated platelet function test, ideally allowing remote analysis of fixed, activated platelets are emerging[27] with the development of reagents to fix platelets for shipping, and assays on 96-well plates that allow for greater standardization and streamline platelet function testing. All of these assays are in research development for the detection of platelet function defects and their use to date has primarily been in the detection of antiplatelet effects of various medications. PFA-100, however, which has been widely used to screen for platelet function disorders, has poor ability to screen for mild platelet function defects and in general performs no better than bleeding time,[28] which has been discarded as a screening tool for the mild platelet function defects. In a review compiling data from approximately 300 patients with platelet function defects compared with 700 control subjects,[28] PFA-100 performed well for detection of severe platelet function defects, especially BSS, but in primary secretion defects and storage pool defects only 50% of patients had an abnormal closure time with epinephrine (C/Epi) and only 25% with ADP (C/ADP). With Hermansky-Pudlak syndrome (HPS), a phenotypically distinct platelet disorder, 80% of patients had an abnormal C/ADP closure time but only 50% of patients had abnormal C/Epi closure time.[28]

Table 1
Genes associated with inherited platelet disorders

Inherited Condition	Gene (Location)	Inheritance	Key Features
Microthrombocytic			
Wiskott-Aldrich syndrome	*WAS* (Xp11)	X-linked	Thrombocytopenia, eczema, severe immunodeficiency, small platelets
X-linked thrombocytopenia	*WAS* (Xp11-exon2)	X-linked	Small platelets, thrombocytopenia, mild immunodeficiency
FYB-related thrombocytopenia	*FYB* (5p13.1)	AR	Small platelets and mild to moderate bleeding
ARCP1B-related thrombocytopenia	*ARCP1B* (7q22.1)	AR	Microthrombocytopenia, eosinophilia, inflammatory disease
Normothrombocytic			
Congenital amegakaryocytic thrombocytopenia	*MPL* (1p34)	AR	Hypomegakaryocytic thrombocytopenia with eventual development of bone marrow failure
Thrombocytopenia with absent radii	*RBM8A* (1q21.1)	AR	Thrombocytopenia that improves with age, limb anomalies (but normal thumbs)
Radioulnar synostosis with amegakaryocytic thrombocytopenia	*HOXA11* (7p15), *MECOM* (3q26.2)	AD	Severe thrombocytopenia that improves with age, skeletal abnormalities (radioulnar synostosis, clinodactyly, syndactyly, hip dysplasia), hearing loss
Familial platelet disorder with predisposition to AML	*RUNX1* (21q22)	AD	Thrombocytopenia, myelodysplasia or even AML, platelet dysfunction
Paris-Trousseau/Jacobsen syndrome	*FLI1* (11p24.3)	AR	Thrombocytopenia with large granules and depending on size of deletion if deleted other symptoms arising from deletion of other genes
Familial thrombocytopenia 2 (THC2)	*ANKRD26* (10p12.1)	AD	Mild to moderate thrombocytopenia with mild bleeding symptoms, cancer predisposition with risk of myeloid malignancy and MDS
ETV6-related thrombocytopenia (THC5)	*ETV6* (12p13.2)	AD	Mild to moderate thrombocytopenia, increased risk of hematologic malignancy including ALL, AML, and MDS

(continued on next page)

Table 1
(continued)

Inherited Condition	Gene (Location)	Inheritance	Key Features
Monoallelic THPO mutation	*THPO* (3q27.1)	AD	Minimal to no bleeding with low platelet count
CYCS-related thrombocytopenia	*CYCS* (7p15)	AD	Thrombocytopenia without significant bleeding caused by abnormal platelet release
SLFN14-related thrombocytopenia	*SLFN14* (17q12)	AD	Variable platelet size (sometimes large) with mild to severe bleeding and impaired platelet function
Stormorken syndrome/ York platelet syndrome	*STIM1* (11p15) or *ORAI1* (12q24.31)	AD	Tubular aggregate myopathy and platelet disorder with decreased α granules, thrombocytopenia and abnormal function and mild to moderate bleeding
Macrothrombocytopenic			
Bernard-Soulier syndrome	*GPIBA* (17p13), *GPIBB* (22q11), *GPIX* (3q21)	AR, AD	Platelet dysfunction with large platelets
Velocardiofacial syndrome (22qDS)	22q11	AD	Cardiac anomalies, cleft palate, hypocalcemia, thymic aplasia, and typical facies; BSS-like thrombocytopenia ± autoimmune
Platelet-type von Willebrand disease	*GPIBA* (17p13)	AD	Decreased high-molecular-weight vWF multimers with thrombocytopenia because of increased platelet affinity for vWF
MYH9-related disease (MYH9-RD)	*MYH9* (22q11.2)	AD	Large platelets, leukocyte inclusions; may have sensorineural hearing loss, cataracts, glomerulonephritis, or renal failure
Gray platelet syndrome	*NBEAL2* (3p21)	AD, AR	Large, pale platelets with absence of α granules
GATA-1 mutation of X-linked thrombocytopenia with thalassemia	*GATA1* (Xp11.23)	X-linked	Thrombocytopenia with variable anemia
TUBB1-related thrombocytopenia	*TUBB1* (20q13.32)	AD	Spherocytic platelets and decreased cardiovascular disease in males

(continued on next page)

Table 1
(continued)

Inherited Condition	Gene (Location)	Inheritance	Key Features
Macrothrombocytopenia with filamin A mutations	FLNA (Xq28)	X-linked	Abnormal granule distribution on EM, mild to moderate thrombocytopenia, impaired aggregation to collagen
GFI1b-related thrombocytopenia	GFI1b (9q24)	AD	Moderate to severe bleeding with gray platelet–like phenotype with absent α granules and variable red cell anisocytosis
TRPM7-related thrombocytopenia	TRPM7 (15q21.2)	AD	Large platelets with aberrant granule distribution and mild bleeding
ACTN1-related thrombocytopenia	ACTN1 (14q24)	AD	Large platelets with absent to mild bleeding
PRKACG-related thrombocytopenia	PRKACG (9q21)	AR	Large platelets with aberrant FLNA expression and impaired function
TPM4-related thrombocytopenia	TPM4 (19p13.1)	AD	Large platelets with mild bleeding
DIAPH1-related thrombocytopenia	DIAPH1 (5q31.3)	AD	Sensorineural hearing loss, large platelets
SRC-related thrombocytopenia	SRC (20q11.23)	AD	Moderate to severe bleeding with hypogranular platelets and impaired platelet function and juvenile-onset myelofibrosis, osteoporosis
ITGA2B/ITGB3-related thrombocytopenia	ITGA2B (17q21) or ITGB3 (17q21)	AD	Moderate bleeding, large platelets, and abnormal function with gain of function variants

Abbreviations: AD, autosomal dominant; ALL, acute lymphoblastic leukemia; AML, acute myeloid leukemia; AR, autosomal recessive; EM, electron microscope; MDS, myelodysplastic syndrome; vWF, von Willebrand factor.

EXPANDING CLINICAL PHENOTYPES
Hereditary Thrombocytopenias

Hereditary thrombocytopenic syndromes are not as rare as once assumed. It is critical that treating physicians maintain a high index of suspicion for these disorders, because patients are often misdiagnosed as having ITP.[29] In about 50% of affected families, at least one family member has had a splenectomy to treat "ITP." Although the literature suggests that approximately 40% of families with inherited thrombocytopenia do not have an identifiable gene defect, this is a rapidly evolving area and most of the novel platelet disorders that have been discovered by NGS have been in the inherited thrombocytopenias.[30]

Thrombocytopenia with Large Platelets

Many inherited thrombocytopenias involve defects in platelet production, with preserved megakaryopoiesis. Impedance-based automated cell counters often underestimate the platelet count because the large particles may be mistaken for red blood cells or even leukocytes, although this may be largely corrected with flow cytometric measurement of platelet count.[31] Although platelet size may be increased in ITP or myeloproliferative neoplasms, a blood smear with a predominance of macrothrombocytes (>60%) suggests a macrothrombocytopenia.[32] The macrothrombocytopenias result generally from defective platelet release and therefore many are caused by variants in genes in the cytoskeleton or cytoskeleton-cell membrane interactions, certain transcription factors, or in the assembly of platelet granules.

The most common of the macrothrombocytopenias, MYH9-related thrombocytopenia, is an autosomal-dominant macrothrombocytopenia that formerly consisted of the May-Hegglin anomaly, Fechtner syndrome, Sebastian syndrome, and Epstein syndromes. All of these are caused by variants in the *MYH9* gene, which codes for nonmuscle myosin IIA. In addition to macrothrombocytopenia, the peripheral blood film may demonstrate Döhle body–like inclusions in neutrophils (which are best detected by immunofluorescence). Associated clinical features including hearing loss, cataracts, and renal failure are present in some patients. Bleeding symptoms are mild to moderate because platelet function is nearly normal apart from a reduction in platelet cytoskeleton contraction with resulting reduced clot stability. About 30% of patients have a de novo mutation and therefore a negative family history. Other macrothrombocytopenias generally also result from variants in genes that affect platelet cytoskeleton genes or membrane-cytoskeleton interactions. Therefore, large platelets are also found in a kindred of patients with von Willebrand disease type IIB (V1316M variant, Montreal platelet syndrome)[33] and in both monoallelic[34,35] and biallelic BSS,[36] which is characterized by the decreased expression of the platelet GPIb-IX complex by flow cytometry, lack of platelet agglutination with high-dose ristocetin, and bleeding. NGS sequencing has demonstrated that inheritance of rare variants in GP1BB in an autosomal-dominant fashion results in macrothrombocytopenia in healthy populations.[34] Furthermore, variants in the platelet cytoskeleton proteins β tubulin (*TUBB1*),[37,38] filamin (*FLNA*),[39] α actinin (*ACTN1*),[40] tropomyosin 4 (*TPM4*),[41] and *DIAPH1*, a member of the formin family, which regulates microtubule assembly, all result in macrothrombocytopenia. DIAPH1 variants are also associated with sensorineural hearing loss.[42,43] Although most often cytoskeletal defects resulting in macrothrombocytopenia are associated with mild to moderate bleeding, more severe bleeding disorders are seen in biallelic BSS and *PRKACG*-related thrombocytopenia.[44] Finally, NGS has identified a subgroup of patients with mild bleeding diathesis and autosomal-dominant macrothrombocytopenia that have specific variants, generally activating mutations, in *ITGA2B/ITGB3* (which cause GT when inherited in an autosomal-recessive form).[45] In addition, altering the platelet membrane, by altering the platelet membrane sterol content as occurs in sitosterolemia, results in macrothrombocytopenia with hemolytic anemia and xanthomas. Patients generally present with elevated plasma sterol levels, stomatocytosis with variable evidence of hemolysis (which can be very mild), and macrothrombocytopenia (which varies with the amount of sitosterolemia) making the diagnosis sometimes difficult. Variants in *ABCG5* and *ABCG8* have been associated with this autosomal-recessive disease that is easily overlooked.[46]

A few hereditary macrothrombocytopenias also occur in association with mutations in specific transcription factors that regulate megakaryocyte and platelet production, including GATA1 (X-linked inheritance, dyserythropoiesis)[47] and FLI-1 (discussed later). Patients with the Paris-Trousseau/Jacobsen syndrome, an autosomal-dominant macrothrombocytopenia, have psychomotor retardation and facial and cardiac abnormalities. This syndrome arises because of deletion of a portion of chromosome 11 (11q23 to 24) that encompasses the gene encoding the transcription factor friend leukemia integration 1 (FLI-1).[48] Autosomal-recessive inheritance of variants in this gene alone reproduce the Paris-Trousseau platelet phenotype without the associated cardiac and developmental abnormalities.[49]

Gray platelet syndrome (deficiency of α granules) results from variants in the NBEAL2 gene (recessive trait) and generally causes a macrothrombocytopenia. Variants in GFI1b have been shown to cause a platelet defect that is similar to gray platelet syndrome with loss of platelet granules and variable alterations in platelet function, which is inherited in an autosomal-dominant fashion.[50] A dominant, gain-of-function variant in SRC causes a juvenile myelofibrosis-associated with a macrothrombocytopenia.[51] Both NBEAL2, inherited in an autosomal-recessive fashion, and SRC, inherited in an autosomal-dominant fashion, have been associated with macrothrombocytopenia and development of myelofibrosis so that patients who present with these symptoms should be tested because identification of variants can have implications for family members.

Thrombocytopenia with Normal-Sized Platelets

The disorders that cause thrombocytopenia with normal-sized platelets are generally disorders that affect megakaryocyte development and platelet development resulting in abnormalities of megakaryocytes and/or stem cells resulting in low platelets. These disorders, therefore, are associated with increased risk of cancer or bone marrow failure, or with skeletal abnormalities caused by abnormalities of the bone marrow milieu and megakaryocyte/osteocyte interactions.

There are currently three autosomal-dominant, inherited thrombocytopenias with associated increased risk of myeloid malignancy: RUNX1 (with variable platelet dysfunction and therefore variable bleeding), ETV6 (mild to no bleeding), and 5'UTR variants in ANKRD26 (mild to no bleeding).[52–54] The risk of malignancy with these disorders is increased but highly variable even within a particular family so genetic counseling and close follow-up are important.[55] Importantly, with RUNX1 defects, the thrombocytopenia is not fully penetrant; therefore, genetic screening should include even those family members with normal platelet counts.

The inherited thrombocytopenias associated with increased risk of bone marrow failure are also generally associated with normal platelet size: congenital amegakaryocytic thrombocytopenia, thrombocytopenia–absent radius syndrome, and radioulnar synostosis with amegakaryocytic thrombocytopenia. Congenital amegakaryocytic thrombocytopenia, a recessive disorder because of mutations in the c-Mpl receptor, is characterized by severe thrombocytopenia, absence of megakaryocytes in the bone marrow, and a risk of trilineage failure. Thrombocytopenia–absent radius syndrome is inherited in a compound fashion with most patients coinheriting a microdeletion of 1q21 encompassing the RBM8A gene and one of two polymorphisms on the other chromosome in RBM8A associated with decreased expression. Radioulnar synostosis with amegakaryocytic thrombocytopenia results from autosomal-dominant inheritance of HOXA11 variants[56] or autosomal-recessive variants in MECOM.[57] The autosomal-recessive form is associated with an increased risk of bone marrow failure and myelodysplastic syndrome.

Thrombocytopenia with Small Platelets

The quintessential small platelet disorder is Wiskott-Aldrich syndrome (WAS), an X-linked disorder characterized by severe immunodeficiency, small platelets, and eczema (discussed later). However, two additional autosomal-recessive disorders with small platelets have been recently described: *FYB*-related thrombocytopenia with isolated small platelets and thrombocytopenia[58–60]; and a rare disorder of inflammation, eosinophilia, and microthrombocytopenia caused by variants in *ARPC1B*.[61]

Disorders of Platelet Function

Disorders of platelet function are characterized by variable mucocutaneous bleeding manifestations and excessive hemorrhage following surgical procedures or trauma. Platelet counts in these disorders are variable. Spontaneous hemarthrosis and deep hematomas are unusual in patients with platelet defects. Intracranial hemorrhage is also rare. Most patients have mild or moderate bleeding; the disorders that cause severe bleeding generally occur as a result of autosomal-recessive inheritance of rare variants. Platelet aggregation and secretion studies provide evidence for the defect, but generally are not predictive of the severity of clinical manifestations.[13]

Despite advances in understanding the molecular biology of platelet disorders, in most patients with inherited abnormalities of platelet function, the molecular defect remains unknown, suggesting that some of these disorders may be the result of coinheritance of multiple hypofunctional variants. Platelet function defects are broken into several categories based on the primary defect encountered in the platelet: adhesion (defects in platelet–vessel wall interactions), aggregation (defects in platelet-platelet interactions), and platelet secretion and signal transduction (a heterogenous group of disorders put together more for convenience than for any underlying similarity in pathobiology).

Disorders of Platelet Adhesion

Bernard-Soulier syndrome

BSS, is classically a rare, autosomal-recessive bleeding disorder that results from an abnormality in the platelet GPIb-IX complex, which mediates the binding of von Willebrand factor to platelets and thus plays a major role in platelet adhesion to the subendothelium, especially at high shear rates. GPIb-IX exists in platelets as a complex consisting of GPIb, GPIX, and GPV, and is reduced or abnormal in BSS. NGS studies and other recent literature has expanded the phenotype to include monoallelic and biallelic forms of BSS depending on the variants inherited and the effect on platelet function and GPIb-IX expression.[36] The platelet count is moderately decreased, and platelets are markedly increased in size on the peripheral smear. Typically, platelet aggregation studies demonstrate normal responses to ADP, epinephrine, thrombin, and collagen but response to ristocetin is decreased or absent. The diagnosis of BSS is established by demonstrating decreased platelet surface GPIb-IX, which is demonstrated using flow cytometry. The most severe phenotype is associated with the biallelic form of BSS where variants are inherited from both parents resulting in markedly reduced expression and/or function of the GPIb/IX complex. Monoallelic forms also have been described with a less severe phenotype, decreased expression of GPIb/IX, and variable response to ristocetin on platelet function testing.

Disorders of Platelet Aggregation

Glanzmann thrombasthenia

GT is a rare autosomal-recessive disorder characterized by markedly impaired platelet aggregation and severe mucocutaneous bleeding manifestations, especially in comparison with other platelet function disorders. GT results from a quantitative or qualitative defect in the integrin αIIb or β3 complex, a heterodimer consisting of αIIb and β3 whose synthesis is governed by distinct genes located on chromosome 17 (*ITGB3* and *IT2AB*). Thus, GT may arise because of compound heterozygous variants. Because fibrinogen plays a critical role in platelet aggregation that is mediated through interaction of αIIb-β3 and fibrinogen, patients with GT have an abnormal LTA to all agonists (except ristocetin) and significantly impaired platelet function in vivo. Expression of αIIb-β3 on the platelet surface is decreased by flow cytometry in patients with variants that affect expression (quantitative variants, which are most common). Parents of patients who carry pathologic variants have approximately 50% expression (heterozygous expression).

A subgroup of disorders of the αIIb-β3 complex are inherited dominantly and result in macrothrombocytopenia. The underlying cause is a mutation in the transmembrane or intracellular part of the integrin, which results in permanent activation of the αIIb-β3 complex and affects membrane-cytoskeleton interactions.[45,62] These variants have been described in *ITGA2B* and *ITGB3* and generally result in a milder bleeding phenotype but significant platelet anisocytosis with macrothrombocytopenia.

Finally, defects in genes downstream of the integrin complex in *FERMT3*[63,64] and *RASGRP2*[65–67] result in Glanzmann-like platelet function defects with severe bleeding phenotype and markedly abnormal platelet responses by LTA but only mild or moderate decrease in expression of αIIb-β3 on the surface of platelets. Patients with the *RASGRP2* variants seem to require higher than normal platelet transfusion volumes to control bleeding, perhaps because of a proposed dominant-negative effect of circulating variant platelets that inhibit platelet aggregation in native clot formation.[68]

Disorders of Platelet Secretion and Signal Transduction

As a unifying theme, patients with these disorders generally demonstrate impaired dense granule secretion and the absence of a second wave of aggregation on stimulation of platelet-rich plasma with ADP or epinephrine; responses to collagen, thromboxane analogue (U46619), and arachidonic acid also may be impaired. The platelet defects result from abnormal platelet granule contents (storage pool deficiency [SPD]) or impaired function of the mechanisms mediating or potentiating aggregation and secretion. These patients are generally the hardest to identify by conventional platelet function assays and to definitively establish whether or not a true bleeding diathesis exists. Likely, these patients exist on a continuum between normal and abnormal that does not have a strict demarcation making differentiation between "normal" and "abnormal" difficult. Inheritance in these disorders, unless associated with the syndromic platelet disorders with SPD, is likely to be mediated in part by multigenic coinheritance of several factors that determine bleeding tendency.

Defects of granule biogenesis

Many of the defects of granule biogenesis result in a common phenotype called SPD. SPD refers to deficiency in platelet content of dense granules (δ-SPD), α granules (α-SPD), or both types of granules ($\alpha\delta$-SPD). Often, the platelet phenotype in these disorders is part of a broader syndromic disease and is recognized by the other systemic manifestations.

Patients with δ-SPD have a mild to moderate bleeding diathesis. In platelet studies, the second wave of aggregation in response to ADP and epinephrine is absent or blunted, and the collagen response is markedly impaired. Normal platelets possess three to eight dense granules (each 200–300 nm in diameter). Under the electron microscope (EM), dense granules are decreased in δ-SPD platelets. By direct biochemical measurements, the total platelet and granule ATP and ADP contents are decreased along with other dense granule constituents including calcium, pyrophosphate, and serotonin. Most confusingly, conventional platelet function studies (LTA and chemiluminescence release assays) are variable in patients with documented abnormalities on EM and determining which correlates best with bleeding scores has been difficult.[16] Classically, δ-SPD is associated with syndromic forms of platelet disorders, HPS, Chédiak-Higashi syndrome, and Griscelli syndrome, but the most common form is actually isolated δ-SPD.

There are at least nine known HPS-causing genes, with most patients having HPS-1 and being from Puerto Rico where HPS affects 1 of every 1800 individuals. HPS is autosomal-recessive and heterozygotes have no clinical findings. In addition to oculocutaneous albinism, many patients have congenital nystagmus and decreased visual acuity; however, the albinism is not always severe or obvious without specialized eye examination. Two additional manifestations associated with certain HPS subtypes are granulomatous colitis and pulmonary fibrosis. With NGS, the phenotype for some HPS variants is expanding and now also includes neutropenia and immunodeficiency.[69]

Patients with gray platelet syndrome have an isolated deficiency of platelet α-granule contents and therefore appear gray on a peripheral blood smear (losing the typical purple staining of granules). These patients have a mild to moderate bleeding diathesis and mild macrothrombocytopenia. The inheritance pattern is variable; autosomal-recessive, autosomal-dominant, and X-linked patterns have been described. Classical gray platelet syndrome (autosomal-recessive) is caused by variants in the *NBEAL2* gene. The autosomal-dominant form is associated with variants in *GFI1b* and is associated in some patients with red cell anisocytosis, whereas the X-linked form has been associated with variants in *GATA1*. Finally, in patients with arthrogryposis-renal dysfunction-cholestasis syndrome, caused by variants in *VPS33B* or *VIPAS39*, there is low α-granule content and platelet dysfunction in a setting of fairly severe systemic disease that is often lethal in early childhood. In all of these disorders, under the EM, platelets and megakaryocytes reveal absent or markedly decreased α-granules. Platelet aggregation responses are variable. Responses to ADP and epinephrine are normal in most patients; in some patients, aggregation responses to thrombin, collagen, and ADP are impaired. Flow cytometry demonstrated decreased P-selectin expression, which typically translocates to platelet surface membranes from α-granules on activation.

Defects in platelet signal transduction and platelet activation

Signal transduction mechanisms encompass processes that are initiated by the interaction of agonists with specific platelet receptors and include such responses as G-protein activation and activation of phospholipase C and phospholipase A_2.

TREATMENT OF INHERITED PLATELET FUNCTION DEFECTS

Because of the wide disparity in bleeding manifestations, management needs to be individualized. Unfortunately, despite significant advances in the diagnosis of IPDs, little progress has been made so far in targeted therapies for specific platelet disorders, although there is hope on the horizon as gene therapy has been successfully used in small cohorts of patients with WAS.

The most important principal for management of patients with IPDs is education of patients and caregivers. Prevention is the best method of management for primary hemostasis, therefore dental hygiene, avoidance of high-risk activities, and appropriate early intervention especially for epistaxis are important.

Platelet transfusions are indicated in the management of significant bleeding and in preparation for surgical procedures. Platelet transfusions are effective in controlling bleeding manifestations but come with potential risks associated with blood products, including alloimmunization in patients lacking platelet GPs. For example, patients with GT and BSS may develop alloantibodies against GPIIb-IIIa and GPIb, respectively, which compromise the efficacy of subsequent platelet transfusions. To minimize the risk of alloimmunization, transfusions in these patients should be leukocyte depleted and, if possible, HLA-matched. Alloimmunization rates have been significantly reduced by leukocyte reduction, but may still be 10% to 25% in patients with GT and BSS. This may be particularly problematic in women of reproductive age because allosensitization may result in neonatal alloimmune thrombocytopenia after transplacental transfer (Siddiq 2011). An alternative to platelet transfusions is administration of desmopressin (DDAVP), which shortens the bleeding time in some patients with platelet function defects, depending on the platelet abnormality. Most patients with GT do not show a shortening of the bleeding time following DDAVP infusion, whereas responses in patients with signaling or secretory defects are variable. Recombinant factor VIIa has been approved for the management of bleeding events in patients with GT and has been used in some other inherited defects. Antifibrinolytic therapies, such as tranexamic acid or aminocaproic acid, are useful adjuncts to treatment or, for some patients, are used as monotherapy, depending on the platelet defect and amount of bleeding. Hormonal contraceptives and/or antifibrinolytic therapy are often effective for management of menorrhagia. Some other mucosal bleeding may respond to intranasal DDAVP or antifibrinolytic agents.

Bone marrow transplant is being used increasingly in the most severe platelet disorders, such as WAS and GT. Successful gene therapy trials in WAS suggest this may also be an option in some of these disorders. Thrombopoietin receptor agonists have been used to increase platelet counts in the congenital thrombocytopenias, particularly those associated with no or minimal platelet dysfunction, and may be used especially around procedures to increase platelet counts and allow for surgical interventions. A basic therapeutic principle in all patients with platelet disorders is to prevent iron-deficiency anemia. Red blood cells are required for sufficient hemostasis. Iron-deficiency anemia is common in this population, especially in women of childbearing age. Oral iron supplementation may be insufficient to normalize iron stores, and intravenous iron therapy may be required.

SUMMARY

Diagnosis of IPD is still a complex task requiring coordinated testing, which may not be available at all centers, and high level of clinical suspicion in patients presenting with isolated thrombocytopenia or mucocutaneous bleeding. The diagnostic tools available to aid in diagnosis are improving and the next decade will likely provide more insight into platelet function and biogenesis. With improved understanding, there will be a future opportunity for the development of targeted therapy to improve the bleeding symptoms in these patients.

REFERENCES

1. McGarry GW. Recurrent epistaxis in children. BMJ Clin Evid 2013;2013:0311.
2. Carpenter RF. The prevalence and distribution of bruising in babies. Arch Dis Child 1999;80(4):363–6.

3. Collins PW, Hamilton M, Dunstan FD, et al. Patterns of bruising in preschool children with inherited bleeding disorders: a longitudinal study. Arch Dis Child 2017; 102(12):1110–7.

4. Downes AJ, Crossland DS, Mellon AF. Prevalence and distribution of petechiae in well babies. Arch Dis Child 2002;86(4):291–2.

5. Soheilifar J, Ahmadi M, Ahmadi M, et al. Prevalence and location of petechial spots in well infants. Arch Dis Child 2010;95(7):518–20.

6. Nava T, Rivard GE, Bonnefoy A. Challenges on the diagnostic approach of inherited platelet function disorders: is a paradigm change necessary? Platelets 2018;29(2):148–55.

7. Zeller B, Rajantie J, Hedlund-Treutiger I, et al. Childhood idiopathic thrombocytopenic purpura in the Nordic countries: epidemiology and predictors of chronic disease. Acta Paediatr 2005;94(2):178–84.

8. Sutor AH, Harms A, Kaufmehl K. Acute immune thrombocytopenia (ITP) in childhood: retrospective and prospective survey in Germany. Semin Thromb Hemost 2001;27(3):253–67.

9. Fiore M, Pillois X, Lorrain S, et al. A diagnostic approach that may help to discriminate inherited thrombocytopenia from chronic immune thrombocytopenia in adult patients. Platelets 2016;27(6):555–62.

10. Lambert MP. What to do when you suspect an inherited platelet disorder. Hematol Am Soc Hematol Educ Program 2011;2011:377–83.

11. Drachman JG. Inherited thrombocytopenia: when a low platelet count does not mean ITP. Blood 2004;103(2):390–8.

12. Gresele P, Subcommittee on Platelet Physiology of the International Society on Thrombosis and Hemostasis. Diagnosis of inherited platelet function disorders: guidance from the SSC of the ISTH. J Thromb Haemost 2015;13(2):314–22.

13. Quiroga T, Goycoolea M, Panes O, et al. High prevalence of bleeders of unknown cause among patients with inherited mucocutaneous bleeding. A prospective study of 280 patients and 299 controls. Haematologica 2007;92(3):357–65.

14. Hayward CP, Pai M, Liu Y, et al. Diagnostic utility of light transmission platelet aggregometry: results from a prospective study of individuals referred for bleeding disorder assessments. J Thromb Haemost 2009;7(4):676–84.

15. Woods GM, Kudron EL, Davis K, et al. Light transmission aggregometry does not correlate with the severity of delta-granule platelet storage pool deficiency. J Pediatr Hematol Oncol 2016;38(7):525–8.

16. Brunet JG, Iyer JK, Badin MS, et al. Electron microscopy examination of platelet whole mount preparations to quantitate platelet dense granule numbers: implications for diagnosing suspected platelet function disorders due to dense granule deficiency. Int J Lab Hematol 2018;40(4):400–7.

17. Siddiq S, Clark A, Mumford A. Haemophilia. A systematic review of the management and outcomes of pregnancy in Glanzmann thrombasthenia. Available at: http://thrombo.cambridgednadiagnosis.org.uk/gene-disorder-list/. Accessed October 1, 2018.

18. Born GV. Aggregation of blood platelets by adenosine diphosphate and its reversal. Nature 1962;194:927–9.

19. Cattaneo M, Cerletti C, Harrison P, et al. Recommendations for the standardization of light transmission aggregometry: a consensus of the working party from the platelet physiology subcommittee of SSC/ISTH. J Thromb Haemost 2013. [Epub ahead of print].

20. Cattaneo M, Hayward CP, Moffat KA, et al. Results of a worldwide survey on the assessment of platelet function by light transmission aggregometry: a report from

the platelet physiology subcommittee of the SSC of the ISTH. J Thromb Haemost 2009;7(6):1029.

21. Hayward CP, Moffat KA, Raby A, et al. Development of North American consensus guidelines for medical laboratories that perform and interpret platelet function testing using light transmission aggregometry. Am J Clin Pathol 2010; 134(6):955–63.

22. Hayward CP, Moffat KA, Pai M, et al. An evaluation of methods for determining reference intervals for light transmission platelet aggregation tests on samples with normal or reduced platelet counts. Thromb Haemost 2008;100(1):134–45.

23. Stissing T, Dridi NP, Ostrowski SR, et al. The influence of low platelet count on whole blood aggregometry assessed by multiplate. Clin Appl Thromb Hemost 2011;17(6):E211–7.

24. van Asten I, Schutgens REG, Baaij M, et al. Validation of flow cytometric analysis of platelet function in patients with a suspected platelet function defect. J Thromb Haemost 2018;16(4):689–98.

25. Rand ML, Reddy EC, Israels SJ. Laboratory diagnosis of inherited platelet function disorders. Transfus Apher Sci 2018;57(4):485–93.

26. Heremans J, Freson K. High-throughput sequencing for diagnosing platelet disorders: lessons learned from exploring the causes of bleeding disorders. Int J Lab Hematol 2018;40(Suppl 1):89–96.

27. Dovlatova N, May JA, Fox SC. Remote platelet function testing: significant progress towards widespread testing in clinical practice. Platelets 2015;26(5): 399–401.

28. Favaloro EJ. Clinical utility of the PFA-100. Semin Thromb Hemost 2008;34(8): 709–33.

29. Arnold DM, Nazy I, Clare R, et al. Misdiagnosis of primary immune thrombocytopenia and frequency of bleeding: lessons from the McMaster ITP Registry. Blood Adv 2017;1(25):2414–20.

30. Noris P, Pecci A. Hereditary thrombocytopenias: a growing list of disorders. Hematol Am Soc Hematol Educ Program 2017;2017(1):385–99.

31. Briggs C. Quality counts: new parameters in blood cell counting. Int J Lab Hematol 2009;31(3):277–97.

32. Fixter K, Rabbolini DJ, Valecha B, et al. Mean platelet diameter measurements to classify inherited thrombocytopenias. Int J Lab Hematol 2018;40(2):187–95.

33. Jackson SC, Sinclair GD, Cloutier S, et al. The Montreal platelet syndrome kindred has type 2B von Willebrand disease with the VWF V1316M mutation. Blood 2009;113(14):3348–51.

34. Sivapalaratnam S, Westbury SK, Stephens JC, et al. Rare variants in GP1BB are responsible for autosomal dominant macrothrombocytopenia. Blood 2017; 129(4):520–4.

35. Ali S, Shetty S, Ghosh K. A novel mutation in GP1BA gene leads to mono-allelic Bernard Soulier syndrome form of macrothrombocytopenia. Blood Coagul Fibrinolysis 2017;28(1):94–5.

36. Savoia A, Kunishima S, De Rocco D, et al. Spectrum of the mutations in Bernard-Soulier syndrome. Hum Mutat 2014;35(9):1033–45.

37. Kunishima S, Kobayashi R, Itoh TJ, et al. Mutation of the beta1-tubulin gene associated with congenital macrothrombocytopenia affecting microtubule assembly. Blood 2009;113(2):458–61.

38. Kunishima S, Nishimura S, Suzuki H, et al. TUBB1 mutation disrupting microtubule assembly impairs proplatelet formation and results in congenital macrothrombocytopenia. Eur J Haematol 2014;92(4):276–82.

39. Nurden P, Debili N, Coupry I, et al. Thrombocytopenia resulting from mutations in filamin A can be expressed as an isolated syndrome. Blood 2011;118(22): 5928–37.

40. Westbury SK, Shoemark DK, Mumford AD. ACTN1 variants associated with thrombocytopenia. Platelets 2017;28(6):625–7.

41. Pleines I, Woods J, Chappaz S, et al. Mutations in tropomyosin 4 underlie a rare form of human macrothrombocytopenia. J Clin Invest 2017;127(3):814–29.

42. Neuhaus C, Lang-Roth R, Zimmermann U, et al. Extension of the clinical and molecular phenotype of DIAPH1-associated autosomal dominant hearing loss (DFNA1). Clin Genet 2017;91(6):892–901.

43. Stritt S, Nurden P, Turro E, et al. A gain-of-function variant in DIAPH1 causes dominant macrothrombocytopenia and hearing loss. Blood 2016;127(23): 2903–14.

44. Manchev VT, Hilpert M, Berrou E, et al. A new form of macrothrombocytopenia induced by a germ-line mutation in the PRKACG gene. Blood 2014;124(16): 2554–63.

45. Nurden AT, Pillois X, Fiore M, et al. Glanzmann thrombasthenia-like syndromes associated with macrothrombocytopenias and mutations in the genes encoding the alphaIIbbeta3 integrin. Semin Thromb Hemost 2011;37(6):698–706.

46. Yoo EG. Sitosterolemia: a review and update of pathophysiology, clinical spectrum, diagnosis, and management. Ann Pediatr Endocrinol Metab 2016;21(1): 7–14.

47. Chou ST, Kacena MA, Weiss MJ, et al. GATA1-related X-linked cytopenia. In: Adam MP, Ardinger HH, Pagon RA, et al, editors. GeneReviews((R)). 1993. Seattle (WA).

48. Favier R, Akshoomoff N, Mattson S, et al. Jacobsen syndrome: advances in our knowledge of phenotype and genotype. Am J Med Genet C Semin Med Genet 2015;169(3):239–50.

49. Shivdasani RA. Lonely in Paris: when one gene copy isn't enough. J Clin Invest 2004;114(1):17–9.

50. Kitamura K, Okuno Y, Yoshida K, et al. Functional characterization of a novel GFI1B mutation causing congenital macrothrombocytopenia. J Thromb Haemost 2016;14(7):1462–9.

51. Turro E, Greene D, Wijgaerts A, et al. A dominant gain-of-function mutation in universal tyrosine kinase SRC causes thrombocytopenia, myelofibrosis, bleeding, and bone pathologies. Sci Transl Med 2016;8(328):328ra330.

52. Perez Botero J, Dugan SN, Anderson MW. ANKRD26-related thrombocytopenia. In: Adam MP, Ardinger HH, Pagon RA, et al, editors. GeneReviews((R)). 1993. Seattle (WA).

53. Feurstein S, Godley LA. Germline ETV6 mutations and predisposition to hematological malignancies. Int J Hematol 2017;106(2):189–95.

54. Schlegelberger B, Heller PG. RUNX1 deficiency (familial platelet disorder with predisposition to myeloid leukemia, FPDMM). Semin Hematol 2017;54(2):75–80.

55. Babushok DV, Bessler M, Olson TS. Genetic predisposition to myelodysplastic syndrome and acute myeloid leukemia in children and young adults. Leuk Lymphoma 2016;57(3):520–36.

56. Thompson AA, Woodruff K, Feig SA, et al. Congenital thrombocytopenia and radio-ulnar synostosis: a new familial syndrome. Br J Haematol 2001;113(4): 866–70.

57. Niihori T, Ouchi-Uchiyama M, Sasahara Y, et al. Mutations in MECOM, encoding oncoprotein EVI1, cause radioulnar synostosis with amegakaryocytic thrombocytopenia. Am J Hum Genet 2015;97(6):848–54.

58. Spindler M, van Eeuwijk JMM, Schurr Y, et al. ADAP deficiency impairs megakaryocyte polarization with ectopic proplatelet release and causes microthrombocytopenia. Blood 2018;132(6):635–46.

59. Hamamy H, Makrythanasis P, Al-Allawi N, et al. Recessive thrombocytopenia likely due to a homozygous pathogenic variant in the FYB gene: case report. BMC Med Genet 2014;15:135.

60. Levin C, Koren A, Pretorius E, et al. Deleterious mutation in the FYB gene is associated with congenital autosomal recessive small-platelet thrombocytopenia. J Thromb Haemost 2015;13(7):1285–92.

61. Kahr WH, Pluthero FG, Elkadri A, et al. Loss of the Arp2/3 complex component ARPC1B causes platelet abnormalities and predisposes to inflammatory disease. Nat Commun 2017;8:14816.

62. Kashiwagi H, Kunishima S, Kiyomizu K, et al. Demonstration of novel gain-of-function mutations of alphaIIbbeta3: association with macrothrombocytopenia and Glanzmann thrombasthenia-like phenotype. Mol Genet Genomic Med 2013;1(2):77–86.

63. Robert P, Canault M, Farnarier C, et al. A novel leukocyte adhesion deficiency III variant: kindlin-3 deficiency results in integrin- and nonintegrin-related defects in different steps of leukocyte adhesion. J Immunol 2011;186(9):5273–83.

64. Kuijpers TW, van de Vijver E, Weterman MA, et al. LAD-1/variant syndrome is caused by mutations in FERMT3. Blood 2009;113(19):4740–6.

65. Westbury SK, Canault M, Greene D, et al. Expanded repertoire of RASGRP2 variants responsible for platelet dysfunction and severe bleeding. Blood 2017; 130(8):1026–30.

66. Lozano ML, Cook A, Bastida JM, et al. Novel mutations in RASGRP2, which encodes CalDAG-GEFI, abrogate Rap1 activation, causing platelet dysfunction. Blood 2016;128(9):1282–9.

67. Sevivas T, Bastida JM, Paul DS, et al. Identification of two novel mutations in RASGRP2 affecting platelet CalDAG-GEFI expression and function in patients with bleeding diathesis. Platelets 2018;29(2):192–5.

68. Piatt R, Paul DS, Lee RH, et al. Mice expressing low levels of CalDAG-GEFI exhibit markedly impaired platelet activation with minor impact on hemostasis. Arterioscler Thromb Vasc Biol 2016;36(9):1838–46.

69. Loredana Asztalos M, Schafernak KT, Gray J, et al. Hermansky-Pudlak syndrome: Report of two patients with updated genetic classification and management recommendations. Pediatr Dermatol 2017;34(6):638–46.

Primary and Secondary Immune Cytopenias
Evaluation and Treatment Approach in Children

Taylor Olmsted Kim, MD[a],*, Jenny M. Despotovic, DO[b]

KEYWORDS

- Autoimmune cytopenias • Thrombocytopenia • ITP • Hemolytic anemia • AIHA

KEY POINTS

- The autoimmune cytopenias include autoimmune hemolytic anemia, immune thrombocytopenia, autoimmune neutropenia, and multilineage conditions in Evans syndrome.
- Autoimmune cytopenias are heterogeneous disorders that may be primary or secondary to infection, malignancy, immunodeficiency, or rheumatologic conditions.
- Treatment selection is based on provider experience and typically involves broad immune suppression. As the understanding of the molecular cause of the autoimmune cytopenias improves, therapies may become more targeted.

INTRODUCTION

Autoimmune cytopenias include autoimmune hemolytic anemia (AIHA), immune thrombocytopenia (ITP), and autoimmune neutropenia (AIN), as well as rarer multilineage disorders. This heterogeneous group of disorders can be challenging to diagnose and treat, as treatments typically involve nonspecific immune suppression. As understanding of the molecular and genetic underpinnings of the autoimmune cytopenias grows, therapies in the future will likely evolve to become more targeted. This review of the autoimmune cytopenias focuses on evaluation and current treatment recommendations for AIHA and ITP.

AUTOIMMUNE HEMOLYTIC ANEMIA

The AIHAs are a spectrum of disorders characterized by autoantibodies directed against endogenous erythrocyte antigens, leading to premature red cell destruction.

Disclosure Statement: The authors have no disclosures to declare.
[a] Pediatric Hematology/Oncology, Baylor College of Medicine, Texas Children's Cancer and Hematology Center, 1102 Bates Avenue, Suite 1025.06, Houston, TX 77030, USA; [b] Pediatric Hematology/Oncology, Baylor College of Medicine, Texas Children's Cancer and Hematology Center, 6701 Fannin Street, Suite 1580, Houston, TX 77070, USA
* Corresponding author.
E-mail address: teolmste@txch.org

Hematol Oncol Clin N Am 33 (2019) 489–506
https://doi.org/10.1016/j.hoc.2019.01.005
0889-8588/19/© 2019 Elsevier Inc. All rights reserved.

hemonc.theclinics.com

These rare disorders affect approximately 0.2 per 10^5 children annually.[1] AIHA is classified by optimal autoantibody binding temperature and reactivity. Warm AIHA (W-AIHA) is the most common subtype affecting children, accounting for approximately 90% of pediatric cases.[2] Cold AIHA (C-AIHA), mixed AIHA, and paroxysmal cold hemoglobinuria (PCH) constitute the remainder of antibody-positive cases. AIHA is further categorized as primary or secondary, with the most common secondary causes being infections and autoimmune and immunodeficiency syndromes.[3]

Warm Autoimmune Hemolytic Anemia

W-AIHA is mediated by polyclonal immunoglobulin G (IgG) antibodies directed, most commonly, at the Rhesus (Rh) protein complex. These autoantibodies demonstrate optimal antibody-antigen interaction at body temperature (37°C). Opsonized red blood cells (RBCs) bind Fc receptors in the reticuloendothelial system and are phagocytized by macrophages, resulting in predominantly extravascular hemolysis.

Presentation

The presentation of W-AIHA is often dramatic and commonly includes a constellation of fatigue, pallor, exertional dyspnea, dizziness, headache, and jaundice. In severe cases, patients may present in extremis with evidence of heart failure. Patients rarely may have a more gradual onset and be minimally symptomatic.

Pertinent complete blood count (CBC) findings include anemia with typically brisk reticulocytosis, although antibody-mediated reticulocyte clearance and/or brisk hemolysis may blunt reticulocytosis initially.[4] The mean corpuscular volume (MCV) may be slightly elevated owing to reticulocytosis and/or mild erythrocyte clumping. Additional expected laboratory findings are general features of hemolysis including indirect hyperbilirubinemia, elevated lactate dehydrogenase, elevated plasma free hemoglobin, and decreased haptoglobin levels. The peripheral smear demonstrates anemia, anisopoikilocytosis, polychromasia, and a dominant abnormal morphology of spherocytes.

The most important test in distinguishing AIHA from other hemolytic anemias is the direct antiglobulin test (DAT).[5] In the case of a positive polyspecific DAT, specific antiglobulin testing can distinguish IgG from C3d-coated erythrocytes. W-AIHA is classically IgG positive and C3d negative. In approximately 5% of cases, patients have a clinical picture consistent with W-AIHA, but the DAT is negative because of a low-affinity or low-titer IgG, IgA, or monomeric IgM antibody.[6]

Management

Corticosteroids are the mainstay of therapy for W-AIHA. Approximately 70% to 85% of children demonstrate an initial respond to steroids, although response may take days to weeks.[1] A variety of dosing regimens including intravenous and oral routes are used (**Fig. 1** shows an example regimen). Relapse during tapering is common, so wean schedules should be prolonged over 4 to 6 months and guided by laboratory parameters and clinical response. Studies demonstrate that those treated on low-dose steroids for longer than 6 months are less likely to relapse and maintain a longer duration of remission.[1]

For steroid nonresponders or relapsed patients, second-line agents should be considered. Before initiation of such therapies, care should be taken to evaluate for underlying immune dysregulation/immunodeficiency, because immunosuppression may increase the risk of life-threatening infection in this setting (see "Secondary Causes of Immune Cytopenias").

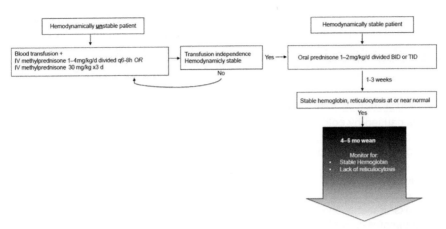

Fig. 1. Algorithm for initial management of warm autoimmune hemolytic anemia. BID, twice a day; TID, 3 times a day; IV, intravenous; q, every.

Rituximab, the preferred second-line agent for steroid refractory or relapsed patients, is an anti-CD20 monoclonal antibody that eliminates antibody-producing B cells from circulation for an average of 6 to 9 months. Rituximab is effective for primary and secondary W-AIHA with an overall response rate of 83% to 87%.[7] Standard rituximab dosing is 375 mg/m^2 weekly for 4 weeks. Adverse events associated with rituximab are rare with the exception of infusion reactions.[8,9] Hypogammaglobulinemia can occur, requiring immunoglobulin replacement. Immunoglobulin levels and full B cell subset panel should be tested before treatment to exclude underlying common variable immunodeficiency (CVID) or other immunodeficiency syndromes. More serious side effects such as serum sickness, progressive multifocal encephalopathy, and hepatitis B reactivation are rare in children.[1] Immunizations should be withheld pending complete B cell recovery (including CD19$^+$27$^+$ memory B cells).

In primary AIHA, splenectomy is often effective but generally delayed in children who have not yet developed humoral immunity, at least until after age 5 years. Children who are splenectomized must be immunized against encapsulated organisms before surgery. Following splenectomy, children need antibiotic prophylaxis to prevent increased risk for sepsis. The risk of postsplenectomy thrombosis is low but above the baseline in children.[1]

There are few data regarding optimal third-line agents for AIHA. Therapeutic options for multirefractory AIHA and ITP are discussed at the end of this review (see "Use of Other Third-Line Agents for Refractory AIHA and ITP").

Cold Autoimmune Hemolytic Anemia

C-AIHA, rare in children, is caused by IgM pentamers, which trigger complement activation and subsequent intravascular hemolysis. Unlike W-AIHA, patients have a C3d-positive and IgG-negative DAT result. Most pediatric cases (50%–75%) develop within 1 to 2 weeks of an infection, most commonly mycoplasma pneumonia.[6] Features are similar to those in W-AIHA with some notable exceptions: patients are generally mildly affected at typical temperatures, have hypocomplementemia, and spherocytes are absent because of predominantly intravascular hemolysis. Significant erythrocyte clumping and rouleaux formation is often evident on peripheral smear. Clumping may impede cell counting, resulting in overestimation of anemia and a falsely elevated or incalculable MCV.

Treatment involves managing the underlying disorder and avoiding cold exposure, including warming blood products and fluids.[2] In some adult patients with C-AIHA rituximab is efficacious, but is rarely needed in children.[2] Plasmapheresis can be used as a temporizing measure to remove intravascular IgM quickly in severely ill patients. Corticosteroids and splenectomy are generally ineffective for C-AIHA.[2]

Paroxysmal Cold Hemoglobinuria

PCH is caused by cold-reacting IgG autoantibodies, known as Donath-Landsteiner antibodies, directed against a common erythrocyte surface polysaccharide, the P antigen.[6] These antibodies are biphasic: they initially fix complement and thereafter, on cooling and rewarming, the complement is amplified and RBCs are hemolyzed.[2]

In children, PCH is associated with viral infections.[6] Antibodies persist for up to 12 weeks. Patients should be managed with supportive care and avoidance of cold. Blood transfusion and intravenous fluids should be warmed.

IMMUNE THROMBOCYTOPENIA

ITP is an autoimmune disorder resulting in platelet destruction. It is the most common acquired bleeding disorder in children with an incidence of 4 to 5 new cases per 100,000 annually.[10] ITP is classified by duration of disease: newly diagnosed (active disease for <3 months), persistent (3 to <12 months), and chronic (>12 months).[11]

ITP is classically described as caused by autoantibodies against platelet glycoproteins, most commonly GPIIb/IIIa and GPIb/IX. However, ITP pathogenesis is much more complex. T cell abnormalities are well described, including shifts toward T-helper cell 1 (Th1), Th0, and Th17 cell types, direct cytotoxic T cell–mediated destruction, and deficiency in number and function of T regulatory cells (Tregs). Abnormalities in B regulatory cells, megakaryocyte maturation and survival, and myeloid-derived suppressor cells have all been demonstrated in ITP.[2]

Presentation

ITP is a diagnosis of exclusion made on the basis of clinical presentation and laboratory findings. Bleeding ranges from mild bruising and petechiae to epistaxis, oral purpura, hematuria, menorrhagia, gastrointestinal hemorrhage, or intracranial bleeding. Patients typically have mild symptoms, and severe life-threatening bleeding is rare.[12] The onset of symptoms is often acute and may be linked to preceding viral illness or vaccination.[13]

Children often present with severe thrombocytopenia with counts less than 20×10^9/L.[2] The mean platelet volume is elevated or variable, indicating that large, new platelets are being generated to compensate for loss.[14] The immature platelet fraction (IPF) is typically elevated in ITP. The IPF can be useful in distinguishing ITP from other thrombocytopenia syndromes, and some studies suggest it is predictive of bleeding risk.[15,16]

Baseline laboratory evaluation should include CBC with differential, reticulocyte count, and peripheral smear review. International Working Group guidelines recommend quantitative immunoglobulin testing to evaluate antibody production and a DAT to assess for anti-RBC antibodies and potential hemolysis risk.[17] Blood typing must be performed if anti-D immunoglobulin therapy is considered.[17] Other testing depends on the clinical scenario and may include an antinuclear antibody test, thyroid function testing, and antiphospholipid antibodies when suspicion for an underlying rheumatologic or immune disorder is high. Bone marrow examination is not necessary in classic ITP, but may be warranted when the clinical picture is not consistent or other concerning features are present.

Management

Most children with ITP have mild bleeding and 70% to 80% experience spontaneous disease resolution. The standard of care is cautious observation for the nonbleeding child.[18] If a child presents with significant bleeding, bleeding risk, or is unable to be followed up closely, treatment to transiently elevate the platelet count is recommended (**Fig. 2**). First-line therapies include a single dose of intravenous IgG (IVIG), or a short course of corticosteroids or Rh immune globulin for those who are Rh(D) positive (**Table 1**).[2]

Second-line agents are reserved for those who fail to respond or relapse after front-line therapy, or who have chronic disease. Splenectomy has favorable efficacy rates, but given the long-term risks in the pediatric population is generally used only when other treatment options are exhausted. Rituximab is well tolerated, but initial response rates are lower for ITP than AIHA (~25%–60%), and long-term remission is rare.[18] Despite this, it is widely used as a nonsurgical attempt at durable remission.[19,20] However, the treatment paradigm has shifted toward increasing use of thrombopoietin receptor agonists (TPO-RAs).[21]

TPO-RAs are commonly used as second-line therapies for primary ITP. Eltrombopag and romiplostim are both approved by the Food and Drug Administration (FDA) for use in children 1 year of age and older with chronic ITP. In phase 2 and 3 randomized, multicenter, placebo-controlled trials, eltrombopag improved platelet counts, reduced bleeding severity, allowed for discontinuation of concomitant medications, and had a favorable side-effect profile.[22–24] Eltrombopag dosing starts at 25 mg daily for those younger than 6 years and 50 mg daily for older children. Reduced starting doses are recommended for patients of East Asian descent. Dosing is titrated based on platelet count with maximum dose of 75 mg per day.[22]

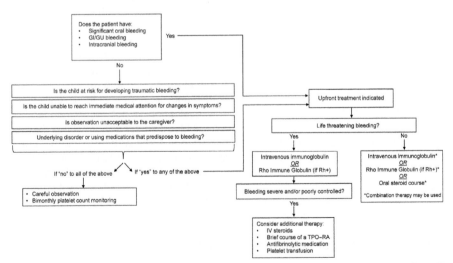

Fig. 2. Decision tree for management of immune thrombocytopenia at presentation. GI, gastrointestinal; GU, genitourinary; IV, intravenous; TPO-RA, thrombopoietin receptor agonist.

Table 1
Suggested dosing for upfront ITP therapies

Medication	Dose	Other Considerations
IVIG	1 g/kg IV × 1 (an additional dose can be given for suboptimal response)	• Antibody and immunodeficiency screens prior (quantitative immunoglobulins, DAT) • *Black box warning*: risk of thrombosis, renal dysfunction, and acute renal failure
Rho immune globulin	50–75 μg/kg IV × 1	• Blood typing required prior, can only be used if Rh+ • Test for signs of hemolysis before dosing (DAT, reticulocyte count) • *Black box warning*: risk for intravascular hemolysis, which can be severe or life-threatening. Monitor patients for minimum 8 h after administration, perform urinalysis to test for hematuria/hemoglobinuria at baseline then every 2 h
Dexamethasone	0.6 mg/kg/d IV × 4 d	• Requires GI prophylaxis because of risk for steroid-induced gastritis
Prednisone[a]	1 mg/kg/d × 1–2 wk + taper 1–2 mg/kg/d × 4 days + taper 4 mg/kg/d × 4-day pulse	• Requires GI prophylaxis because of risk for steroid-induced gastritis • Treatment course should not exceed 2 wk. If unable to wean, consider initiating second-line agents

Abbreviations: GI, gastrointestinal; IV, intravenous.
[a] No standard dosing regimen.

Romiplostim was approved for use in children in December 2018, but was previously widely used off-label in pediatric ITP. It is dosed weekly by subcutaneous injection starting at 1 μg/kg/wk and titrated to achieve hemostasis or a platelet count greater than 50×10^9/L. Whereas romiplostim has not been directly compared with eltrombopag in children, in adults success rates of 74% to 88% were achieved when switching sequentially between different TPO-RAs. Patients who fail to respond to one agent may successfully switch to the other.[25]

Both eltrombopag and romiplostim require regular laboratory monitoring. The platelet count is monitored to guide dosing adjustments. Bone marrow fibrosis has been reported following prolonged exposure to eltrombopag and romiplostim. However, bone marrow reticulin deposition was mild and did not result in clinically significant cytopenias.[26,27] Routine bone marrow evaluation is not recommended, but should be considered if cytopenias or peripheral blood smear abnormalities develop. Thrombosis risk does not seem to be increased in children without comorbid conditions. Additional considerations for eltrombopag therapy include monitoring of liver function because of a transient transaminitis seen in clinical trials.[22] In addition eltrombopag chelates iron, and patients should be monitored for iron deficiency if anemia or microcytosis develops. Because eltrombopag binds other divalent cations such as calcium and magnesium, dietary precautions are indicated.

SECONDARY CAUSES OF IMMUNE CYTOPENIAS

Box 1 lists systemic autoimmune disorders, immunodeficiencies, rheumatologic conditions, infections, and malignancies associated with autoimmune cytopenias. Recommended testing for these disorders is also indicated in **Box 1**.

Box 1
Conditions associated with autoimmune cytopenias

Lymphoproliferative disorders

Autoimmune lymphoproliferative syndrome[a]

Rosai-Dorfman disease

Castleman disease

Ras-associated leukoproliferative disorder

Immunodeficiency syndromes

Common variable immune deficiency[a]

Selective IgA deficiency

Chromosome 22q11.2 deletion (DiGeorge syndrome, velocardiofacial syndrome)

Severe combined immunodeficiency[a]

Rheumatologic conditions

SLE[a]

Antiphospholipid antibody syndrome[a]

Juvenile idiopathic arthritis/Juvenile rheumatoid arthritis

Sjögren syndrome

Sarcoid

Malignancies

Non-Hodgkin lymphoma

Acute lymphoblastic leukemia

Myelodysplastic syndrome

Hodgkin lymphoma

Chronic infections

Epstein-Barr virus

HIV[b]

Helicobacter pylori

Cytomegalovirus

Hepatitis C virus

Other

Celiac disease

Inflammatory bowel disease

Recommended evaluation for children with chronic single-lineage autoimmune cytopenias or multilineage autoimmune cytopenias[a]

Flow cytometry for double-negative T cells (ALPS)

ANA (SLE)

Antiphospholipid antibodies

Quantitative immunoglobulins (CVID)

Disease associated with autoimmune cytopenias in children

Specific antibody titers (CVID)

T cell subsets (CD3/CD4, CD3/CD8)

HIV[b]

[a] Consider screening for these conditions in children with chronic single-lineage autoimmune cytopenias or multilineage autoimmune cytopenias.

[b] Consider also screening for HIV in adolescents with chronic single-lineage or multilineage autoimmune cytopenias. Other diseases should be considered if the history or physical are suggestive of the underlying condition. It is extremely rare for the other conditions to present with autoimmune cytopenias and no other signs or symptoms suggestive of the underlying disease. Thus, the utility of routine screening is low.

Adapted from Teachey DT, Lambert MP. Diagnosis and management of autoimmune cytopenias in childhood. Pediatr Clin N Am 2013;60(6):1496–7; with permission.

Drug-Induced Autoimmune Hemolytic Anemia

Approximately 150 different drugs are reported to induce immune hemolysis.[3] Cephalosporins are the most important cause in children, causing 70% of drug-induced AIHA in this age group.[28] If the diagnosis is uncertain, testing can be done for specific drug-related antibodies.[3] In cases driven by haptenization, removal of the offending agent improves symptoms.[3]

Post-transplant Cytopenias

Following hematopoietic stem cell transplantation (HSCT) and solid organ transplantation, patients can develop autoimmune cytopenias. AIHA occurs in 1.37% of patients while ITP is reported in 0.76% of patients after HSCT.[29] In addition to viral infections, delayed immune reconstitution, and graft-versus-host disease, alteration of T cell immunity via use of calcineurin inhibitors such as tacrolimus contributes substantially to post-transplant AIHA.[30] Treatment begins with lowering the dose of these drugs or switching to an alternative immunosuppressant. Addition of steroids and/or rituximab may be required.[31] Autoimmune cytopenias are strongly associated with increased morbidity and mortality in this population.[31]

EVANS SYNDROME

Evans syndrome (ES) is defined as autoimmune cytopenias affecting at least 2 cell lineages. Initially described as ITP accompanied by AIHA, the recent definition of ES is 2 autoimmune cytopenias occurring together or developing over time. The cytopenias may include ITP, AIHA, or AIN.[32,33] Disease presentation depends on the cell lines affected and is often a combination of anemia and mucosal bleeding.

Diagnosis

ES is a diagnosis of exclusion. Previously defined as idiopathic, improvements in genetic sequencing technology have facilitated improved identification of causative defects, leading to the broad immune dysregulation characteristic of ES. Initial workup and management for ES is the same as that for ITP and AIHA. Following upfront symptom management, further workup for ES involves broad evaluation for rheumatologic disorders, immunodeficiencies, and infectious etiologies (**Fig. 3**).

Immunodeficiencies Associated with Evans Syndrome

Patients with ES may have underlying immunologic abnormalities such as autoimmune lymphoproliferative disorder (ALPS), CVID, or systemic autoimmune disorders

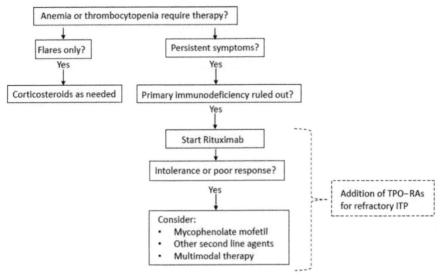

Fig. 3. Suggested algorithm for management of primary Evans syndrome. ITP, immune thrombocytopenia; TPO-RA, thrombopoietin receptor agonist.

such as systemic lupus erythematosus (SLE). Advances in genomics have increasingly identified causative novel genetic aberrations in ES. These include cytotoxic T lymphocyte–associated protein 4 (CTLA4) haploinsufficiency, lipopolysaccharide-responsive beige-like anchor (LRBA) protein deficiency, signal transducer and activator of transcription (STAT) gain-of-function mutations, and activated phosphoinositide 3-kinase δ (PI3KD) syndrome (**Table 2**).[33] The elucidation of the underlying molecular defects in these cases has led to identification of targeted therapies.

Autoimmune lymphoproliferative syndrome

Autoimmune lymphoproliferative syndrome (ALPS) is characterized by uncontrolled lymphocytic proliferation in the absence of a malignancy or inciting infection.[34] ALPS is caused by *FAS* apoptotic pathway defects leading to impaired cellular apoptosis and inability to regulate activated lymphocytes.[34] Patients present with lymphadenopathy, splenomegaly, and/or hepatomegaly in conjunction with cytopenias.[2] These patients are at increased risk for secondary cancers.[35,36]

Diagnosing ALPS requires:

1. Chronic nonmalignant lymphoproliferation defined as lymphadenopathy or splenomegaly for longer than 6 months
2. Elevated peripheral blood double-negative T (DNT) cells (CD3$^+$/CD4$^-$/CD8$^-$ and positive for T cell receptor α/β).[37]

Abnormal Fas-mediated apoptosis testing is supportive of the diagnosis but is not part of the formal diagnostic criteria.

IVIG is ineffective for ALPS patients. Rituximab and splenectomy are contraindicated in ALPS. ALPS patients treated with rituximab may not recover their B cell population and could require indefinite IVIG replacement. If splenectomized, patients with ALPS are at dramatically increased risk for pneumococcal sepsis.[2] Though a chronic disease, ALPS symptoms may occur in acute flares, commonly managed with corticosteroids. Sirolimus, an mammalian target of rapamycin (mTOR) inhibitor, is now

Table 2
Genetic causes of secondary Evans syndrome with targeted therapies

Diagnosis	Molecular Defect	Targeted Therapy	Proposed Mechanism of Action
ALPS	DNT with hyperactivation of PI3K/Akt/mTOR signaling pathway	Sirolimus	mTOR inhibitor. Inhibits hyperactivated PI3K/Akt/mTOR signaling pathway
CTLA-4 haploinsufficiency	Loss of CTLA-4, a negative regulator of immune responses	Abatacept	Immunoglobulin-CTLA-4 fusion protein. Restores CTLA-4 insufficiency
LRBA deficiency	Loss of LRBA, a possible regulator of CTLA-4	Abatacept	Restoration of CTLA-4 insufficiency
PI3KD syndrome	Gain-of-function mutation in PI3K/Akt/mTOR signaling pathway	Sirolimus, rapamycin	mTOR inhibitor. Inhibits hyperactivated PI3K/Akt/mTOR signaling pathway
		Leniolisib (CDZ173)	Decreased Alt phosphorylation
STAT1 gain-of-function	Excess STAT1 activation, hyperresponsiveness to IFN-γ and abnormal T-helper responses	Ruxolitinib	Inhibits JAK1/2, an upstream IFN-γ receptor
STAT3 gain-of-function	Excess STAT3 activation: represses FAS signaling, promotes IL-6 signaling, promotes antiapoptotic protein Bcl2	Tocilizumab ABT-737	IL-6 inhibitor Bcl-2 inhibitor
Ras-associated autoimmune leukoproliferative disorder (RALD)	NRAS and KRAS mutations lead to RAF/MEK/ERK signaling	Farnesyltransferase inhibitors	Inhibition of RAS
Dianzani autoimmune lymphoproliferative disease (DALD)	Defective Fas-dependent apoptosis, elevated IL-17 levels	Anti-IL-17 antibody	IL-17 neutralization

Abbreviations: IFN, interferon; IL, interleukin; PI3K, phosphoinositide 3-kinase.

regarded as an optimal first-line therapy.[2,33,38] Mycophenolate mofetil, which inhibits purine synthesis, is also an appropriate choice.[2] Both of these drugs modulate cellular immunity, specifically targeting B and T cells.[2]

Common variable immunodeficiency

CVID is strongly associated with ES; an estimated 10% of ES patients have underlying CVID and more than half present with autoimmune cytopenias.[33] These patients have frequent infections, which may be severe or refractory to treatment. Patients also lack response to vaccines. CVID patients have paradoxic autoimmunity including autoimmune cytopenias. There is increased risk for malignancy in adulthood, most typically lymphoma.[39] ES patients should be at minimum screened for hypogammaglobulinemia characteristic of CVID.[33]

Systemic autoimmune disease

Many primary autoimmune disorders are associated with ES, including antiphospholipid antibody syndrome, Hashimoto thyroiditis, Sjögren disease, and, most commonly, SLE.[33] Approximately 50% of SLE patients develop AIHA and/or ITP months to years before developing features of SLE.[40,41] Providers should be vigilant for the development of additional manifestations suggestive of SLE over time.

Management of Primary Evans Syndrome

Corticosteroids are commonly the first-line treatment of acute exacerbations of ES with AIHA. For some, no treatment is required between disease relapses, and for others chronic therapy is necessary.

Treatments for ES follow standard therapies for the respective immune cytopenias, with some caveats. Splenectomy is frequently ineffective in ES and imparts a high risk for sepsis in those patients with underlying immune dysregulation. Rituximab has demonstrated an initial response rate of 75% to 80% in pediatric ES patients with 36% to 65% remaining relapse free at 6 years.[42,43] The presence of an immunodeficiency disorder must be ruled out before therapy with rituximab, which may induce permanent hypogammaglobulinemia in a subset of patients.

Treatment with mycophenolate mofetil or sirolimus shows a response in 80% of ES patients and these drugs are generally well tolerated.[38,44] The response to these therapies may be sustained, thereby avoiding additional immunosuppressive medications.

USE OF OTHER THIRD-LINE AGENTS FOR REFRACTORY AUTOIMMUNE HEMOLYTIC ANEMIA, IMMUNE THROMBOCYTOPENIA

Considerations for Third-Line Agents

Common initial and second-line therapies for the autoimmune cytopenias have been well described earlier. However, the choice of subsequent therapies for refractory patients is less clear. There are a multitude of drugs used off-label in refractory disease, including alemtuzumab, mercaptopurine, azathioprine, methotrexate, calcineurin inhibitors, sirolimus, cyclophosphamide, and vincristine. **Table 3** details second-line agents used in the treatment of autoimmune cytopenias. In considering the risk associated with these immunosuppressants, it is important to realize that the doses used to treat autoimmune cytopenias are much lower than those used in cancer therapy. At lower doses and as monotherapy, many of these immunosuppressants have a more favorable side-effect profile than commonly used first-line agents such as corticosteroids.[2] In addition, for multirefractory ITP patients, a single immunosuppressant used in conjunction with a TPO-RA may have a synergistic effect, suggesting a role for multimodal therapy in this patient cohort.[45]

Factors in Treatment Decision Making

There are no randomized controlled trials directly comparing second-line therapies for autoimmune cytopenias. When selecting medications, side effects, cost, route of administration, and speed of response should be considered. When providers cite reasons for selecting particular second-line agents in childhood ITP, the most common reasons for treatment choice included the possibility of long-term remission, parental/patient preference, and side-effect profile.[19] There are also physician and treatment center biases that affect treatment selection.[19]

Table 3
Summary of third-line treatments for AIHA and ITP

	Acute or Chronic Treatment	Mechanism of Action	Target Cell Population	Route of Administration	Side Effects and Monitoring Considerations	Infection Risk
Alemtuzumab	Chronic	Anti-CD52 antibody	B and T cells, monocytes, macrophages, NK cells, granulocytes	IV, SC	Significant immune suppression, requires prophylactic antifungal and antiviral treatment	High
Anti-D immunoglobulin	Acute	Saturates reticuloendothelial Fc receptors with anti-D coated RBCs bound to macrophages	B cells (antibody interference)	IV	Risk for hemolytic anemia. Infusion-related headache, fever, chills, rare DIC. Can only be used for Rh+ blood types	None
Antithymocyte globulin	Chronic	Antibodies against T cell antigens	T cells	IV	Significant immune suppression, infusion reactions, and rare serum sickness	High if used in combination
Calcineurin inhibitors(tacrolimus, cyclosporine)	Chronic	Prevents T cell activation	T cells	PO	Cause autoimmune cytopenias, nephrotoxicity, electrolyte disturbances, require drug level monitoring. Risk for PML	Low
Corticosteroids	Acute, chronic	Decreased leukocyte trafficking, depletes T and B cells, decreased inflammatory cytokine productions	B, T, and NK cells, monocytes, macrophages, neutrophils, eosinophils	PO, IV	Hypertension, hyperglycemia, weight gain, mood changes, loss of bone density, growth delay, cataracts	Low if used as monotherapy. high if used in combination therapy
Cyclophosphamide	Chronic	DNA alkylator	B, T, and NK cells, Tregs	PO	Dose-dependent myelosuppression, GI toxicity, and alopecia. Infertility, increased risk of Monosomy 7 MDS/AML. Risk for PML	Low (dose-dependent)

Drug	Acute/Chronic	Mechanism	Cell target	Route	Adverse effects/notes	Risk
Eltrombopag	Chronic	Stimulates platelet production and megakaryopoiesis	N/A	PO	Requires routine lab testing, transaminitis, chelates calcium, cannot be given around dairy intake, possible risk for bone marrow fibrosis (not reported as clinically relevant fibrosis)	None
IVIG	Acute, chronic	Interferes with reticuloendothelial Fc receptors	B cells (antibody interference)	IV	Headache, aseptic meningitis, nausea, vomiting, allergic reactions	None
Methotrexate	Chronic	Inhibits thymidine synthesis	B, T, and NK cells	PO	Myelosuppression, hepatic and renal toxicity rare at low doses	Low
mTOR inhibitors (sirolimus)	Chronic	Inhibits PI3K/Akt/mTOR signaling	B and T cells, spares Tregs	PO	Requires routine monitoring of drug levels, requires liver enzyme monitoring. Can cause hyperlipidemia	Low
Mycophenolate mofetil	Chronic	Inhibits purine synthesis	B, T, and NK cells	PO, IV	Diarrhea, neutropenia, risk for PML, teratogenic	Low
Plasmapheresis	Acute	Mechanical removal of autoantibodies	N/A	N/A	Requires central line insertion, hypotension, hypocalcemia. Ineffective for IgG-mediated disease.	Moderate, line-related risk only
Purine analogs (mercaptopurine, azathioprine, thioguanine)	Chronic	Inhibits purine synthesis	B, T, and NK cells	PO	Genetic polymorphisms may alter drug metabolism. Myelosuppression and hepatotoxicity rare at low doses. Azathioprine: risk for PML	Low

(continued on next page)

Table 3
(continued)

	Acute or Chronic Treatment	Mechanism of Action	Target Cell Population	Route of Administration	Side Effects and Monitoring Considerations	Infection Risk
Rituximab	Chronic	Anti-CD20 antibody	B cells	IV	Infusion-related fever, nausea, headache, pruritus. Rare serum sickness, PML. Risk of prolonged hypogammaglobulinemia	Low if used as monotherapy
Romiplostim	Chronic	Stimulates platelet production and megakaryopoiesis	N/A	SC	Requires routine lab testing. Given as weekly injection. Side effects of transaminitis, possible risk for bone marrow fibrosis (not reported as clinically relevant fibrosis)	None
Splenectomy	Chronic	Removes site of platelet destruction, antibody production	N/A	N/A	Requires surgical procedure. Subsequent risk of encapsulated bacterial sepsis, venous thromboembolism, pulmonary hypertension. Contraindicated in ALPS	Moderate, specific for encapsulated organisms

Abbreviations: AML, acute myeloid leukemia; DIC, disseminated intravascular coagulation; IV, intravenous; MDS, myelodysplastic syndrome; N/A, not applicable; NK, natural killer; PML, progressive multifocal leukoencephalopathy; PO, oral; SC, subcutaneous.

Adapted from Teachey DT, Lambert MP. Diagnosis and management of autoimmune cytopenias in childhood. Pediatr Clin North Am 2013;60(6):1501–6; with permission.

Table 4
Novel agents in development for autoimmune cytopenia management

Drug	Mechanism of Action	Status of Drug Trials
Toralizumab, ruplizumab	Inhibition of CD40-CD154 interaction between T and B cells	Thromboembolic events in early trials halted use. Newer agents are currently being tested
Rozrolimupab	Anti-RhD monoclonal antibody	Currently in clinical trials. Preliminary results demonstrate efficacy. Adverse events include hemolytic anemia
Fostamatinib	Spleen tyrosine kinase (SYK) inhibitor. Impedes phagocytosis of Fc receptor-bound platelets	FDA approved April 2018 as second-line agent for adult chronic ITP patients
Rozanolixizumab	Antineonatal Fc receptor (FcRn). Decreases recycling of circulating IgG	Interim analysis of phase 2 trials in 2017 demonstrate efficacy and tolerable safety profile
Avatrombopag	Novel thrombopoietin receptor agonist	Approved for management of thrombocytopenia in preoperative liver disease patients in May 2018. Adverse events reported of thromboembolic events and gastric problems
Amifostine	Increases platelet production	Two small studies completed, which showed improved platelet count and several patients with disease resolution

Novel Treatments

There are novel agents in development for ITP and AIHA, including monoclonal antibodies targeting T and B cell interactions, Fc receptor blockade, spleen tyrosine kinase (SYK) inhibitors, and new thrombopoietin agonists (**Table 4**). These agents are currently being studied in adults with ITP and have not been tested in children.[46,47]

THE FUTURE OF AUTOIMMUNE CYTOPENIA THERAPY

Owing to limitations in our understanding of the underlying cause of these conditions, the ability to make a selection based on the disease biology remains limited. Elucidating the role of the mTOR pathway in ALPS, leading to identification of sirolimus as an efficacious targeted first-line treatment, is a promising model for the future of autoimmune cytopenia management. Genetic sequencing technologies, investigations on the biological changes induced by TPO-RAs, and continued molecular immunology research is poised to transform the diagnostic pathway and introduce targeted treatment in the coming decades.

SUMMARY

The autoimmune cytopenias represent a broad spectrum of hematologic disease. These conditions vary in presentation, severity, and underlying cause. Despite these differences, treatments have significant overlap and cause broad immune suppression. As research in the field continues to grow, our understanding of each of these conditions will improve and allow for more directed therapies.

REFERENCES

1. Zanella A, Barcellini W. Treatment of autoimmune hemolytic anemias. Haematologica 2014;99(10):1547–54.
2. Teachey DT, Lambert MP. Diagnosis and management of autoimmune cytopenias in childhood. Pediatr Clin North Am 2013;60(6):1489–511.
3. Bass GF, Tuscano ET, Tuscano JM. Diagnosis and classification of autoimmune hemolytic anemia. Autoimmun Rev 2014;13(4–5):560–4.
4. Liesveld JL, Rowe JM, Lichtman MA. Variability of the erythropoietic response in autoimmune hemolytic anemia: analysis of 109 cases. Blood 1987;69(3):820–6.
5. Coombs RR, Mourant AE, Race RR. A new test for the detection of weak and incomplete Rh agglutinins. Br J Exp Pathol 1945;26:255–66.
6. Qasim S. Background, presentation and pathophysiology of autoimmune hemolytic anemia. In: Despotovic JM, editor. Immune hematology. Diagnosis and management of immune cytopenias. Cham (Switzerland): Springer International Publishing AG; 2018. p. 83–102.
7. Dierickx D, Verhoef G, Van Hoof A, et al. Rituximab in auto-immune haemolytic anaemia and immune thrombocytopenic purpura: a Belgian retrospective multicentric study. J Intern Med 2009;266(5):484–91.
8. Zecca M, Nobili B, Ramenghi U, et al. Rituximab for the treatment of refractory autoimmune hemolytic anemia in children. Blood 2003;101(10):3857–61.
9. Rao A, Kelly M, Musselman M, et al. Safety, efficacy, and immune reconstitution after rituximab therapy in pediatric patients with chronic or refractory hematologic autoimmune cytopenias. Pediatr Blood Cancer 2008;50(4):822–5.
10. Lilleyman JS. Management of childhood idiopathic thrombocytopenic purpura. Br J Haematol 1999;105(4):871–5.
11. Rodeghiero F, Stasi R, Gernsheimer T, et al. Standardization of terminology, definitions and outcome criteria in immune thrombocytopenic purpura of adults and children: report from an international working group. Blood 2009;113(11):2386–93.
12. Neunert CE, Buchanan GR, Imbach P, et al. Severe hemorrhage in children with newly diagnosed immune thrombocytopenic purpura. Blood 2008;112(10):4003–8.
13. Cines DB, Bussel JB, Liebman HA, et al. The ITP syndrome: pathogenic and clinical diversity. Blood 2009;113(26):6511–21.
14. Tang YT, He P, Li YZ, et al. Diagnostic value of platelet indices and bone marrow megakaryocytic parameters in immune thrombocytopenic purpura. Blood Coagul Fibrinolysis 2017;28(1):83–90.
15. Adly AA, Ragab IA, Ismail EA, et al. Evaluation of the immature platelet fraction in the diagnosis and prognosis of childhood immune thrombocytopenia. Platelets 2015;26(7):645–50.
16. Frelinger AL 3rd, Grace RF, Gerrits AJ, et al. Platelet function tests, independent of platelet count, are associated with bleeding severity in ITP. Blood 2015;126(7):873–9.
17. Provan D, Stasi R, Newland AC, et al. International consensus report on the investigation and management of primary immune thrombocytopenia. Blood 2010;115(2):168–86.
18. Neunert C, Lim W, Crowther M, et al. The American Society of Hematology 2011 evidence-based practice guideline for immune thrombocytopenia. Blood 2011;117(16):4190–207.

19. Grace RF, Despotovic JM, Bennett CM, et al. Physician decision making in selection of second-line treatments in immune thrombocytopenia in children. Am J Hematol 2018;93(7):882–8.

20. Cuker A. Transitioning patients with immune thrombocytopenia to second-line therapy: challenges and best practices. Am J Hematol 2018;93(6):816–23.

21. Ghanima W, Khelif A, Waage A, et al. Rituximab as second-line treatment for adult immune thrombocytopenia (the RITP trial): a multicentre, randomised, double-blind, placebo-controlled trial. Lancet 2015;385(9978):1653–61.

22. Kim TO, Despotovic J, Lambert MP. Eltrombopag for use in children with immune thrombocytopenia. Blood Adv 2018;2(4):454–61.

23. Bussel JB, de Miguel PG, Despotovic JM, et al. Eltrombopag for the treatment of children with persistent and chronic immune thrombocytopenia (PETIT): a randomised, multicentre, placebo-controlled study. Lancet Haematol 2015;2(8): e315–25.

24. Grainger JD, Locatelli F, Chotsampancharoen T, et al. Eltrombopag for children with chronic immune thrombocytopenia (PETIT2): a randomised, multicentre, placebo-controlled trial. Lancet 2015;386(10004):1649–58.

25. Gonzalez KJ, Zuluaga SO, DaRos CV, et al. Sequential treatment with thrombopoietin-receptor agonists (TPO-RAs) in immune thrombocytopenia (ITP): experience in our center. Ann Hematol 2017;96(3):507–8.

26. Brynes RK, Wong RS, Thein MM, et al. A 2-year, longitudinal, prospective study of the effects of eltrombopag on bone marrow in patients with chronic immune thrombocytopenia. Acta Haematol 2017;137(2):66–72.

27. Saleh MN, Bussel JB, Cheng G, et al. Safety and efficacy of eltrombopag for treatment of chronic immune thrombocytopenia: results of the long-term, open-label EXTEND study. Blood 2013;121(3):537–45.

28. Garratty G, Arndt PA. An update on drug-induced immune hemolytic anemia. Immunohematology 2007;23(3):105–19.

29. Neunert CE, Despotovic JM. Autoimmune hemolytic anemia and immune thrombocytopenia following hematopoietic stem cell transplant: a critical review of the literature. Pediatr Blood Cancer 2018;e27569. https://doi.org/10.1002/pbc. 27569.

30. Park JA, Lee HH, Kwon HS, et al. Sirolimus for refractory autoimmune hemolytic anemia after allogeneic hematopoietic stem cell transplantation: a case report and literature review of the treatment of post-transplant autoimmune hemolytic anemia. Transfus Med Rev 2016;30(1):6–14.

31. Sanz J, Arriaga F, Montesinos P, et al. Autoimmune hemolytic anemia following allogeneic hematopoietic stem cell transplantation in adult patients. Bone Marrow Transplant 2007;39(9):555–61.

32. Evans RS, Takahashi K, Duane RT, et al. Primary thrombocytopenic purpura and acquired hemolytic anemia; evidence for a common etiology. AMA Arch Intern Med 1951;87(1):48–65.

33. Grimes AB. Evans syndrome: background, clinical presentation, pathophysiology, and management. In: Despotovic JM, editor. Immune hematology. Diagnosis and management of immune cytopenias. Cham (Switzerland): Springer International Publishing AG; 2018. p. 125–50.

34. Rieux-Laucat F, Le Deist F, Fischer A. Autoimmune lymphoproliferative syndromes: genetic defects of apoptosis pathways. Cell Death Differ 2003;10(1): 124–33.

35. Sneller MC, Wang J, Dale JK, et al. Clinical, immunologic, and genetic features of an autoimmune lymphoproliferative syndrome associated with abnormal lympho-cyte apoptosis. Blood 1997;89(4):1341–8.

36. Straus SE, Jaffe ES, Puck JM, et al. The development of lymphomas in families with autoimmune lymphoproliferative syndrome with germline Fas mutations and defective lymphocyte apoptosis. Blood 2001;98(1):194–200.

37. Bleesing JJ, Brown MR, Dale JK, et al. TcR-alpha/beta(+) CD4(-)CD8(-) T cells in humans with the autoimmune lymphoproliferative syndrome express a novel CD45 isoform that is analogous to murine B220 and represents a marker of altered O-glycan biosynthesis. Clin Immunol 2001;100(3):314–24.

38. Bride KL, Vincent T, Smith-Whitley K, et al. Sirolimus is effective in relapsed/re-fractory autoimmune cytopenias: results of a prospective multi-institutional trial. Blood 2016;127(1):17–28.

39. Patuzzo G, Barbieri A, Tinazzi E, et al. Autoimmunity and infection in common var-iable immunodeficiency (CVID). Autoimmun Rev 2016;15(9):877–82.

40. Zhang L, Wu X, Wang L, et al. Clinical features of systemic lupus erythematosus patients complicated with evans syndrome: a case-control, single center study. Medicine 2016;95(15):e3279.

41. Miescher PA, Tucci A, Beris P, et al. Autoimmune hemolytic anemia and/or throm-bocytopenia associated with lupus parameters. Semin Hematol 1992;29(1):13–7.

42. Ducassou S, Leverger G, Fernandes H, et al. Benefits of rituximab as a second-line treatment for autoimmune haemolytic anaemia in children: a prospective French cohort study. Br J Haematol 2017;177(5):751–8.

43. Bader-Meunier B, Aladjidi N, Bellmann F, et al. Rituximab therapy for childhood Evans syndrome. Haematologica 2007;92(12):1691–4.

44. Miano M, Ramenghi U, Russo G, et al. Mycophenolate mofetil for the treatment of children with immune thrombocytopenia and Evans syndrome. A retrospective data review from the Italian association of paediatric haematology/oncology. Br J Haematol 2016;175(3):490–5.

45. Mahevas M, Gerfaud-Valentin M, Moulis G, et al. Characteristics, outcome, and response to therapy of multirefractory chronic immune thrombocytopenia. Blood 2016;128(12):1625–30.

46. Lambert MP, Gernsheimer TB. Clinical updates in adult immune thrombocyto-penia. Blood 2017;129(21):2829–35.

47. Despotovic JM. Emerging therapies in immune thrombocytopenia. The Hematol-ogist ASH News and Reports 2018;15(4):1–6.

New Approaches and Trials in Pediatric Transfusion Medicine

Cyril Jacquot, MD, PhD[a,b,c,d,*], Yunchuan Delores Mo, MD, MSc[a,b,c,d], Naomi L.C. Luban, MD[a,b,c,d]

KEYWORDS

- Pediatric transfusion practice • Pathogen reduction technology
- Platelet additive solutions • Hemoglobin-based oxygen carriers • Blood substitutes

KEY POINTS

- Pathogen reduction technologies hold promise in improving blood safety by proactively targeting known and emerging pathogens.
- Concerns exist about the safety profile and increased costs and complexity of pathogen reduction technologies in children.
- Platelet additive solutions help reduce allergic reactions and alloimmune hemolysis by reducing plasma content.
- Hemoglobin-based oxygen carriers are currently in various stages of investigation, but none is Food and Drug Administration approved; these may benefit patients for whom allogeneic blood transfusion is not an option.

INTRODUCTION

Transfusions are among the most common medical interventions and are frequently lifesaving in critically ill patients. In the past decades, there has been a growing recognition of the infectious and noninfectious adverse events associated with blood transfusions. The former have been addressed by years of incremental improvements in

Disclosure Statement: The authors have no relevant disclosures to report.
[a] Division of Laboratory Medicine, Center for Cancer and Blood Disorders, Children's National Health System, Sheikh Zayed Campus for Advanced Children's Medicine, 111 Michigan Avenue Northwest, Washington, DC 20010, USA; [b] Division of Hematology, Center for Cancer and Blood Disorders, Children's National Health System, Sheikh Zayed Campus for Advanced Children's Medicine, 111 Michigan Avenue Northwest, Washington, DC 20010, USA; [c] Department of Pediatrics, George Washington University School of Medicine and Health Sciences, Washington, DC, USA; [d] Department of Pathology, George Washington University School of Medicine and Health Sciences, Washington, DC, USA
* Corresponding author. Division of Laboratory Medicine, Children's National Health System, 111 Michigan Avenue Northwest, Washington, DC 20010.
E-mail address: cjacquot@childrensnational.org

donor screening for infection risk factors and laboratory detection of pathogens. One example of risk mitigation for the latter has been a deferral policy for previously pregnant women with respect to plasma and platelet donations. These donors have a higher incidence of antibodies to human leukocyte antigens, which have been implicated in transfusion-related acute lung injury.

Discussion of risks and benefits is central to consenting patients to blood transfusions. Like adults, children and neonates are affected by transfusion complications. In one recent study, pediatric patients were found to have a higher incidence of transfusion reactions. Of note, adults and children had a similar rate of severe or life-threatening transfusion reactions.[1] Patient blood management, which has become widespread in adult transfusion practice, is gradually being applied to pediatric practice. Although alternatives to transfusions should always be considered, many scenarios arise whereby blood use is crucial to treatment.

Efforts are underway to continue improving blood safety by implementing pathogen reduction (PR) systems and platelet additive solutions (PAS). Blood substitutes, which remain limited in scope, have been successfully used in patients for whom allogeneic blood use is not possible, either due to religious beliefs or due to alloimmunization to red blood cell (RBC) antigens. With any new practices and investigational products, it is important to be alert for adverse events in vulnerable patient populations. This article aims to summarize some of the newer developments in transfusion medicine with a focus on the neonatal and pediatric population.

IMPROVING PLATELET SAFETY BY ENHANCING BACTERIAL TESTING

Platelets have the highest risk of bacterial contamination because they are stored at room temperature. As a result, their shelf-life is limited to 5 days. Platelets may be collected from a single donor via apheresis or by pooling platelet fractions (eg, buffy coats) from 4 to 6 whole blood donors; both preparations provide a typical adult dose. The residual risk of a bacterially contaminated platelet unit is about 1 in 6000, whereas the risk of septic transfusion reaction is 1 in 100,000 apheresis platelets.[2,3] In comparison, transmissions of the higher profile viral infections have much lower occurrence risks (**Table 1**). Bacterial septic reactions can be severe and fatal, especially in patients who are critically ill and/or immunocompromised.

Most pathogens implicated in platelet contamination are constituents of normal skin flora, which may be introduced into the product at the time of donor venipuncture or when sterile technique is not closely followed. To counter this, the donor's arm is thoroughly cleaned before phlebotomy with an antiseptic scrub to reduce bacterial density. In addition, the first 30 to 50 mL of the collection, which frequently contain the

Table 1	
Current infectious disease transmission residual risks	
Test	**Residual Risk of Transfusion**
HIV	1:1,467,000
Hepatitis C virus (HCV)	1:1,149,000
Hepatitis B virus (HBV)	1:750,000
Human T-lymphotropic virus (HTLV)	1:2,993,000
Bacteria	1:6000 (contaminated platelet unit) 1:100,000 (septic reaction from platelet unit)

Data from Refs [2,3,53–55]

skin plug with commensal bacteria flora, are routed to a separate diversion pouch before blood enters the sterile collection bag.[4]

After collection, all platelets are cultured to monitor for bacteria growth. Before testing, the bag is held for 24 hours to increase culture sensitivity by allowing additional time for contaminating bacteria to grow. After inoculation, the culture must remain negative for 12 hours before the platelets are released for transfusion. If the culture turns positive at any point, the corresponding products and cocomponents (for example, RBCs and plasma) in inventory are quarantined and discarded. If transfusion has already occurred, the ordering physician is notified to monitor the patient for signs of infection and possibly initiate empiric antibiotic treatment.

One limitation of the current platelet surveillance approach is detection of bacteria with a long lag phase. In such circumstances, the culture inoculated at 24 hours may be negative, but the product transfused 4 days later may have a clinically significant bacterial burden. To address this possibility, some centers repeat the culture at a later time (eg, day 3 or day 4) to detect such occurrences.[5] The most recent Food and Drug Administration (FDA) draft guidance proposes the use of point-of-issue testing (eg, Verax Biomedical, Marlborough, MA, USA) as an additional "safety measure."[6] In this scenario, the platelet unit is tested to identify bacterial markers, such as lipopolysaccharide or lipoteichoic acid, before release from the blood bank. If positive, the unit is quarantined and cultured. The use of Verax to prolong platelet storage up to 7 days was pioneered at Dartmouth-Hitchcock Medical Center and is now gaining more acceptance.[7] Blood banks wishing to implement this process for their in-house inventory must be registered with the FDA and notify the agency. Other options to improve surveillance include increasing the inoculum volume or adding an anaerobic culture bottle; both interventions should improve bacterial detection sensitivity. Although high sensitivity is desirable to prevent transfusion of contaminated products, care must also be taken to ensure high specificity in order to prevent unnecessary donor anxiety and wastage of products because of false positives.

PATHOGEN REDUCTION: A PROACTIVE APPROACH TO INFECTION PREVENTION

PR is an all-encompassing term for a variety of methods, including photochemical activation, that may be applied to blood following collection to confer broad protection against multiple infectious agents.[8] Many of these technologies are effective across different classes of pathogens (eg, viruses, bacteria, and parasites), offering the ability to interdict agents that are known to be transfusion transmissible as well as emerging pathogens that pose uncertain risks to the blood supply (**Table 2**).

The appeal of PR is that it is a proactive approach that inactivates pathogens instead of only screening for their presence. PR technologies broadly destroy pathogens by targeting their genetic material or cell membranes. Proponents also argue that PR could replace some of the current infectious disease testing and could reduce the number of donor deferrals due to disease risk factors. PR also prevents transfusion-associated graft-versus-host disease (TA-GVHD) by blocking leukocyte proliferation. PR technologies may therefore replace gamma- or X-ray irradiation for abrogating TA-GVHD.[9,10]

At this time, 3 different methodologies of photochemical activation have been developed: INTERCEPT (psoralen/UV-A), Mirasol (riboflavin/UV-B), and Theraflex (UV-C). This article focuses on the first 2 more extensively studied processes. Thus far, PR has only been applied to platelets, because of the heightened contamination risk, and plasma. RBCs present an obstacle due to hemoglobin's light absorption; although a different non-light-dependent PR process is being investigated for RBCs, it is not currently approved.[11]

Table 2
Blood product screening, testing, and treatments to improve safety

Method	Donor Questionnaire	Laboratory Screening Tests	Pathogen Reduction Technology	Solvent/Detergent Technique
Targeted organisms	• General infection (fever) • Malaria, dengue, chikungunya (travel history) • Prion diseases (residence in Europe) • Risk factors (incarceration, intravenous drug use, prostitution, close contact with infected people)	• HIV • HBV • HCV • HTLV • West Nile virus • Chagas • Syphilis • Zika • Babesia (certain regions) • Bacteria (only platelets)	• Broad activity against viruses, bacteria, parasites (results vary slightly among 3 most studied platforms)	• Enveloped viruses
Limitations	Broad screening tool, but lacks sensitivity and specificity	High sensitivity and specificity, but does not detect emerging diseases	Breakthrough infections due to spore-forming bacteria or fast-growers is possible	Nonenveloped viruses (hepatitis A, parvovirus B19) are relatively resistant

INTERCEPT

INTERCEPT (Cerus, Concord, CA, USA) is widely used for platelets and plasma. It has been approved in the European Union and United States; it is the only FDA-approved PR process at this time.[12,13] INTERCEPT is effective against viruses, bacteria, and protozoans. However, breakthrough transmission has been reported with naked viruses and certain spore-forming and/or fast-growing bacteria.[14,15] The technique uses amotosalen, which can intercalate between DNA bases. Upon UV-A light activation, this molecule irreversibly cross-links with the DNA, thus preventing transcription and cellular reproduction.[16] After INTERCEPT treatment, an adsorption step removes excess amotosalen, leaving only a minute residual amount.[17] Extensive animal studies have shown no toxicologically relevant effects of platelet concentrates prepared by this technology; the residual amount is much lower than the toxic threshold.[18,19]

Among published studies with INTERCEPT platelets, few children are included. Rasonglès and colleagues[20] reported on the use of such platelets in Ile de la Réunion during a Chikungunya epidemic. Over the course of 1 year, 1950 INTERCEPT platelets were transfused to 224 adults, 51 children (1–18 years), and 41 infants (<1 year). Adverse event and acute transfusion reaction occurrences were higher in children than adults (2.7% and 1.6%, compared with 0.4% and 0.1%, respectively) and predominantly classified as grade 1 severity. No infants experienced adverse events or reactions. No sepsis, acute lung injury, or death occurred as a result of transfusion. More recently, a large European prospective hemovigilance study of INTERCEPT-treated platelets following 19,175 transfusions in 2441 patients demonstrated a low incidence of acute transfusion reactions and a safety profile comparable with conventional platelet components. Only 46 of the patients were neonates (<28 days of age), whereas 242 were children (<18 years of age). No adverse events occurred in the neonatal patients. Pediatric patients experienced similar rates of acute transfusion reactions (3.7%, $P = .179$) and severe adverse events (0.4%, $P = .550$) compared with adults. None of the latter was judged to be related to INTERCEPT-treated platelets.[21]

Following FDA approval, Cerus is performing a postmarketing active surveillance study entitled the Phase IV INTERCEPT Platelets Entering Routine use (PIPER) Study. PIPER is a prospective, open-label study designed to evaluate the transfusion of conventional and INTERCEPT-treated platelets in hematology/oncology patients including children and will monitor outcomes related to respiratory adverse events.[22] The PIPER design arose in part due to increased rates of lung injury in patients who received treated platelets in a randomized controlled trial.[23] Long-term longitudinal studies have not been conducted.

MIRASOL

The Mirasol system (TerumoBCT, Lakewood, CO, USA) uses riboflavin as a photosensitizer compound with UV-B light. Riboflavin readily traverses lipid membranes and then intercalates nonspecifically with nucleic acids. Upon exposure to UV-B light, intercalated riboflavin modifies guanine residues and promotes the generation of oxygen radicals.[24–26] Because riboflavin and its by-products are naturally occurring, no additional steps for removal following treatment are thought to be necessary.[27] Mirasol has shown efficacy against a wide variety of pathogens that pose a risk of transfusion transmission.[12,26,28,29]

The single full-length publication describing the use of PR platelets in children included only 51 patients receiving 141 Mirasol platelets and 86 controls receiving 291 control platelets (100% plasma or 40% plasma and 60% additive solution [SSP1, MacoPharma, Lyon, France]) who were retrospectively compared at a single center.[30] The study and control groups were similar with respect to age (mean 11 years), type of cancer diagnosis, and mean number of transfused platelet doses (2.3×10^{11} platelets/μL). Measures of transfusion efficacy and rates of adverse events were similar between the 2 groups, although the small study may not have provided enough power to detect a difference.

Regarding clinical effectiveness of the 2 systems described above, a Cochrane review that evaluated 12 randomized control trials of pathogen-reduced platelets (9 with INTERCEPT, 3 with Mirasol) showed no difference in clinically significant bleeding or severe bleeding between recipients of pathogen-reduced platelets compared with control platelets. The studies included a total of 2075 patients. When evaluated, all-cause mortality, product utilization, and adverse events were also not increased.[31] Children younger than 16 years accounted for 5% of the total study populations.

TerumoBCT is currently sponsoring the MIPLATE (Efficacy of Mirasol-treated Apheresis Platelets in Patients With Hypoproliferative Thrombocytopenia) study, which is a prospective, randomized controlled noninferiority study comparing Mirasol-treated to standard apheresis platelets. The primary outcome measure is the number of days of grade 2 or higher bleeding up to 28 days following the first transfusion or until transfusion independence. Adults and children (>10 kg in weight) requiring 2 or more platelet transfusions will undergo daily bleeding assessments.[32]

PATHOGEN REDUCTION: CAUSE FOR CONCERN IN CHILDREN?

Children and neonates may particularly be at risk of transfusion complications because of lower total blood volume, immature immune systems, and susceptibility to metabolic derangements from additives. Patients with hematologic or oncologic disorders, as well as those receiving massive blood transfusions, will have even higher exposures. In addition, younger recipients are at risk of long-term effects due to ongoing neurocognitive development and the longest life expectancy after medical intervention. Long-term outcomes from possible genotoxicity, carcinogenesis, exocrine disruption, or metabolic dysfunction arising from blood product modification and manipulation therefore are of concern to some transfusion practitioners.

In humans, photosensitizing psoralen and psoralen-derivative compounds have been used in ultraviolet (psoralen UV-A [PUVA]) treatments for psoriasis and in extracorporeal photopheresis (ECP). A Swedish study of mothers treated with PUVA therapy during pregnancy (504 infants born to mothers treated before pregnancy and 14 infants born to mothers treated during pregnancy) found no congenital malformations in the 14 exposed to PUVA in utero and a rate of 3.6% of those with mothers exposed before pregnancy, which is lower than the population norm of 4.8%.[33] ECP uses 8-methoxypsoralen (methoxsalen), a compound similar but not identical to the amotosalen in INTERCEPT. It is FDA approved for treatment of refractory cutaneous T-cell lymphoma, but is also used extensively off-label for GVHD, including in children. Despite regular clinical use, a 2015 Cochrane review confirmed that there are no randomized controlled trials of ECP in pediatric patients assessing either its efficacy or its harmful effects. Therefore, current understanding is based only on retrospective and observational studies.[34] Contraindications to ECP and methoxsalen exposure include aphakia, systemic lupus erythematosus, and diseases causing photosensitivity (eg, porphyria, xeroderma pigmentosum, and albinism), suggesting phototherapy in conjunction with psoralen exposure may be contraindicated. Neonatologists have raised theoretic concerns about photosensitization exacerbation in neonates receiving both photochemically treated blood products and phototherapy.

As PR technology has become more widely available, multiple studies have reported an increased risk of platelet refractoriness secondary to human leukocyte antigens alloimmunization in patients receiving pathogen-inactivated platelet concentrates. Most observations have been described with use of the INTERCEPT system, although similar findings were also noted in a Mirasol study,[35] and alloimmunization rates continue to be monitored as secondary outcomes in ongoing clinical trials. The exact cause is unclear, although higher rates of alloimmunization may be related to smaller posttransfusion increments and therefore increased numbers of platelet transfusions and donor exposures in patients receiving PR versus standard platelets. Increased demand for platelet products may strain the blood supply's ability to support patient need.

In addition, PR implementation brings additional complexity and costs.[36,37] These estimates depend on whether other infectious disease screening tests can be eliminated due to redundancy. Although costs will be lower if PR is not universally implemented, transfusion services will then be challenged with dual inventories and the need to triage products to different patients.

On the other hand, proponents argue that children and neonates have much to gain from these technologies if they can protect against blood-borne infections that might cause severe sequelae. The use of PR blood products is slowly increasing throughout the world. The benefits of reduction in transfusion-transmitted pathogens through PR must be weighed against the potential toxicities of the technologies. As the United States and other parts of the world are contemplating bringing in PR products into their inventory, transfusion medicine groups must grapple with questions about the safety of the products.

PLATELET ADDITIVE SOLUTIONS: REDUCTION OF TRANSFUSION REACTIONS

PAS were developed in the 1980s. Their composition varies depending on the manufacturer. Some formulations improve the duration of allowable platelet storage.[38] The appeal of PAS solution is that by reducing plasma content by about 65% in the platelet product, the incidence of allergic reactions (due to donor allergens in plasma) and immune hemolytic anemia (due to donor isohemagglutinins in incompatible plasma) is reduced. In addition, the replacement of plasma by PAS increases the availability of plasma for other purposes, such as fractionation.[39] PAS also help mitigate platelet damage caused by PR techniques, for example, by providing additional buffering capacity upon introduction of the chemical, amotosalen.

Corrected count increments, a quantitative measure of platelet effectiveness, have generally been lower in PAS platelets, but newer solutions appear to have closed the gap.[39] There is scarce information available on bleeding differences between patients receiving various platelet products. Platelets in PAS appear more susceptible to bacterial contamination, possibly because of removal of bactericidal plasma proteins.[39] However, faster growth likely improves the chances that a contaminated unit will be detected, quarantined, and discarded. Theoretically, the depletion of plasma and associated clotting factors could have a deleterious effect on coagulopathic patients receiving PAS platelets.[40] This effect would be particularly pronounced in patients receiving massive transfusions whereby the entire volume of blood is replaced by transfused products.

Similar concerns apply to smaller patients as well. Despite increasing availability of PAS in the United States, the efficacy and safety in neonates or pediatric patients have not been widely published with a few exceptions analyzing small sample sizes.[41,42]

HEMOGLOBIN-BASED OXYGEN CARRIERS: AN ALTERNATIVE WHEN BLOOD IS NOT AVAILABLE

Hemoglobin-based oxygen carriers (HBOCs) initially garnered interest during the human immunodeficiency virus (HIV) crisis of the 1980s as a potentially safer alternative to the blood supply. Infectious disease screening and testing have since markedly improved. However, in certain settings such as the military, there is growing recognition of the limitations of donated blood, including stringent storage conditions, storage lesion development, short shelf-lives (especially platelets), and need for pretransfusion compatibility testing.[43] In the civilian population, blood substitute use may benefit Jehovah's Witnesses, who refuse blood transfusions, or patients with multiple antibodies to high-frequency antigens (eg, sickle cell disease), for whom it is challenging to find compatible blood.

Cell-free hemoglobin presents the advantage of minimal antigenicity and the ability to off-load oxygen in plasma more efficiently because of the lack of interference from the cell membrane.[43] Unfortunately, free hemoglobin is a nitric oxide (NO) scavenger, lacks 2,3-diphosphoglycerate to facilitate oxygen release to tissue, and can also alter blood osmolarity, leading to fluid shifts. In the absence of a cell membrane, free hemoglobin tetramers rapidly disintegrate and undergo clearance from the bloodstream through the kidneys. It should be noted that free hemoglobin is nephrotoxic. Stabilization efforts have been attempted through chemical modification and macromeric bioconjugation (eg, with polyethylene glycol [PEG]). Enzymatic attachments aim to prevent iron auto-oxidation, because this can catalyze further redox reactions associated with subsequent globin dysfunction and instability. Encapsulated HBOC systems aim to mimic the RBC environment.

No HBOCs are clinically FDA approved for human applications in the United States at this time. Several human trials conducted in a variety of indications, including trauma and elective surgeries, have provided mixed results. Of note, a large meta-analysis, published in 2008, of 16 clinical trials investigating 5 different RBC surrogates found that HBOCs were associated with higher rates of myocardial ischemia and death.[44] These adverse events have been attributed in part to scavenging of NO by free hemoglobin, which leads to vasoconstriction and blood pressure elevation. Additional mechanisms include oversupply of oxygen and heme-mediated oxidative reactions.[45] As a result of these findings, HBOC research and development slowed considerably.

Other researchers have argued that the meta-analysis had drawbacks, such as comparing several compounds with different concentrations and properties, including data from non-peer-reviewed sources, and using flawed mortality analysis. Mackenzie and colleagues[46] also highlight major physiologic differences between HBOCs and RBCs that should be taken into account when evaluating effectiveness. For example, HBOCs contain 13 g/dL of iron compared with 25 to 30 g/dL in RBCs. Thus, similar doses of the 2 would not be expected to provide comparable oxygen delivery.

Currently, HBOC availability for transfusion is limited to FDA-approved expanded access. In recent years, HBOC applications have also evolved into using them for ex vivo preservation and oxygen perfusion of transplant tissues and organs. HBOCs may help patients for whom allogeneic blood is not available. Patients with sickle cell disease and other aplastic and hemolytic anemias often require transfusions, which may be complicated by alloimmunization or hyperhemolysis syndrome. In the latter scenario, a dangerous immune response occurs whereby the recipient destroys both transfused and autologous cells, leading to precipitous decrements in hemoglobin below pretransfusion levels.[47] In addition to minimal immunogenicity, HBOCs

Table 3
Summary of selected hemoglobin-based oxygen carriers

Brand Name	Manufacturer	Product Description	Approval/Trial Status	References
SANGUINATE	Prolong Pharmaceuticals (South Plainfield, NJ, USA)	PEGylated bovine carboxy-hemoglobin	Phase 2 clinical trials underway; available for expanded access only	DeSimone et al,[56] 2018
Hemopure (HBOC-201)	HbO$_2$ Therapeutics (Souderton, PA, USA) (previously Biopure)	Cell-free polymerized bovine hemoglobin	Approved in South Africa; phase 3 clinical trial in United States; available for expanded access only	Davis et al,[50] 2018; Weiskopf et al,[57] 2017
Hemolink	LPBP Inc (Toronto, Canada)	o-Raffinose cross-linked human hemoglobin	Phase 2 (suspended)	[58]
PolyHeme	Northfield Laboratories (Evanston, IL, USA) (defunct)	Polymerized HBOC manufactured from expired human blood	Phase 3	Dube et al,[59] 2017
Hemospan	Sangart Inc (San Diego, CA, USA)	Oxygenated PEG-modified human hemoglobin	Phase 2	Olofsson et al,[60] 2011
HEMOXYCarrier	Hemarina (Morlaix, France)	Large-molecular-weight extracellular hemoglobin isolated from marine invertebrates	Animal studies	Le Gall et al,[61] 2014

exhibit smaller molecular sizes, which could facilitate their ability to deliver oxygen despite vessel narrowing or obstruction. On the other hand, hemoglobin S has decreased oxidative stability and higher rates of auto-oxidization. Concerns exist about whether HBOCs would accelerate this detrimental oxidation process, making their use in sickle cell disease questionable.

Clinical studies of various HBOCs are underway at different stages (**Table 3**). SANGUINATE, a purified bovine hemoglobin conjugated with PEG residues and ligated to carbon monoxide, has completed a phase 1 trial in which 3 cohorts of 8 healthy volunteers received single ascending doses (80, 120, or 160 mg/kg, respectively) without adverse events. A phase 1b study completed in stable patients with sickle cell disease demonstrated an acceptable safety profile.[48] Hemopure, a polymerized bovine hemoglobin (also known as HBOC-201), has been studied in adult patients with sickle cell disease who were not in crisis (n = 18). None experienced toxicity, and there was significant improvement in heart rate response to aerobic exercise workload. Case reports have also described HBOC-201 use in critically ill patients during sickle cell crisis and in a Jehovah's Witness patient with critical anemia and cardiac hypoxia.[49,50] A clinical trial investigating the use of HBOC-201 in patients aged 18 to 80 years with life-threatening anemia for whom allogeneic blood is not an option is underway.[51] Of note, HBOCs have been reported to interfere with certain laboratory analyzers, including hemoglobin quantification, which can complicate monitoring in patients.[52]

SUMMARY

Several new blood products and derivatives are under investigation or have recently been introduced for clinical use and aim to improve the safety profile of blood by mitigating infectious and noninfectious complications. Blood collection centers and national blood services are attempting to estimate and prepare for the impacts of additional costs, process complexities, and potential increased platelet demand. Although adult studies have demonstrated advantages, the lack of pediatric data renders it challenging to weigh risks and benefits in this vulnerable population. As newer technologies, in particular PR, become more widespread, short- and long-term monitoring of pediatric transfusion recipients remains extremely important to detect adverse events.

REFERENCES

1. Oakley FD, Woods M, Arnold S, et al. Transfusion reactions in pediatric compared with adult patients: a look at rate, reaction type, and associated products. Transfusion 2015;55:563–70.
2. Hong H, Xiao W, Lazarus HM, et al. Detection of septic transfusion reactions to platelet transfusions by active and passive surveillance. Blood 2016;127:496–502.
3. Dumont LJ, Kleinman S, Murphy JR, et al. Screening of single-donor apheresis platelets for bacterial contamination: the PASSPORT study results. Transfusion 2010;50:589–99.
4. Eder AF, Kennedy JM, Dy BA, et al. Bacterial screening of apheresis platelets and the residual risk of septic transfusion reactions: the American Red Cross experience (2004-2006). Transfusion 2007;47:1134–42.
5. Bloch EM, Marshall CE, Boyd JS, et al. Implementation of secondary bacterial culture testing of platelets to mitigate residual risk of septic transfusion reactions. Transfusion 2018;58:1647–53.

6. FDA. Draft guidance for industry: bacterial risk control strategies for blood collection establishments and transfusion serivces to enhance the safety and availability of platelets for transfusion [monograph on the internet]. Silver Spring (MD): Center for Biologics Evaluation and Research, Food and Drug Administration; 2016. Available at: https://www.fda.gov/downloads/BiologicsBloodVaccines/GuidanceComplianceRegulatoryInformation/Guidances/Blood/UCM425952.pdf.

7. Dunbar NM, Dumont LJ, Szczepiorkowski ZM. How do we implement Day 6 and Day 7 platelets at a hospital-based transfusion service? Transfusion 2016;56: 1262–6.

8. Webert KE, Cserti CM, Hannon J, et al. Proceedings of a Consensus Conference: pathogen inactivation-making decisions about new technologies. Transfus Med Rev 2008;22:1–34.

9. Ooley PW, editor. Standards for blood banks and transfusion services. 31st edition. Bethesda (MD): AABB Press; 2018.

10. Kleinman S, Stassinopoulos A. Transfusion-associated graft-versus-host disease reexamined: potential for improved prevention using a universally applied intervention. Transfusion 2018;58(11):2545–63.

11. Brixner V, Kiessling AH, Madlener K, et al. Red blood cells treated with the amustaline (S-303) pathogen reduction system: a transfusion study in cardiac surgery. Transfusion 2018;58:905–16.

12. Musso D, Richard V, Broult J, et al. Inactivation of dengue virus in plasma with amotosalen and ultraviolet A illumination. Transfusion 2014;54:2924–30.

13. Irsch J, Seghatchian J. Update on pathogen inactivation treatment of plasma, with the INTERCEPT Blood System: current position on methodological, clinical and regulatory aspects. Transfus Apher Sci 2015;52:240–4.

14. Hauser L, Roque-Afonso AM, Beyloune A, et al. Hepatitis E transmission by transfusion of Intercept blood system-treated plasma. Blood 2014;123:796–7.

15. Schmidt M, Hourfar MK, Sireis W, et al. Evaluation of the effectiveness of a pathogen inactivation technology against clinically relevant transfusion-transmitted bacterial strains. Transfusion 2015;55:2104–12.

16. Kaiser-Guignard J, Canellini G, Lion N, et al. The clinical and biological impact of new pathogen inactivation technologies on platelet concentrates. Blood Rev 2014;28:235–41.

17. Ciaravino V, McCullough T, Cimino G. The role of toxicology assessment in transfusion medicine. Transfusion 2003;43:1481–92.

18. Ciaravi V, McCullough T, Dayan AD. Pharmacokinetic and toxicology assessment of INTERCEPT (S-59 and UVA treated) platelets. Hum Exp Toxicol 2001;20: 533–50.

19. Ciaravino V, Hanover J, Lin L, et al. Assessment of safety in neonates for transfusion of platelets and plasma prepared with amotosalen photochemical pathogen inactivation treatment by a 1-month intravenous toxicity study in neonatal rats. Transfusion 2009;49:985–94.

20. Rasonglès P, Angelini-Tibert MF, Simon P, et al. Transfusion of platelet components prepared with photochemical pathogen inactivation treatment during a Chikungunya virus epidemic in Ile de La Reunion. Transfusion 2009;49:1083–91.

21. Knutson F, Osselaer J, Pierelli L, et al. A prospective, active haemovigilance study with combined cohort analysis of 19,175 transfusions of platelet components prepared with amotosalen-UVA photochemical treatment. Vox Sang 2015;109:343–52.

22. Rico S, Carter K, Benjamin RJ, et al. Piper study rationale and design: characterizing the incidence of acute respiratory distress syndrome in hematology-

oncology patients following the transfusion of conventional or pathogen-reduced platelet components. Biol Blood Marrow Transplant 2016;22:S173–4.

23. Snyder E, McCullough J, Slichter SJ, et al. Clinical safety of platelets photochemically treated with amotosalen HCl and ultraviolet A light for pathogen inactivation: the SPRINT trial. Transfusion 2005;45:1864–75.

24. Cardo LJ, Salata J, Mendez J, et al. Pathogen inactivation of Trypanosoma cruzi in plasma and platelet concentrates using riboflavin and ultraviolet light. Transfus Apher Sci 2007;37:131–7.

25. Li J, de Korte D, Woolum MD, et al. Pathogen reduction of buffy coat platelet concentrates using riboflavin and light: comparisons with pathogen-reduction technology-treated apheresis platelet products. Vox Sang 2004;87:82–90.

26. Goodrich RP, Edrich RA, Li J, et al. The Mirasol PRT system for pathogen reduction of platelets and plasma: an overview of current status and future trends. Transfus Apher Sci 2006;35:5–17.

27. Perez-Pujol S, Tonda R, Lozano M, et al. Effects of a new pathogen-reduction technology (Mirasol PRT) on functional aspects of platelet concentrates. Transfusion 2005;45:911–9.

28. Prowse CV. Component pathogen inactivation: a critical review. Vox Sang 2013; 104:183–99.

29. Aubry M, Richard V, Green J, et al. Inactivation of Zika virus in plasma with amotosalen and ultraviolet A illumination. Transfusion 2016;56:33–40.

30. Trakhtman P, Karpova O, Balashov D, et al. Efficacy and safety of pathogen-reduced platelet concentrates in children with cancer: a retrospective cohort study. Transfusion 2016;56(Suppl 1):S24–8.

31. Estcourt LJ, Malouf R, Murphy MF. Pathogen-reduced platelets for the prevention of bleeding in people of any age. JAMA Oncol 2018;4:571–2.

32. Efficacy of mirasol-treated apheresis platelets in patients with hypoproliferative thrombocytopenia (MIPLATE) [monograph on the internet]. Available at: https://www.clinicaltrials.gov/ct2/show/NCT02964325. Accessed October 27, 2018.

33. Gunnarskog JG, Kallen AJ, Lindelof BG, et al. Psoralen photochemotherapy (PUVA) and pregnancy. Arch Dermatol 1993;129:320–3.

34. Weitz M, Strahm B, Meerpohl JJ, et al. Extracorporeal photopheresis versus alternative treatment for chronic graft-versus-host disease after haematopoietic stem cell transplantation in paediatric patients. Cochrane Database Syst Rev 2015;(12):CD009898.

35. Estcourt LJ, Malouf R, Hopewell S, et al. Pathogen-reduced platelets for the prevention of bleeding. Cochrane Database Syst Rev 2017;(7):CD009072.

36. Cicchetti A, Coretti S, Sacco F, et al. Budget impact of implementing platelet pathogen reduction into the Italian blood transfusion system. Blood Transfus 2018;16(6):483–9.

37. Prioli KM, Karp JK, Lyons NM, et al. Economic implications of pathogen reduced and bacterially tested platelet components: a US Hospital budget impact model. Appl Health Econ Health Policy 2018;16(6):889–99.

38. Slichter SJ, Corson J, Jones MK, et al. Exploratory studies of extended storage of apheresis platelets in a platelet additive solution (PAS). Blood 2014;123:271–80.

39. van der Meer PF, de Korte D. Platelet additive solutions: a review of the latest developments and their clinical implications. Transfus Med Hemother 2018;45:98–102.

40. Mays JA, Hess JR. Modelling the effects of blood component storage lesions on the quality of haemostatic resuscitation in massive transfusion for trauma. Blood Transfus 2017;15:153–7.

41. Honohan A, van't Ende E, Hulzebos C, et al. Posttransfusion platelet increments after different platelet products in neonates: a retrospective cohort study. Transfusion 2013;53:3100–9.

42. Yanagisawa R, Shimodaira S, Kojima S, et al. Replaced platelet concentrates containing a new additive solution, M-sol: safety and efficacy for pediatric patients. Transfusion 2013;53:2053–60.

43. Gupta AS. 2017 military supplement: hemoglobin-based oxygen carriers: current state-of-the-art and novel molecules. Shock 2017. [Epub ahead of print].

44. Natanson C, Kern SJ, Lurie P, et al. Cell-free hemoglobin-based blood substitutes and risk of myocardial infarction and death: a meta-analysis. JAMA 2008;299: 2304–12.

45. Alayash AI. Hemoglobin-based blood substitutes and the treatment of sickle cell disease: more harm than help? Biomolecules 2017;7 [pii:E2].

46. Mackenzie CF, Pitman AN, Hodgson RE, et al. Are hemoglobin-based oxygen carriers being withheld because of regulatory requirement for equivalence to packed red blood cells? Am J Ther 2015;22:e115–21.

47. Danaee A, Inusa B, Howard J, et al. Hyperhemolysis in patients with hemoglobinopathies: a single-center experience and review of the literature. Transfus Med Rev 2015;29:220–30.

48. Misra H, Bainbridge J, Berryman J, et al. A Phase Ib open label, randomized, safety study of SANGUINATE™ in patients with sickle cell anemia. Rev Bras Hematol Hemoter 2016;39:20–7.

49. Fitzgerald MC, Chan JY, Ross AW, et al. A synthetic haemoglobin-based oxygen carrier and the reversal of cardiac hypoxia secondary to severe anaemia following trauma. Med J Aust 2011;194:471–3.

50. Davis JM, El-Haj N, Shah NN, et al. Use of the blood substitute HBOC-201 in critically ill patients during sickle crisis: a three-case series. Transfusion 2018;58: 132–7.

51. HBOC-201 expanded access protocol for life-threatening anemia for whom allogeneic blood transfusion is not an option [monograph on the internet]. Available at: https://www.clinicaltrials.gov/ct2/show/NCT02934282. Accessed October 27, 2018.

52. Korte EA, Pozzi N, Wardrip N, et al. Analytical interference of HBOC-201 (Hemopure, a synthetic hemoglobin-based oxygen carrier) on four common clinical chemistry platforms. Clin Chim Acta 2018;482:33–9.

53. Stramer SL, Krysztof DE, Brodsky JP, et al. Comparative analysis of triplex nucleic acid test assays in United States blood donors. Transfusion 2013;53:2525–37.

54. Zou S, Dorsey KA, Notari EP, et al. Prevalence, incidence, and residual risk of human immunodeficiency virus and hepatitis C virus infections among United States blood donors since the introduction of nucleic acid testing. Transfusion 2010;50:1495–504.

55. Katz L, Dodd R. Transfusion-transmitted diseases. In: Shaz BH, Hillyer CD, Roshal M, et al, editors. Transfusion medicine and hemostasis, clinical and laboratory aspects. 2nd edition. Philadelphia: Elsevier; 2013.

56. DeSimone RA, Berlin DA, Avecilla ST, et al. Investigational use of PEGylated carboxyhemoglobin bovine in a Jehovah's Witness with hemorrhagic shock. Transfusion 2018;58:2297–300.

57. Weiskopf RB, Beliaev AM, Shander A, et al. Addressing the unmet need of life-threatening anemia with hemoglobin-based oxygen carriers. Transfusion 2017; 57:207–14.

58. Phase II Study To Evaluate The Safety and Efficacy of Hemoglobin Raffimer in Patients Undergoing First Time CABG Surgery [monograph on the internet]. 2018. Available at: https://www.clinicaltrials.gov/ct2/show/NCT00038454. Accessed October 27, 2018.

59. Dube GP, Pitman AN, Mackenzie CF. Relative efficacies of HBOC-201 and polyheme to increase oxygen transport compared to blood and crystalloids. "2017 Military Supplement". Shock 2017. [Epub ahead of print].

60. Olofsson CI, Gorecki AZ, Dirksen R, et al. Evaluation of MP4OX for prevention of perioperative hypotension in patients undergoing primary hip arthroplasty with spinal anesthesia: a randomized, double-blind, multicenter study. Anesthesiology 2011;114:1048–63.

61. Le Gall T, Polard V, Rousselot M, et al. In vivo biodistribution and oxygenation potential of a new generation of oxygen carrier. J Biotechnol 2014;187:1–9.

Updates in Neonatal Hematology

Causes, Risk Factors, and Management of Anemia and Thrombocytopenia

Isabelle M.C. Ree, MD[a,b], Enrico Lopriore, MD, PhD[a,*]

KEYWORDS

- Anemia • Thrombocytopenia • Erythrocytes • Platelets • Transfusion

KEY POINTS

- There is no international consensus regarding red blood cell and platelet transfusion thresholds, resulting in widely varying practices.
- The identification of suitable biomarkers for red blood cell and platelet transfusion may contribute to a more individualized and effective transfusion practice.
- Two large randomized controlled trials (ETTNO and TOP) are currently assessing safe and effective red blood cell transfusion thresholds, taking into account long-term neurodevelopment.
- A recent randomized controlled trial showed that restrictive platelet transfusion may be preferable to liberal guidelines in preterm neonates with thrombocytopenia.
- Prevention of neonatal anemia can partly be achieved using delayed cord clamping and by minimizing iatrogenic blood loss.

INTRODUCTION

Anemia and thrombocytopenia are common hematologic disorders in neonates, particularly in (very) preterm neonates. Blood products, either red blood cells (RBC) or platelets to correct anemia and thrombocytopenia, respectively, are frequently administered in neonates admitted to neonatal intensive care units (NICU). With the advances in neonatal care and related increase of survival of neonates and especially of preterm neonates, the overall rate of transfusions has increased exponentially over the last years.[1]

Disclosures: The authors have no financial support or relationships that may pose potential conflict of interest. No honorarium, grant, or other form of payment was given to anyone to produce the article.

[a] Department of Pediatrics, Division of Neonatology, Leiden University Medical Center, Albinusdreef 2, 2333 ZA Leiden, Zuid-Holland, the Netherlands; [b] Center for Clinical Transfusion Research, Sanquin Research, Plesmanlaan 1A, 2333 BZ Leiden, Zuid-Holland, the Netherlands
* Corresponding author.
E-mail address: e.lopriore@lumc.nl

Hematol Oncol Clin N Am 33 (2019) 521–532
https://doi.org/10.1016/j.hoc.2019.01.013
0889-8588/19/© 2019 Elsevier Inc. All rights reserved.

hemonc.theclinics.com

Up to 90% of (very) low-birth-weight and/or (very) preterm neonates require at least one RBC transfusion during admission due to anemia,[1,2] whereas thrombocytopenia is reported to occur in 20% to 35% of neonates admitted to a NICU, with again even higher incidences in the more fragile subpopulations of preterm neonates.[2–4] Anemia and thrombocytopenia are traditionally treated with transfusions. However, current transfusion practices are heavily discussed, not so much because of safety issues (blood products in developed countries are nowadays in general considered safe), but mostly in regard to effectiveness and the optimal transfusion thresholds. Transfusion thresholds are largely based on expert opinion rather than scientific evidence, and the great variance in available transfusion guidelines reflects the lack of consensus on this topic.

This review aims to provide a brief overview of the causes, risk factors, and management of neonatal anemia and thrombocytopenia, focusing mainly on the recent developments in transfusion practices and outlining several expected future developments.

ANEMIA
Causes and Risk Factors

Anemia is defined as a hemoglobin level below the lower limit of the reference range adjusted for age and is a common finding in neonatal populations. All neonates show a physiologic postnatal decline in hemoglobin in the first weeks after birth, resulting in varying degrees of (relative) anemia. In term infants, hemoglobin levels decrease from 14.6 to 22.5 g/dL at birth to 10.0 to 12.0 g/dL by 8 to 10 weeks of age, the physiologic nadir. Thereafter, hemoglobin levels gradually increase toward adult hemoglobin values within the first 2 years of life. This physiologic anemia, or "early anemia of infancy," is more pronounced in preterm and low-birth-weight neonates than in term neonates. It is a reflection of the transition from fetal hemoglobin with a high oxygen affinity, because the fetal circulation is relatively hypoxic, to adult hemoglobin after birth and a transitional decline in plasma erythropoietin (EPO).[5]

Nevertheless, the physiologic hemoglobin decline after birth is not the main cause of anemia in hospitalized neonates. Its effect is outweighed by nonphysiologic factors, such as obstetric complications, clinical conditions, such as sepsis, inadequate nutrition, and cardiorespiratory disease, and in particular, iatrogenic blood loss accompanying frequent laboratory testing. Estimates of iatrogenic blood loss due to laboratory testing in the NICU in the first 6 weeks of life vary, but may amount up to 15% to 30% of an infant's total blood volume. Neonatal anemia can also be caused by conditions such as HDFN caused by maternal erythrocyte antibodies against the various blood group systems.[5,6]

Treatment: Erythrocyte Transfusions

Thresholds
There is no international consensus regarding optimal hemoglobin thresholds for RBC transfusions. A summary of guidelines is shown in **Table 1**, stressing the great international variation in transfusion hemoglobin thresholds. Symptomatic signs of anemia, such as apnea, bradycardia, and increased oxygen need, often occur when there is an imbalance between oxygen consumption and delivery.[7] These symptoms are nonspecific, and simultaneous conditions, including sepsis and lung conditions, may obscure the symptomatic course of anemia. The hemoglobin level at which these symptoms occur is therefore not well defined and is also likely to vary between neonates of similar and varying gestational ages.

Table 1
Overview of international guidelines for red blood cell transfusions

Postnatal week	British Committee for Standards in Haematology 2016[50]		Australian National Blood Authority 2016[51]		Canadian Blood Services 2017[52]		Dutch Guidelines Quality Council (Concept) 2018[53]	
	Respiratory support[a]	No respiratory support	Respiratory support	No respiratory support	Respiratory support	No respiratory support	Respiratory support	No respiratory support
Week 1	10–12 g/dL	<10 g/dL	11–13 g/dL	10–12 g/dL	<11.5 g/dL	<10 g/dL	<11.5 g/dL	<10 g/dL
Week 2	9.5–10 g/dL	<7.5 g/dL	10–12.5 g/dL	8.5–11 g/dL	<10 g/dL	<8.5 g/dL	<10 g/dL	<8.5 g/dL
Week ≥3	8.5–10 g/dL	<7.5 g/dL	8.5–11 g/dL	7–10 g/dL	<8.5 g/dL	<7.5 g/dL	<8.5 g/dL	<7.5 g/dL

[a] For example, supplemental oxygen, high-flow nasal cannula, CPAP (continuous positive airway pressure), positive-pressure ventilation.

The decision to transfuse is made based on clinical judgment of the caregiver and national or local guidelines. Reviews have reported on the variation in guidelines and postulated hemoglobin thresholds between and within countries and geographic areas.[8,9] To date, only a few randomized controlled trials compared different transfusion hemoglobin thresholds in very low-birth-weight neonates (<1000 g) in regard to safety and effectiveness. As shown in the latest Cochrane review,[10] no significant differences were found between liberal and restrictive transfusion groups, on both short- and long-term outcome parameters. In terms of noninferiority, this would favor a restrictive attitude toward transfusion in clinically stable patients, but conclusions have to be drawn cautiously. Comparison of these trials and adequate interpretation of their results are complicated because these trials did not use the same definitions of "liberal" and "restrictive" in terms of RBC transfusion, which resulted in a variety of hemoglobin thresholds. Two ongoing trials in this field may shed further light in the near future on the safety and effectiveness of liberal versus restrictive thresholds for RBC transfusions. The transfusion of prematures (TOP trial; NCT01702805) will include 1824 low-birth-weight infants, and the primary outcome is death or significant neurodevelopment impairment in surviving infants at 22 to 26 months of age. The study is expected to complete at the end of 2019 (including the long-term assessment). The ETTNO trial (effects of transfusion thresholds on neurocognitive outcome of extremely low-birth-weight infants; NCT01393496) will include 920 very low-birth-weight infants, and the primary outcome measure of this study is death or significant neurodevelopmental impairment determined at 24 months of age. As the study recently reached completion, the results are expected in the course of 2019.

Transfusion markers

A major step toward reaching consensus on clearly defined transfusion thresholds may be the identification of better markers for anemia and the need of transfusion.[11] Currently, decisions are based on a combination of clinical signs, laboratory findings, such as hemoglobin levels, and cardiorespiratory or ventilation status. The relationship between pretransfusion peripheral hemoglobin values and actual tissue perfusion and oxygenation has been questioned,[12,13] whereas other markers of oxygenation and perfusion have gained much interest. Serum lactate, for example, is an end product of anaerobic metabolism and decreases significantly after transfusion.[14] However, lactate is also elevated in conditions, such as sepsis and asphyxia, and may therefore be too nonspecific for clinical use. Various other laboratory and bedside measures are under investigation as potential markers of anemia in neonates. A tool of particular interest due to its noninvasive nature is near-infrared spectroscopy (NIRS), which measures regional tissue oxygen saturation by using the difference in light absorption of oxygenated and deoxygenated hemoglobin. NIRS has mostly been evaluated in neonates for cerebral measurements with encouraging results,[15] but the gut and splanchnic oxygenation has gained increased interest and, it is hoped, will identify an optimal trigger for transfusion.[11] Despite its promising features, NIRS has yet to be validated for neonates of different gestational age groups. As a secondary study in the aforementioned TOP trial, the differences in cerebral oxygenation and fractional tissue oxygen extraction with NIRS will be determined between high- and low-hemoglobin value threshold groups during RBC transfusions, which will help to evaluate the role of NIRS in transfusion practice.

Type of product

RBC products in the neonatal population are often leukocyte depleted and irradiated for infants weighing less than 1200 g, and the RBC transfusion volumes vary between

10 and 20 mL/kg. Some concerns were raised over the age of RBC products at the time of transfusion, but a trial addressing whether older stored RBCs are harmful to neonates showed no benefit of fresher RBC products. In this study, 377 preterm neonates were randomized to RBC products stored less than or equal to 7 days, compared with standard RBC products (storage time 2–42 days). No differences were seen in death or neonatal morbidities, such as intraventricular hemorrhage (IVH), necrotizing enterocolitis (NEC), and retinopathy of prematurity (ROP).[16]

Complications

All blood component transfusions come with similar risks, such as clinical errors in administration and incorrect blood component transfusion. In general, transfusions are regarded as safe. Transmission of infectious agents is rare in developed countries with extensive screening and processing protocols of human blood products, but some complications might be underrecognized in the neonatal population and especially in (very) preterm neonates. It is unclear how various risks reported in adults undergoing transfusion translate to a neonatal population. For example, conditions such as transfusion-related lung injury (TRALI) and transfusion-associated circulatory overload (TACO) may be difficult to differentiate in the sick neonate with prematurity-related respiratory failure.[17] However, typical neonatal conditions may be associated with transfusion, as several studies have suggested associations with RBC transfusions and IVH,[18] NEC (so-called TANEC, transfusion-associated necrotizing enterocolitis),[19] ROP,[20] and iron overload.[21] The pathophysiologic explanations for these associations are unknown and are likely multifactorial. In addition, the evidence for a causal association between RBC transfusions and various neonatal complications is lacking and remains speculative. Last, multiple transfusions may theoretically suppress the endogenous erythropoiesis and cause a delay in natural recovery of anemia.

Treatment: Alternatives

Erythropoietin administration

The physiologic decline of hemoglobin after birth is accompanied by a transient deficiency of endogenous EPO, a hormone that stimulates erythropoiesis. Administration of synthetic EPO or darbepoetin, a long-acting form of EPO, may theoretically reduce neonatal anemia.[6] Many studies have investigated the role of EPO in the prevention of anemia and the reduction RBC transfusions in preterm and/or low-birth-weight neonates as well as evaluated its role as a neuroprotective agent. Two separate, recently updated Cochrane reviews assessed the effectiveness and safety of early EPO administration (at or before 7 days after birth, 34 randomized controlled trials, enrolling 3643 preterm infants)[22] and late EPO administration (after 7 days, 30 randomized controlled trials, enrolling 1591 preterm infants), respectively.[23] Overall, EPO treatment caused a reduction in RBC transfusions and the volume of RBCs transfused, although the results vary and the overall effect is reported to be of limited clinical importance. In recent trials, the incidence of ROP was no longer a topic of concern and did not differ between treatment groups, although late administration of EPO still showed a trend in increased risk for ROP. A meta-analysis specifically addressing the issue of ROP in EPO treatment showed no increased risk for any stage of ROP.[24,25] Furthermore, early EPO treatment significantly decreased rates of IVH and NEC, although these effects were not observed after late EPO treatment. The effect of EPO on neurodevelopment is more difficult to assess, because long-term follow-up is limited. To date, the neurodevelopmental outcomes at 18 to 22 months vary greatly, and although results seem promising and suggest a neuroprotective effect of EPO,[26] further long-term assessment of these infants is necessary. An ongoing trial on the effect of EPO as a neuroprotective agent (the PENUT trial, preterm EPO neuroprotection trial; NCT01378273) is particularly interesting in this regard and is expected to complete at the end of 2018. At the moment, routine administration of EPO is not recommended as treatment of neonatal anemia. The reported benefits are too limited, and the evidence on potentially severe side effects is inconclusive.

In the specific case of hemolytic disease of the fetus and newborn (HDFN), EPO treatment might be beneficial to treat the anemia, which can be ongoing for several months after birth. HDFN is not a registered indication for EPO treatment, but off-label use has been reported.[27,28] The potential effect of EPO in neonates with HDFN was shown in small studies and case reports, showing overall an increased hemoglobin level and decreased transfusion need. An ongoing trial in this specific neonatal population is expected to clarify the role of EPO (the EPO-4-Rh trial; NCT03104426), and the trial is planned to complete in 2020.

Reduction of iatrogenic phlebotomy

Neonatal anemia is, in hospitalized infants, mostly caused by iatrogenic blood loss accompanying frequent laboratory testing.[29] Neonates with arterial lines or central venous catheters are at highest risk, because collecting blood is more convenient and accessible. Samples drawn from central venous catheters also have greater overdraw volumes compared with peripheral venous catheters.[30] Iatrogenic blood loss should be reduced to a minimum, and critical assessment of the need for laboratory testing is one of the major steps toward prevention of neonatal anemia. Significant reductions in anemia by phlebotomy can further be achieved by microtechnique laboratory procedures, which allow for smaller sampling volumes, the development of noninvasive monitoring methods, and consequent use of fetal blood from the placenta for all NICU baseline laboratory blood tests.[30] Mathematical modeling has been used to develop algorithms to predict when blood values are necessary based on clinical findings.[31]

Delayed umbilical cord clamping

In recent years, the effect of delayed umbilical cord clamping has regained much interest with regard to the prevention of neonatal anemia. Delayed cord clamping by at least 30 to 60 seconds after birth allows for a prolonged placental transfusion and is now recommended in preterm and full-term neonates, as stated in a guideline by the World Health Organization.[32] In preterm neonates, it is associated with fewer RBC transfusions, better circulatory stability, and possibly a lower risk for IVH and NEC compared with early or direct cord clamping.[33] In full-term neonates, the beneficial effect is less apparent. Overall, delayed clamping is associated with higher hemoglobin levels after birth, but not with significantly fewer RBC transfusions, with an increase in iron stores at 4 to 6 months of age,[34] and improved neurodevelopmental outcomes at 12 months[35] and 4 years of age.[36] In full-term neonates, delayed umbilical cord clamping may cause an increase in hyperbilirubinemia and phototherapy.[34]

THROMBOCYTOPENIA
Causes and Risk Factors

In the late fetal and neonatal period, megakaryocytes are smaller and generate fewer platelets per megakaryocyte compared with adult megakaryocytes.[37] To compensate, the fetal megakaryocytes have a higher proliferation rate and are more sensitive to thrombopoietin, the most potent stimulating agent of megakaryocyte production and differentiation.[38]

From the end of the first trimester, the mean platelet count is considered greater than 150×10^9/L, regardless of gestational age. However, reference values for normal platelet counts are debated. In neonates, "reference values" are limited because healthy neonates generally do not undergo blood sampling, and there is a wide normal range of platelet counts for neonates of different gestational ages.[39] There is no clear correlation between platelet cutoff values and individual bleeding risk,[40,41] as was also the conclusion of a recent systematic review on this matter.[42] Platelets counts less than 20×10^9/L are still generally considered high risk for bleeding, although the clinical significance of platelet count cutoff values remains controversial.

The *mechanisms* of thrombocytopenia in neonates can be divided into the classical categories of either decreased production, increased platelet consumption, increased extravascular loss, or a combination of these factors. The *causes* of thrombocytopenia in neonates vary according to the underlying disease and can be classified according to the age of onset in early- (within 3 days after birth) and late-onset (more than 3 days after birth) thrombocytopenia. Early-onset thrombocytopenia is generally associated with prenatal factors, such as maternal disease (preeclampsia), intrauterine growth restriction, perinatal asphyxia, or fetal/neonatal alloimmune thrombocytopenia, whereas late-onset thrombocytopenia is often caused by bacterial sepsis or NEC, or thrombotic events associated with the use of central lines.[2,43]

Treatment: Platelet Transfusions

Thresholds

Thrombocytopenia is generally treated with transfusions to prevent or treat major hemorrhages, such as IVH or lung bleeding. Although bleeding in association with marked thrombocytopenia is a clear indication for immediate platelet transfusion, the relationship between the severity of thrombocytopenia and the occurrence of hemorrhages is not clear cut. A prospective observational study showed that 81% of platelet transfusions in neonates are given prophylactically (ie, when transfusions are indicated by a predefined platelet threshold and not by bleeding signs). Of the 194 neonates in this study with platelet counts less than 60×10^9/L, 73% were reported to have minor hemorrhages, but only 9% developed severe hemorrhage. Among the most severe thrombocytopenic neonates in this study, with a platelet count less than 20×10^9/L (n = 58), just 9% developed major hemorrhage.[4] Only one randomized trial compared higher ($<150 \times 10^9$/L) versus a lower ($<50 \times 10^9$/L) platelet count threshold for prophylactic transfusion in preterm thrombocytopenic neonates. The primary outcome was the incidence of intracranial hemorrhage, which did not significantly differ between the 2 treatment groups (26 vs 28%, $P = .73$).[44] Several national guidelines on platelet transfusion thresholds are summarized in **Table 2**.

Table 2
Overview of international guidelines for platelet transfusions

	British Committee for Standards in Haematology 2016[54]	Australian National Blood Authority 2016[51]	Canadian Blood Services 2017[52]	Dutch Guidelines Quality Council (Concept) 2018[53]
Prophylactic in stable infant	25×10^9/L	$10\text{-}20 \times 10^9$/L	$<20 \times 10^9$/L	$<25 \times 10^9$/L
Bleeding or invasive procedure	$50\text{--}100 \times 10^9$/L	50×10^9/L	$<50 \times 10^9$/L	$<50 \times 10^9$/L

In a recently published international randomized trial, 660 preterm neonates with severe thrombocytopenia were randomized to receive platelet transfusions at platelet count thresholds of 50×10^9/L or 25×10^9/L. Mortality of major bleeding within 28 days of randomization was significantly higher in the less than 50×10^9/L group compared with the less than 25×10^9/L group, respectively, 26% (85/324) versus 19% (61/329) (odds ratio 1.57, 95% confidence interval 1.06–2.32, $P = .02$). This study suggests that platelet transfusions may cause harm in preterm neonates. Restrictive platelet transfusion guidelines may thus be preferable compared with liberal transfusion guidelines.[45]

Transfusion markers

A novel laboratory parameter may be of use in the clinical assessment of neonatal thrombocytopenia, the immature platelet fraction (IPF). Platelets, when newly released from the liver or bone marrow, are reticulated (ie, contain RNA that can be detected by vital stains or thiazole orange) and can be measured in this immature precursor state. The quantification of these reticulated platelets is called the IPF and may be a reliable measure of the platelet production rate, comparable to the reticulocyte count in the assessment of anemia. An increase in IPF precedes rising platelet counts and could provide additional information about the thrombocytopenia in the neonate. However, currently there are not yet defined reference ranges for neonates of different gestational ages and clinical conditions.[46]

Complications

Similar to RBC transfusions, platelet transfusions also have the risk of "human" errors in practical administration of the transfusions as well as a risk of transmission of bacterial or viral infections, risks of allergic reaction, and a risk of causing TACO or TRALI.[17] In a study by Baer and colleagues,[47] in 1600 thrombocytopenic neonates admitted to the NICU, an association was found between multiple platelet transfusions and mortality in neonates. However, some of this association was ascribed to unmeasured factors, such as level of illness. It is therefore unclear whether increased neonatal death was a consequence or a cause of thrombocytopenia and platelet transfusions.

Treatment: Alternatives

Thrombopoietic agents

Exogenous administration of recombinant human thrombopoietin was tested in healthy volunteers, but led to formation of antithrombopoietin antibodies and severe hyporegenerative thrombocytopenia.[48] Currently, research has switched focus to thrombopoietin receptor agonists, such as eltrombopag and romiplostim. These agonists act through binding to the thrombopoietin receptor, simulating the effect of thrombopoietin. Although approved for use in children, these agents have not been tested in neonates. The pharmacodynamics and pharmacokinetics properties of these agents in neonates are unclear and need further investigation, especially because thrombopoietin receptors have also been identified on nonhematopoietic cells, including the brain.[49]

SUMMARY

Anemia and thrombocytopenia are very common in (very) preterm neonates. Up to 90% of (very) low-birth-weight and/or (very) preterm neonates require at least one RBC transfusion due to anemia, and thrombocytopenia is reported to occur in 20% to 35% of neonates admitted to the NICU.

Anemia in neonates can be physiologic, but is mostly caused by iatrogenic blood sampling in hospitalized neonates. There is no international consensus regarding optimal hemoglobin thresholds for RBC transfusion, and studies comparing liberal and restrictive hemoglobin thresholds are not conclusive. Prevention of neonatal anemia in preterm neonates can partly be achieved by implementing inexpensive measures, such as delayed cord clamping and minimization of iatrogenic blood loss. RBC transfusions are generally considered safe, but some complications of transfusions may be underreported in neonatal populations.

Thrombocytopenia can be caused by perinatal factors, such as intrauterine growth restriction, but is most commonly seen in sepsis or NEC. There is no clear correlation between platelet cutoff values and individual bleeding risk, and most platelet transfusions are given as prophylactic treatment. However, the benefit of these prophylactic transfusions is unclear in nonbleeding neonates, and a recent randomized controlled trial shows a higher rate of mortality or major bleeding if a higher platelet level threshold is used compared with a lower threshold.

FUTURE PERSPECTIVES

Although anemia and thrombocytopenia are frequent neonatal complications, there is great uncertainty in transfusion practice. Assessment of transfusion need could be improved by biomarkers complementary to the serum hemoglobin level and platelet count, such as NIRS measures or the IPF. In addition, international consensus guidelines would help to decrease the variability in transfusion practice. To optimize transfusion guidelines, the results of ongoing randomized controlled trials need to be carefully evaluated, and further research is needed in specific neonatal subpopulations to ascertain appropriate thresholds.

The greatest advances in transfusion practice are preventive and supportive measures. Further reduction of iatrogenic phlebotomy, delayed cord clamping, and timely recognition and treatment of underlying conditions, such as infection, may prevent a significant number of transfusions. Furthermore, supportive measures, such as the administration of EPO in anemia and thrombopoietin receptor agonists in thrombocytopenia, may prove of great future value and need to be investigated in the neonatal population.

REFERENCES

1. Keir AK, Yang J, Harrison A, et al. Temporal changes in blood product usage in preterm neonates born at less than 30 weeks' gestation in Canada. Transfusion 2015;55(6):1340–6.
2. Christensen RD, Henry E, Wiedmeier SE, et al. Thrombocytopenia among extremely low birth weight neonates: data from a multihospital healthcare system. J Perinatol 2006;26(6):348–53.
3. Roberts I, Stanworth S, Murray NA. Thrombocytopenia in the neonate. Blood Rev 2008;22(4):173–86.
4. Stanworth SJ, Clarke P, Watts T, et al. Prospective, observational study of outcomes in neonates with severe thrombocytopenia. Pediatrics 2009;124(5): e826–34.
5. Widness JA. Pathophysiology of anemia during the neonatal period, including anemia of prematurity. Neoreviews 2008;9(11):e520.
6. Widness JA, Madan A, Grindeanu LA, et al. Reduction in red blood cell transfusions among preterm infants: results of a randomized trial with an in-line blood gas and chemistry monitor. Pediatrics 2005;115(5):1299–306.

7. Alverson DC. The physiologic impact of anemia in the neonate. Clin Perinatol 1995;22(3):609–25.

8. Murray NA, Howarth LJ, McCloy MP, et al. Platelet transfusion in the management of severe thrombocytopenia in neonatal intensive care unit patients. Transfus Med 2002;12(1):35–41.

9. Von Lindern JS, Lopriore E. Management and prevention of neonatal anemia: current evidence and guidelines. Expert Rev Hematol 2014;7(2):195–202.

10. Whyte R, Kirpalani H. Low versus high haemoglobin concentration threshold for blood transfusion for preventing morbidity and mortality in very low birth weight infants. Cochrane Database Syst Rev 2011;(11):CD000512.

11. Banerjee J, Aladangady N. Biomarkers to decide red blood cell transfusion in newborn infants. Transfusion 2014;54(10):2574–82.

12. Bailey SM, Hendricks-Munoz KD, Wells JT, et al. Packed red blood cell transfusion increases regional cerebral and splanchnic tissue oxygen saturation in anemic symptomatic preterm infants. Am J Perinatol 2010;27(6):445–53.

13. Seidel D, Blaser A, Gebauer C, et al. Changes in regional tissue oxygenation saturation and desaturations after red blood cell transfusion in preterm infants. J Perinatol 2013;33(4):282–7.

14. Takahashi D, Matsui M, Shigematsu R, et al. Effect of transfusion on the venous blood lactate level in very low-birthweight infants. Pediatr Int 2009;51(3):321–5.

15. van Hoften JC, Verhagen EA, Keating P, et al. Cerebral tissue oxygen saturation and extraction in preterm infants before and after blood transfusion. Arch Dis Child Fetal Neonatal Ed 2010;95(5):F352–8.

16. Fergusson DA, Hebert P, Hogan DL, et al. Effect of fresh red blood cell transfusions on clinical outcomes in premature, very low-birth-weight infants: the ARIPI randomized trial. JAMA 2012;308(14):1443–51.

17. Stainsby D, Jones H, Wells AW, et al. Adverse outcomes of blood transfusion in children: analysis of UK reports to the serious hazards of transfusion scheme 1996-2005. Br J Haematol 2008;141(1):73–9.

18. Baer VL, Lambert DK, Henry E, et al. Among very-low-birth-weight neonates is red blood cell transfusion an independent risk factor for subsequently developing a severe intraventricular hemorrhage? Transfusion 2011;51(6):1170–8.

19. Mohamed A, Shah PS. Transfusion associated necrotizing enterocolitis: a meta-analysis of observational data. Pediatrics 2012;129(3):529–40.

20. Hesse L, Eberl W, Schlaud M, et al. Blood transfusion. Iron load and retinopathy of prematurity. Eur J Pediatr 1997;156(6):465–70.

21. Hirano K, Morinobu T, Kim H, et al. Blood transfusion increases radical promoting non-transferrin bound iron in preterm infants. Arch Dis Child Fetal Neonatal Ed 2001;84(3):F188–93.

22. Ohlsson A, Aher SM. Early erythropoiesis-stimulating agents in preterm or low birth weight infants. Cochrane Database Syst Rev 2017;(11):CD004863.

23. Aher SM, Ohlsson A. Late erythropoietin for preventing red blood cell transfusion in preterm and/or low birth weight infants. Cochrane Database Syst Rev 2014;(4):CD004868.

24. Xu XJ, Huang HY, Chen HL. Erythropoietin and retinopathy of prematurity: a meta-analysis. Eur J Pediatr 2014;173(10):1355–64.

25. Chou HH, Chung MY, Zhou XG, et al. Early erythropoietin administration does not increase the risk of retinopathy in preterm infants. Pediatr Neonatol 2017;58(1):48–56.

26. Ohls RK, Kamath-Rayne BD, Christensen RD, et al. Cognitive outcomes of pre-term infants randomized to darbepoetin, erythropoietin, or placebo. Pediatrics 2014;133(6):1023–30.

27. Zuppa AA, Alighieri G, Calabrese V, et al. Recombinant human erythropoietin in the prevention of late anemia in intrauterine transfused neonates with Rh-isoim-munization. J Pediatr Hematol Oncol 2010;32(3):e95–101.

28. Nicaise C, Gire C, Casha P, et al. Erythropoietin as treatment for late hyporege-nerative anemia in neonates with Rh hemolytic disease after in utero exchange transfusion. Fetal Diagn Ther 2002;17(1):22–4.

29. Bateman ST, Lacroix J, Boven K, et al. Anemia, blood loss, and blood transfu-sions in North American children in the intensive care unit. Am J Respir Crit Care Med 2008;178(1):26–33.

30. Valentine SL, Bateman ST. Identifying factors to minimize phlebotomy-induced blood loss in the pediatric intensive care unit. Pediatr Crit Care Med 2012; 13(1):22–7.

31. Rosebraugh MR, Widness JA, Nalbant D, et al. A mathematical modeling approach to quantify the role of phlebotomy losses and need for transfusions in neonatal anemia. Transfusion 2013;53(6):1353–60.

32. World Health Organization. WHO guideline: delayed umbilical cord clamping for improved maternal and infant health and nutrition outcomes. Geneva (Switzerland): World Health Organization; 2014.

33. Rabe H, Diaz-Rossello JL, Duley L, et al. Effect of timing of umbilical cord clamp-ing and other strategies to influence placental transfusion at preterm birth on maternal and infant outcomes. Cochrane Database Syst Rev 2012;(8):CD003248.

34. McDonald SJ, Middleton P, Dowswell T, et al. Effect of timing of umbilical cord clamping of term infants on maternal and neonatal outcomes. Cochrane Data-base Syst Rev 2013;(7):CD004074.

35. Rana N, Kc A, Malqvist M, et al. Effect of delayed cord clamping of term babies on neurodevelopment at 12 months: a randomized controlled trial. Neonatology 2018;115(1):36–42.

36. Andersson O, Lindquist B, Lindgren M, et al. Effect of delayed cord clamping on neurodevelopment at 4 years of age: a randomized clinical trial. JAMA Pediatr 2015;169(7):631–8.

37. Mattia G, Vulcano F, Milazzo L, et al. Different ploidy levels of megakaryocytes generated from peripheral or cord blood CD34+ cells are correlated with different levels of platelet release. Blood 2002;99(3):888–97.

38. Debili N, Wendling F, Katz A, et al. The Mpl-ligand or thrombopoietin or megakar-yocyte growth and differentiative factor has both direct proliferative and differen-tiative activities on human megakaryocyte progenitors. Blood 1995;86(7): 2516–25.

39. Wiedmeier SE, Henry E, Sola-Visner MC, et al. Platelet reference ranges for neo-nates, defined using data from over 47,000 patients in a multihospital healthcare system. J Perinatol 2009;29(2):130–6.

40. Bonifacio L, Petrova A, Nanjundaswamy S, et al. Thrombocytopenia related neonatal outcome in preterms. Indian J Pediatr 2007;74(3):269–74.

41. Von Lindern JS, Van den Bruele T, Lopriore E, et al. Thrombocytopenia in neo-nates and the risk of intraventricular hemorrhage: a retrospective cohort study. BMC Pediatr 2011;11:16.

42. Fustolo-Gunnink SF, Huijssen-Huisman EJ, van der Bom JG, et al. Temporary removal: are thrombocytopenia and platelet transfusions associated with major

bleeding in preterm neonates? A systematic review. Blood Rev 2018. [Epub ahead of print].

43. Sola-Visner M, Saxonhouse MA, Brown RE. Neonatal thrombocytopenia: what we do and don't know. Early Hum Dev 2008;84(8):499–506.

44. Andrew M, Vegh P, Caco C, et al. A randomized, controlled trial of platelet transfusions in thrombocytopenic premature infants. J Pediatr 1993;123(2):285–91.

45. Curley A, Stanworth SJ, Willoughby K, et al. Randomized trial of platelet-transfusion thresholds in neonates. N Engl J Med 2019;380(3):242–51.

46. Cremer M, Paetzold J, Schmalisch G, et al. Immature platelet fraction as novel laboratory parameter predicting the course of neonatal thrombocytopenia. Br J Haematol 2009;144(4):619–21.

47. Baer VL, Lambert DK, Henry E, et al. Do platelet transfusions in the NICU adversely affect survival? Analysis of 1600 thrombocytopenic neonates in a multi-hospital healthcare system. J Perinatol 2007;27(12):790–6.

48. Li J, Yang C, Xia Y, et al. Thrombocytopenia caused by the development of antibodies to thrombopoietin. Blood 2001;98(12):3241–8.

49. Sallmon H, Gutti RK, Ferrer-Marin F, et al. Increasing platelets without transfusion: is it time to introduce novel thrombopoietic agents in neonatal care? J Perinatol 2010;30(12):765–9.

50. New HV, Berryman J, Bolton-Maggs PH, et al, British Committee for Standards in Haematology. Guidelines on transfusion for fetuses, neonates and older children. Br J Haematol 2016;175(5):784–828.

51. Australian National Blood Authority. Patient blood management guidelines: module 6 neonatal and paediatrics. 2016. Available at: https://www.blood.gov.au/pbm-module-6. Accessed October 23, 2018.

52. Lau W. Chapter 13: neonatal and pediatric transfusion. In: Canadian Blood services, clinical guide to transfusion. 2017. Available at: https://professionaleducation.blood.ca/en/transfusion/clinical-guide/neonatal-and-pediatric-transfusion.

53. Dutch Guidelines Quality Council, 3rd revision, in press.

54. Estcourt LJ, Birchall J, Allard S, et al, British Committee for Standards in Haematology. Guidelines for the use of platelet transfusions. Br J Haematol 2017;176(3):365–94.

Congenital Neutropenia and Rare Functional Phagocyte Disorders in Children

Kelly Walkovich, MD[a],*, James A. Connelly, MD[b]

KEYWORDS

- Neutropenia • Phagocytes • Granulocyte colony-stimulating factor (G-CSF)
- *ELANE* • Oxidative burst

KEY POINTS

- Many congenital neutropenia disorders have a propensity to develop myelodysplasia/leukemia. At-risk patients should be monitored with annual bone marrow evaluations and quarterly blood counts.
- Diagnosis of the functional phagocyte disorders relies on the recognition of clinical manifestations correlating to the functional defect.
- Both classic neutropenia and phagocyte functional disorders are increasingly being recognized as a feature of broader primary immunodeficiency diseases.

INTRODUCTION

The term phagocyte is derived from the Greek phagein, meaning to eat or devour, and cyte meaning cell. Phagocytes, namely monocytes, macrophages, and neutrophils, are hematopoietic cells capable of engulfing and digesting microorganisms, foreign particles, and cellular debris. The term granulocytes, although often used interchangeably with phagocytes, specifically refers to white blood cells (WBCs), characterized by the presence of granules in their cytoplasm (ie, neutrophils, eosinophils, basophils, and mast cells). Phagocytes play a critical role in innate immune function to protect children from bacterial and fungal infections. The absence of neutrophils

Disclosure: K. Walkovich is the local principal investigator for X4P-001 in Patients with WHIM Syndrome, an industry-supported clinical trial for evaluating the safety and efficiency of a novel CXCR4 antagonist; J.A. Connelly has no disclosures.
[a] Pediatric Hematology/Oncology, Department of Pediatrics, University of Michigan Medical School, 1500 E. Medical Center Drive, D4202 Medical Professional Building, SPC 5718, Ann Arbor, MI 48109-5718, USA; [b] Pediatric Hematopoietic Stem Cell Transplant, Department of Pediatrics, Vanderbilt University Medical Center, 2220 Pierce Avenue, 397 PRB, Nashville, TN 37232-6310, USA
* Corresponding author.
E-mail address: kwalkovi@med.umich.edu

or dysfunctional phagocytes poses significant risk for recurrent, unusual, and/or overwhelming infections most often in the blood, lungs, liver, oropharynx, and skin. Many patients with such disorders present in infancy to early childhood, although the diagnosis may be delayed to adulthood.

DEFINITION OF NEUTROPENIA IN CHILDREN

Neutropenia is a decrease in the absolute number of segmented neutrophils and bands in the peripheral blood. The absolute neutrophil count (ANC) is calculated by multiplying the sum of the percentage of segmented neutrophils and bands by the total WBC count. Mild neutropenia is an ANC between 1001 and 1500 cells/μL, moderate is between 501 and 1000 cells/μL, and severe is less than 500 cells/μL. However, ANC values must be considered in the context of age and race.

Normal values for ANCs vary significantly by age, especially in the neonatal period because of the surge of neutrophils released from the marrow during delivery and the subsequent decrease in the marrow proliferative pool.[1] The lower limit of normal for an ANC during the first 24 hours after birth is 6000 cells/μL, then 5000 cells/μL during the second week, followed by 1000 cells/μL between 2 weeks and 1 year.[2] After 1 year, the lower limit of normal for the ANC is 1500 cells/μL.

Many healthy individuals of African descent along the malarial belt have a lower ANCs compared with patients of white European or Asian heritage. The lower ANC is linked to a polymorphism in the Duffy antigen receptor chemokine (DARC) gene, which encodes the Duffy antigen (FyA/B), a chemokine receptor expressed on the surface of red blood cells (RBCs) used by *Plasmodium vivax* to infect RBCs. Patients with homozygous DARC null polymorphism are often regarded as having benign ethnic neutropenia (BEN), although Duffy null status is not required for the diagnosis of BEN. Patients with BEN are not at risk for infection or malignancy. Heterozygous patients have normal mean neutrophil counts.

COMMON BENIGN CAUSES OF NEUTROPENIA IN CHILDREN

Transient neutropenia is common in childhood and can most often be attributed to infections, medications, nutrition, or immune-mediated causes. Viruses are the most common trigger for neutropenia with neutropenia occurring during the first 24 to 48 hours of illness and persisting during the period of viremia, which is generally 3 to 8 days. Various bacteria, protozoa, rickettsial, and fungal infections also cause neutropenia through decreased granulocyte production or increased destruction with accelerated turnover. The pathogenesis of drug-induced neutropenia is poorly understood, with immune-mediated, direct/indirect toxicity, hypersensitivity, and idiosyncratic mechanisms known. Common drugs resulting in neutropenia include anticonvulsants (eg, valproic acid), antibiotics, and antipsychotic agents (eg, clozapine). The neutropenia often resolves with withdrawal of the suspected offending drug, although recombinant granulocyte colony-stimulating factor (G-CSF) can be used when drug removal is not an option. Several nutritional deficiencies, including folate, vitamin B_{12}, and copper deficiency, can contribute to neutropenia. Alloimmune neutropenia develops during the first pregnancy from transplacental passage of maternally derived immunoglobulin (Ig) G antibodies, with the ANC improving as the maternal IgG clears, whereas autoimmune neutropenia of infancy (AIN) commonly presents around age 12 months. Children with AIN often are identified incidentally. The presence of antineutrophil antibodies may support the diagnosis of AIN but is fraught with both false-negatives and false-positives, so the absence of a detectable antibody does not exclude the diagnosis and a positive result does not exclude other conditions. Treatment is generally not required for AIN because it is only rarely associated with serious infection because of the marrow being functional and spontaneously remits with a median of 7 to 30 months from diagnosis. However, low-dose G-CSF can be used for recurrent infections, to promote wound healing following surgery and/or avert emergency room visits or hospitalizations for febrile illnesses.

Although transient neutropenia is common in childhood, vigilance must be maintained for presentations concerning for the more rare congenital neutropenia disorders. Patients who present with a combination of recurrent fevers, oral ulcers, gingivitis, periodontitis, skin infections (including folliculitis and omphalitis), deep tissue abscesses (eg, perirectal abscesses), and/or associated syndromic findings warrant further investigation. The diagnostic evaluation often includes repeating complete blood count with platelets and differential (CBCPDs), a bone marrow aspirate and biopsy, interrogation of the immune system, imaging for physical anomalies, and confirmatory genetic testing. The comprehensive list of congenital neutropenia disorders continues to expand (**Table 1**), with a major distinguishing feature being the risk, or documented lack thereof, for leukemogenesis. Selected disorders are described in more detail later.

Severe Congenital Neutropenia

Severe congenital neutropenia (SCN) is a genetically heterogeneous condition with a prevalence estimated to be 3 to 8.5 cases per million individuals.[3,4] The SCN phenotype was initially described in the 1950s in a Swedish population with mutations in the recessively inherited *HAX1* gene (ie, Kostmann syndrome). Now more than 24 genes are known to be associated with congenital neutropenia with autosomal dominant, recessive, and X-linked forms recognized. Despite the expansion of genetic causes, in 25% of cases, the genetic basis remains elusive. Mutations in the neutrophil elastase gene, *ELANE*, which encodes neutrophil elastase and is inherited in an autosomal dominant fashion, account for 45% to 60% of the germline mutations in SCN from the Severe Chronic Neutropenia International Registry.[5,6]

Clinically, SCN is characterized by ANCs consistently less than 500 cells/μL and often less than 200 cells/μL present from birth. Patients have a high risk for bacterial and fungal infections and present with recurrent fevers, oral ulcers, skin infections (including omphalitis), and deep tissue abscesses within the first few months of life. Patients with mutations in *ELANE*, *HAX1*, *CLPB*, *G6PC3*, or *GCSF3R* have the classic promyelocyte arrest visualized on inspection of the bone marrow. Many mutated genes also give these patients a marked propensity to develop myelodysplasia and acute myeloid leukemia (AML).

Primary treatment of SCN is administration of G-CSF. Most patients (~90%–95%) have an adequate response to G-CSF, eliminating the risk of severe infection. Patients with no response to G-CSF should proceed to curative hematopoietic stem cell transplant (HSCT). Development of myelodysplastic syndrome (MDS) and AML is a common occurrence in SCN, with a cumulative incidence of 22% at 15 years.[7] Patients who require higher doses of G-CSF with poor neutrophil response have a higher incidence of malignant transformation. HSCT is necessary for all patients who develop MDS or AML, with survival outcomes reported at 82%,[8] better than seen in children with de novo MDS or AML.

Cyclic Neutropenia

Cyclic neutropenia is an autosomal dominant disorder with variable expression and an estimated incidence of 1 to 2 per million. More than 90% of the cases are attributed to mutations in *ELANE*. The disorder is characterized by regular, periodic oscillations in

Table 1
Congenital neutropenia

Disease	Gene	Inheritance Pattern	Other Hematologic Manifestations	Nonhematologic Manifestations
			Disorders with Near-universal Congenital Neutropenia	
Severe congenital neutropenia	*ELANE*	AD	Monocytosis, eosinophilia, high risk of transformation to MDS/AML	Osteopenia
	CSF3R[47]	Mixed	None	None
	GFI1	AD	Lymphopenia, increased number of immature myeloid cells in peripheral blood, risk of transformation to MDS/AML	None
	HAX1[48]	AR	Risk of transformation to MDS/AML	Seizures, developmental delay
	JAGN1[49]	AR	Risk of transformation to MDS/AML	Short stature, bone and teeth defects
	G6PC3[50,51]	AR	Thrombocytopenia, promyelocyte maturation arrest in the bone marrow, myelokathexis, rare risk of transformation to MDS/AML	Increased visibility of superficial veins, congenital heart defects, urogenital malformations, pulmonary hypertension, cognitive impairment, endocrine abnormalities
	TCIRG1[52]	AD	None	Hemangiomas with increased prominence with G-CSF administration
Cyclic neutropenia	*ELANE*	AD	Reciprocal monocytosis, cyclic platelet counts, rare risk of transformation to MDS/AML	None
Reticular dysgenesis[53]	*AK2*	AR	SCID, bone marrow maturation arrest at the promyelocyte stage, anemia, thrombocytopenia	Sensorineural hearing loss, premature birth, small for gestational age, very early onset of bacterial infections
Shwachman-Diamond syndrome[15]	*SBDS*	AR	Anemia, thrombocytopenia, bone marrow failure, risk of transformation to MDS/AML	Pancreatic exocrine insufficiency, steatorrhea, skeletal abnormalities, short stature, increased transaminases
SRP54 related neutropenia[12]	*SRP54*	AR	Failure of neutropenia to respond to G-CSF, neutrophil migration defect	Pancreatic exocrine insufficiency, possible language or autistic disorder

Disorder	Gene	Inheritance	Features	Associated findings
VPS45 related neutropenia[54]	VPS45	AR	Bone marrow fibrosis, extramedullary hematopoiesis, lack of response to G-CSF, decreased neutrophil chemotaxis with impaired migration and NADPH oxidase dysfunction, progressive anemia, thrombocytopenia, hypergammaglobulinemia	Nephromegaly, hepatosplenomegaly, possible neurologic deficits
WHIM syndrome[29]	CXCR4	AD	Lymphopenia, dysgammaglobulinemia, myelokathexis	Warts, HPV-related anogenital dysplasia and invasive cancer, tetralogy of Fallot
Disorders with Variable Congenital Neutropenia				
Barth syndrome[55]	TAZ	XL	Frequent cytoplasmic vacuoles in neutrophils, bone marrow maturation arrest at the myelocyte stage	Dilated cardiomyopathy, skeletal myopathy, increased urinary 3-methylglutuaconic acid and 2-ethylhydracrylic acid
Bruton agammaglobulinemia[56]	BTK	XL	Marked B-cell lymphopenia, dysgammaglobulinemia, reduced serum antibodies	Increased susceptibility to encapsulated bacteria and enteroviruses
Cartilage-hair hypoplasia[57-59]	RMRP	AR	Humoral or combined immunodeficiency, non-Hodgkin lymphoma, rare risk of leukemia, anemia, thrombocytopenia	Short stature, metaphyseal chondrodysplasia, sparse hair, increased susceptibility to VZV infection, celiac disease, basal cell carcinoma
Chédiak-Higashi syndrome[60]	LYST	AR	Large lysosomal inclusion bodies in granulocytes, decreased phagocyte chemotaxic response, defective NK cell function, mild coagulation defect with platelet aggregation defect, risk of hemophagocytic lymphohistiocytosis	Oculocutaneous albinism, progressive neurologic dysfunction, recurrent infections
CLPB deficiency[61,62]	CLPB	AR	Risk of evolution to MDS/AML	3-Methylglutaconic acid, progressive brain atrophy, intellectual disability, cataracts, movement disorder
Clericuzio-type poikiloderma[63]	USB1	AR	Risk of progression to MDS/AML	Inflammatory eczematous rash, reactive airway disease, nonhealing ulcers, sinopulmonary infections, bronchiectasis,

(continued on next page)

Table 1
(continued)

Disease	Gene	Inheritance Pattern	Other Hematologic Manifestations	Nonhematologic Manifestations
Cohen syndrome[64]	VPS13B	AR	None	FTT, progressive retinochoroidal dystrophy, myopia, hypotonia, developmental delay, cheery disposition
CXCR2-related neutropenia	CXCR2	AR	Myelokathexis	None
DADA2 deficiency[65,66]	CECR1	AR	Pure red blood cell aplasia, bone marrow failure, dysgammaglobulinemia	Fevers, polyarteritis nodosa, livedo racemose, vasculitis, early-onset stroke, lymphoproliferation
DNAJC21-related neutropenia[67,68]	DNAJC21	AR	Bone marrow failure	Growth retardation, FTT, developmental delay, recurrent infections, skin/teeth/nail abnormalities, pancreatic sufficiency, liver cirrhosis
EFL1 related neutropenia[14]	EFL1	AR	Progressive normocytic anemia, thrombocytopenia	Pancreatic exocrine dysfunction, skeletal abnormalities, FTT, short stature, developmental delay
GATA2 haploinsufficiency[69]	GATA2	AD	Monocytopenia, NK and B-cell lymphopenia, bone marrow failure, risk of evolution to MDS/AML	Mycobacterial infections, warts, pulmonary alveolar proteinosis, lymphedema, sensorineural hearing loss
Glycogen storage disease type 1b[70,71]	SLC37A4	AR	Neutrophil dysfunction, anemia, platelet dysfunction (caused by dyslipidemia), rare evolution to MDS/AML	Hypoglycemia, increased triglycerides, lactic acidosis, Crohn-like colitis, recurrent infections, short stature, hepatic adenoma, thyroid autoimmunity
Griscelli syndrome[72]	RAB27A	AR	NK cell dysfunction, variable T-cell and B-cell defects, thrombocytopenia	Partial albinism, progressive neurologic dysfunction, hepatosplenomegaly, recurrent infections

Disorder	Gene	Inheritance	Hematologic Findings	Clinical Features
Hermansky-Pudlak, type 2[73]	AP3B1	AR	Bleeding diathesis, immunodeficiency	Oculocutaneous albinism, pulmonary fibrosis
Hyper IgM syndrome[74]	CD40LG	XL	Decreased B-cell class switching; markedly low IgG, IgA, and IgE; combined immunodeficiency	Recurrent sinopulmonary infections with encapsulated bacteria, opportunistic infections (eg, PJP), chronic diarrhea, cryptococcal infection, liver disease, solid tumors, osteopenia
p14 deficiency[75]	LAMTOR2	AR	B-cell and cytotoxic T-cell deficiency	Oculocutaneous albinism, short stature
Pearson syndrome[76]	mt DNA deletion	mt DNA	Refractory sideroblastic anemia, vacuolization of marrow precursors	Mitochondrial myopathy, neuromuscular degeneration, endocrine abnormalities, pancreatic exocrine dysfunction, renal dysfunction
PGM3 deficiency[77]	PGM3	AR	T and B lymphopenia, congenital leukemia	Increased IgE, recurrent infections, skeletal anomalies, intellectual disability
STK4 deficiency[78]	STK4	AR	Monocytopenia, T-cell and B-cell lymphopenia	Atrial septal defects, warts, recurrent bacterial infections, mucocutaneous candidiasis
Transcobalamin II deficiency[79]	TCN2	AR	Megaloblastic anemia, pancytopenia	Failure to thrive, mental retardation and neurologic abnormalities, recurrent infections, methylmalonic aciduria, homocystinuria
Wolcott-Rallison syndrome[80]	EIF2AK3	AR	None	Early-onset insulin-dependent diabetes in infancy, skeletal dysplasia, growth retardation
X-linked neutropenia[81,82]	WAS	XL	Lymphopenia, decreased number of NK cells, risk of transformation to MDS/AML	None

Abbreviations: AD, autosomal dominant; AML, acute myeloid leukemia; AR, autosomal recessive; CLPB, caseinolytic peptidase B protein homolog; FTT, failure to thrive; HPV, human papilloma virus; MDS, myelodysplastic syndrome; mt, mitochondria; NK, natural killer; PJP, *Pneumocystis jiroveci* pneumonia; SCID, severe combined immunodeficiency; VZV, varicella-zoster virus; XL, X linked.

the ANC, ranging from normal to less than 200 cells/μL, accompanied by a reciprocal monocytosis. Cycling of the other cell lines (ie, platelets and reticulocyte count) is often noted. Cycle length ranges between 14 and 35 days; however, almost all patients cycle every 21 days with 7 to 10 days of profound neutropenia during the cycle.[9] The diagnosis of cyclic neutropenia is made by obtaining CBCPDs 2 to 3 times per week for 6 to 8 weeks to document the periodicity of the ANC and reciprocal monocytosis. The diagnosis can be further confirmed by identifying a mutation in ELANE, which may be sent at initial suspicion to avoid frequent venipuncture in young children to track neutrophil count oscillations.

Patients present with recurrent fevers often associated with malaise, stomatitis, gingivitis, and/or bacterial infections that occur during the period of neutropenia. Although most of the infections are minor and self-resolve, more serious infections, such as pneumonia, mastoiditis, and intestinal perforation with peritonitis leading to life-threatening clostridial sepsis, occasionally occur. Before the availability of G-CSF, 10% of patients with cyclic neutropenia died of clostridial or gram-negative sepsis. As such, patients with an ANC nadir less than 200 cells/μL are recommended to be treated with G-CSF to minimize the risk of infection and reduce inflammation. Patients typically require a dose of 1 to 5 μg/kg/d to achieve ANCs greater than 1000 cells/μL, although some patients are able to achieve ANC goals on alternate-day dosing.[9] Of note, administration of G-CSF does not completely eliminate the neutropenic nadir but instead hastens the cycle and shortens the length of profound neutropenia to 1 to 3 days.

Long-term follow-up of patients with the cyclic neutropenia phenotype, including those treated with G-CSF, has not shown a risk for leukemogenesis.[10] Patients are not routinely followed with annual bone marrows. However, a recent report described 2 patients with cyclic neutropenia who developed CSF3R mutations, 1 of whom developed AML.[11]

Shwachman-Diamond Syndrome

Shwachman-Diamond syndrome (SDS) is an autosomal recessive disorder most commonly caused by proapoptotic mutations in the SBDS gene, which encodes a protein involved in ribosome biogenesis and RNA processing. Roughly 90% of patients with SDS have a mutation in SBDS identified, although additional genes associated with ribosome assembly or protein translation (DNAJC21, ELF1, and SRP54) are reported to recapitulate an SDS-like phenotype.[12–14]

Patients without an identified gene are diagnosed from their clinical manifestations per consensus guidelines.[15,16] Typically, patients present with neutropenia detected incidentally or in association with recurrent infections that may progress to bone marrow failure, exocrine pancreatic insufficiency, and skeletal abnormalities. However, many of the classic features, in particular the exocrine pancreatic dysfunction, may be subtle and not readily clinically apparent, and the absence of pancreatic lipomatosis or skeletal anomalies on imaging does not rule out the diagnosis.[17] Patients with SDS also frequently have hepatic abnormalities[17] and/or cardiac, endocrine, or neurocognitive defects.

The neutropenia associated with SDS generally develops in the first year of life, but can be delayed in onset until adulthood. The ANC may range in severity from mild to severe and be persistent or intermittent. Besides neutropenia, other immunologic dysfunction, including mild neutrophil chemotaxis defects, low number of B cells with suboptimal immunoglobulin production, and abnormal T-cell proliferation, have been noted in patients with SDS,[18] likely compounding their risk for infection, especially secondary to viruses.[19]

Patients with SDS frequently show myelodysplasia in the setting of cytogenetic abnormalities, including monosomy 7, isochromosome 7, and deletion of 20q, with occasional self-resolution of the abnormal clone reported.[20] In addition, patients with SDS are at risk for leukemic transformation, with a reported incidence of 1% per year of MDS/AML and an overall incidence of 8.1% over 10 years.[21] Mutations in *TP53*, a tumor suppressor gene, may contribute to the development of MDS/AML because clonal hematopoiesis with *TP53* mutations was frequently identified in patients with SDS but not in patients with SCN or healthy controls.[22] Progression to bone marrow failure also occurs. The only curative therapy for patients with SDS with malignant transformation or severe aplastic anemia is HSCT, particularly because patients with SDS may not tolerate standard chemotherapy well. Reduced-intensity regimens have improved the historically dismal outcomes for such patients.[23] Otherwise, patients benefit from routine surveillance for progression to aplasia and malignancy with regular CBCPDs and annual bone marrows.[15] Many patients also benefit from low-dose G-CSF.

WHIM Syndrome

The syndrome of warts, hypogammaglobulinemia, infections and myelokathexis (WHIM) is extremely rare, with an estimated incidence of 0.23 cases per million births.[24] Mechanistically, nearly all patients with WHIM syndrome have an autosomal dominant gain-of-function mutation in *CXCR4*, which encodes for a G protein–coupled chemokine receptor that is highly expressed on progenitor cells of the hematopoietic, cardiovascular, nervous, and reproductive systems.[25]

Patients present with chronic severe neutropenia with an ANC less than 500 cells/μL in infancy or early childhood. The peripheral neutropenia is caused by the exaggerated response of the chemokine ligand, CXCL12, binding to CXCR4 and leading to failed downregulation/internalization of CXCR4[26,27] and subsequent myelokathexis with retention of mature of neutrophils and other leukocyte subsets in the bone marrow. The bone marrow is hypercellular with an increased myelocyte to erythroid ratio and a plethora of bands and mature neutrophils. The retained neutrophils have a characteristic apoptotic appearance with vacuolization and a hypersegmented pyknotic nucleus with very long filaments connecting the nuclear lobes.[28] Although an increase in apoptosis of neutrophils has been documented in WHIM syndrome,[29] neutrophil function is normal. Note that the neutropenia may be obscured during periods of infection or other stressors when the marrow proliferative drive temporarily overcomes the issue of defective marrow release.

Besides neutropenia, patients with WHIM syndrome generally have concurrent monocytopenia, severe lymphopenia complicated by hypogammaglobulinemia, and inconsistent antibody responses to vaccination. Repeated infections often begin in infancy and include extracellular bacterial pathogens affecting the ear, skin, oral cavity, and sinopulmonary tract[30] leading to bronchiectasis. Warts secondary to human papilloma virus (HPV) infection are often extensive or treatment refractory and can progress to dysplasia and invasive cancer, although some patients do not experience warts. Tetralogy of Fallot is associated with 10% of patients with WHIM.[31] Patients with WHIM syndrome are not as susceptible to fungal and opportunistic infections (eg, *Pneumocystis jiroveci*) as would be expected based on the degree of neutropenia and lymphopenia. Treatment with intravenous immunoglobulin replacement is common to mitigate the risk for bronchiectasis, whereas the use of prophylactic antibiotics, G-CSF, and granulocyte-monocyte colony-stimulating factor (GM-CSF) and reversible antagonists that block the capacity of CXCl12 to sustain permanent activation of CXCR4 is more variable.[31]

NORMAL PHAGOCYTE FUNCTION IN CHILDREN

Following the egress of mature phagocytes from the bone marrow to the peripheral blood, several key steps must be successfully navigated for optimal phagocytic function. First, the phagocytes must sense chemoattractants, such as lipid mediators or cytokines, and attach to activated vascular endothelium through the processes of rolling and adhesion via selectins, integrins, intracellular adhesion molecules, and other glycoproteins. Once adhered to the endothelium, phagocytes must then pass through the endothelium to the tissue space via diapedesis and migrate through orchestration of their actin cytoskeleton to the targeted area. Activation of the phagocyte occurs through direct contact of the foreign material or recognition of pathogen-associated molecular patterns resulting in engulfment and digestion of the target through phagocytosis, triggering degranulation of functional cytoplasmic granules and generation of the oxidative burst to create toxic oxygen metabolites. Neutrophils also participate in a nonphagocytosis method of killing, neutrophil extracellular traps, wherein the neutrophil extrudes chromatin and neutrophil granule content into the extracellular space. This scaffold entraps microbes and provides a high concentration of antimicrobial components.[32] Similar to the quantitative neutrophil defects, qualitative defects in phagocytes result in a substantial risk for recurrent, unusual, and deep-seated/severe infections. The spectrum of phagocyte functional disorders continues to grow (**Table 2**). Selected disorders are detailed further here.

Chronic Granulomatous Disease

Chronic granulomatous disease (CGD) is a multigenic disorder that occurs with an estimated frequency of 1 in 200,000 live births,[33] characterized by mutations in any of the genes (ie, CYBB, CYBA, NFC1, NFC2, NFC4) that encode the 5 subunits (ie, gp91phox, p22phox, p47phox, p67phox, p40phox, respectively) of the phagocyte nicotinamide adenine dinucleotide phosphate (NADPH) oxidative complex. The NADPH oxidative complex is responsible for the generation of the oxidative burst in phagocytes and its dysfunction results in failure of neutrophils, monocytes, and macrophages to kill certain organisms, particularly catalase-positive bacteria, including *Staphylococcus aureus*, *Burkholderia cepacia*, *Serratia marcescens*, and *Nocardia*, and fungi such as *Aspergillus*. Clinical suspicion of CGD can be confirmed through the dihydrorhodamine 123 (DHR) oxidation test and gene sequencing.

Most patients present in infancy or childhood with severe or recurrent infections, frequently affecting the skin, lungs, liver, and lymph nodes, although the clinical presentation of the patient may be underwhelming even if there is extensive infection. Fungal infections are the most common cause of death and carry a higher mortality risk than bacterial infections.[34] Patients with the X-linked CGD or the autosomal recessive form affecting p22phox generally present with more severe disease, as do those patients with completely absent or lower residual superoxide production.[35] Besides infections, patients with CGD are prone to inflammatory complications, including granulomas and inflammatory bowel disease.[36,37]

The treatment of CGD relies on the prophylactic antimicrobials, such as trimethoprim-sulfamethoxazole, and antifungals, such as itraconazole,[38] used with or without interferon gamma,[39] and aggressive management of infectious complications. HSCT is a curative therapy for CGD[40] but the decision to proceed to transplant is often based on the degree of disease severity and quality of the donor match. A limited number of patients with CGD have been treated with gene therapy.

Table 2
Functional phagocyte disorders

Disease	Gene	Inheritance Pattern	Phagocyte Functional Defect	Clinical Manifestations
CARD9 deficiency[83]	CARD9	AR	Selective Candida albicans neutrophil killing defect, decreased IL-8 production by neutrophils, reduced production of IL-6 and IL-1β by monocytes	Invasive fungal infections, meningoencephalitis caused by Candida, chronic mucocutaneous candidiasis, deep and disseminated dermatophytosis
Chédiak-Higashi syndrome[84]	LYST	AR	Impaired intracellular killing of bacteria caused by failure of delivery of peroxidase to the phagosome, large lysosomal inclusion bodies in granulocytes	Oculocutaneous albinism, progressive neurologic dysfunction, recurrent infections, bleeding diathesis, risk of hemophagocytic lymphohistiocytosis
Chronic granulomatous disease[85,86]	CYBB CYBA NCF1 NCF2 NCF4	XL AR AR AR AR	Neutrophils unable to produce superoxide, failure to activate granule proteases, with ineffective microbial killing, decreased expression of TLR5, CD18, and CXCR1 affecting neutrophil activation and chemotaxis, abnormal neutrophil extracellular traps	Recurrent bacterial and function infections particularly with catalase-positive organisms, colitis, granuloma formation
IRAK4 deficiency[87]	IRAK4	AR	Monocytes fail to produce proinflammatory cytokines (TNF-α, IL-1, IL-6), impaired priming and activation of NADPH oxidase	Lack of fever, unexpectedly low CRP in setting of infection, recurrent invasive bacterial infections, inadequate polysaccharide vaccine response
IRF8 deficiency[88]	IRF8	AR	Reduced neutrophil oxidative respiratory	Severe monocytopenia and lack of dendritic cells, disseminated BCG infection
Job syndrome (STAT3 LOF)[89,90]	STAT3	AD	Intermittent chemotaxic defects of neutrophils	Recurrent "cold" skin abscesses (especially Staphylococcus aureus), eczema, retained primary teeth, coarse facial features, vascular anomalies, increased IgE, fractures, allergies
Leukocyte adhesion deficiency[91]	ITGB2	AR	Marked defect in adhesion, transmigration and chemotaxis secondary to lack of CD18 expression	Leukocytosis, delayed umbilical cord separation, impaired wound healing, severe periodontitis, ulcerative skin lesions, colitis, HPV infections
	SLC35C1	AR	Defect in adhesion and migration caused by granulocytes unable to bind selectins on vascular endothelium	Leukocytosis, recurrent infections, intellectual disability, depressed nasal bridge, Bombay blood phenotype
	RASGRP2	AR	Poor neutrophil migration caused by defective integrin activation	Leukocytosis, recurrent infections, bleeding, osteoporosislike bone abnormalities

(continued on next page)

Table 2
(continued)

Disease	Gene	Inheritance Pattern	Phagocyte Functional Defect	Clinical Manifestations
Myeloperoxidase deficiency[92]	*MPO*	mixed	Impaired respiratory burst from defective hypochlorous acid production	Generally asymptomatic, candida infections in the setting of diabetes
MyD88 deficiency[93]	*MYD88*	AR	Monocytes fail to produce proinflammatory cytokines (TNF-α, IL-1, IL-6), impaired priming and activation of NADPH oxidase	Recurrent infections, especially pneumococcal
NEMO deficiency[87]	*IKBKG*	XL	Impaired priming and activation of NADPH oxidase	Immunodeficiency, ectodermal dysplasia
Papillon-Lefèvre syndrome[94]	*CTSC*	AR	Impaired neutrophil chemotaxis	Severe destructive periodontal disease, redness and thickening of palms and soles, intellectual disability, recurrent infections
Rac2 deficiency[95]	*RAC2*	AD	Abnormal neutrophil chemotaxis, defective respiratory burst, impaired neutrophil degranulation	Neutrophilia, recurrent infections, nonhealing abscesses, delayed umbilical cord separation
Shwachman-Diamond syndrome[15]	*SDBS*	AR	Impaired neutrophil chemotaxis	Pancreatic exocrine insufficiency, steatorrhea, skeletal abnormalities, short stature, increased transaminases, bone marrow failure, risk for MDS/AML
Specific granule defect[96]	*CEBPE*	AR	Defective bactericidal activity	Increased pyogenic infections, absence of specific granules, frequent bilobed neutrophils, risk of MDS/AML
Wiskott-Aldrich syndrome[97]	*WAS*	XL	Defects in adhesion, migration, and phagocytosis	Bleeding, immunodeficiency, eczema, malignancy

Abbreviations: BCG, bacille Calmette-Guérin; CRP, C-reactive protein; IL, interleukin; NADPH, nicotinamide adenine dinucleotide phosphate, reduced form; NEMO, nuclear factor-κB Essential Modulator; TNF-α, tumor necrosis factor alpha.

Leukocyte Adhesion Defect Type 1

First described in 1974 by Boxer and colleagues,[41] leukocyte adhesion deficiency type 1 (LAD-1) is a rare autosomal recessive immunodeficiency characterized by defective immune cell migration and estimated to occur in 1 in 1 million live births.[42] Genetically, LAD-1 is defined by biallelic mutations in *ITGB2*, the gene encoding the beta2 (β2) integrin CD18, which lead to impairment in β2 integrin expression or heterodimer formation with an α integrin subunit.

Normal integrin expression is essential for an appropriate inflammatory response. Phagocytes with defective CD18 aggregate suboptimally and have impaired binding to intercellular adhesion molecules and iC3b on activated endothelial cells, rendering the leukocytes incapable of egressing from the vasculature to sites of microbial entry and injury.[43] The absence of tissue neutrophils in the oropharynx and gastrointestinal tract also results in a lack of inhibition of the interleukin (IL)-23/IL-17 axis, precipitating an upregulated chronic hyperinflammatory response.[44]

As expected, patients with LAD-1 show a lack of pus formation at sites of infection, poor wound healing, and a basal leukocytosis that is greatly exacerbated during infection. Many patients also present with delayed umbilical cord detachment, nonhealing ulcers, periodontitis, HPV infection, and inflammatory bowel disease. Management relies on aggressive oral hygiene and treatment of active infections.

Caspase Recruitment Domain–containing Protein 9 Deficiency

Caspase recruitment domain–containing protein 9 (CARD9) deficiency is a rare autosomal recessive neutrophil function defect caused by mutations in CARD9.[45] CARD9 is an intracellular myeloid signaling molecule downstream of C-type lectin and Toll-like receptors, which are critical for defense against *Candida* and other invasive fungal infections.

Activation of the C-type lectin or Toll-like receptors via recognition of fungal cell wall components leads to phosphorylation of CARD9 and formation of a trimeric complex with B-cell lymphoma 10 (BCL10) and mucosa-associated lymphoid tissue lymphoma translocation gene 1 (MALT1). This trimeric complex then actives nuclear factor-κB and promotes a proinflammatory response with IL-6 and IL-1β production, which is critical for antifungal innate immunity, particularly against *Candida*. In addition, CARD9 is important for the induction of IL-17 production by T-helper cells, which also plays a major role in the clearance of *Candida*.[46]

Patients with CARD9 deficiency present with a selective heightened susceptibility to fungal diseases, particularly to central nervous system and gastrointestinal tract infections with *Candida*, invasive *Exophiala* infections, and persistent mucocutaneous candidiasis. The killing defect of neutrophils in patients with *CARD9* deficit likely contributes to the invasive nature of the fungal disease. Treatment relies on antifungal therapy in combination with G-CSF and GM-CSF.

SUMMARY

Phagocytes, particularly neutrophils, play a critical role in the innate immune system, as shown by the clinical consequences of both quantitative and qualitative defects. The expanding list of congenital neutrophil disorders are typified by a risk for overwhelming infection that can generally be mitigated by the use of G-CSF to augment neutrophil numbers; however, many of the congenital neutropenia disorders have a risk for leukemogenesis that is not modified by therapy. Similarly, the spectrum of functional phagocyte disorders continues to grow with more nuanced recognition of flaws in the key elements of phagocyte function relating to clinical manifestations of bacterial and/or fungal infection and inflammation. In addition, both classic neutropenia and phagocyte functional disorders are increasingly being recognized as a feature of broader primary immunodeficiency diseases.

REFERENCES

1. Lawrence SM, Corriden R, Nizet V. Age-appropriate functions and dysfunctions of the neonatal neutrophil. Front Pediatr 2017;5:23.
2. Segel GB, Halterman JS. Neutropenia in pediatric practice. Pediatr Rev 2008; 29(1):12–23 [quiz: 24].
3. Carlsson G, Fasth A, Berglof E, et al. Incidence of severe congenital neutropenia in Sweden and risk of evolution to myelodysplastic syndrome/leukaemia. Br J Haematol 2012;158(3):363–9.
4. Donadieu J, Beaupain B, Mahlaoui N, et al. Epidemiology of congenital neutropenia. Hematol Oncol Clin North Am 2013;27(1):1–17, vii.
5. Skokowa J, Dale DC, Touw IP, et al. Severe congenital neutropenias. Nat Rev Dis Primers 2017;3:17032.
6. Donadieu J, Beaupain B, Fenneteau O, et al. Congenital neutropenia in the era of genomics: classification, diagnosis, and natural history. Br J Haematol 2017; 179(4):557–74.
7. Rosenberg PS, Zeidler C, Bolyard AA, et al. Stable long-term risk of leukaemia in patients with severe congenital neutropenia maintained on G-CSF therapy. Br J Haematol 2010;150(2):196–9.
8. Fioredda F, Iacobelli S, van Biezen A, et al. Stem cell transplantation in severe congenital neutropenia: an analysis from the European Society for Blood and Marrow Transplantation. Blood 2015;126(16):1885–92 [quiz: 1970].
9. Dale DC, Bolyard AA, Aprikyan A. Cyclic neutropenia. Semin Hematol 2002; 39(2):89–94.
10. Dale DC, Bolyard A, Marrero T, et al. Long-term effects of G-CSF therapy in cyclic neutropenia. N Engl J Med 2017;377(23):2290–2.
11. Klimiankou M, Mellor-Heineke S, Klimenkova O, et al. Two cases of cyclic neutropenia with acquired CSF3R mutations, with 1 developing AML. Blood 2016; 127(21):2638–41.
12. Carapito R, Konantz M, Paillard C, et al. Mutations in signal recognition particle SRP54 cause syndromic neutropenia with Shwachman-Diamond-like features. J Clin Invest 2017;127(11):4090–103.
13. Dhanraj S, Matveev A, Li H. Biallelic mutations in DNAJC21 cause Shwachman-Diamond syndrome. Blood 2017;129(11):1557–62.
14. Stepensky P, Chacon-Flores M, Kim KH, et al. Mutations in EFL1, an SBDS partner, are associated with infantile pancytopenia, exocrine pancreatic insufficiency and skeletal anomalies in aShwachman-Diamond like syndrome. J Med Genet 2017;54(8):558–66.
15. Nelson AS, Myers KC. Diagnosis, treatment, and molecular pathology of Shwachman-Diamond syndrome. Hematol Oncol Clin North Am 2018;32(4): 687–700.
16. Rothbaum R, Perrault J, Vlachos A, et al. Shwachman-Diamond syndrome: report from an international conference. J Pediatr 2002;141(2):266–70.
17. Myers KC, Bolyard AA, Otto B, et al. Variable clinical presentation of Shwachman-Diamond syndrome: update from the North American Shwachman-Diamond Syndrome Registry. J Pediatr 2014;164(4):866–70.

18. Dror Y, Ginzberg H, Dalal I, et al. Immune function in patients with Shwachman-Diamond syndrome. Br J Haematol 2001;114(3):712–7.
19. Grinspan ZM, Pikora CA. Infections in patients with Shwachman-Diamond syndrome. Pediatr Infect Dis J 2005;24(2):179–81.
20. Dror Y, Durie P, Ginzberg H, et al. Clonal evolution in marrows of patients with Shwachman-Diamond syndrome: a prospective 5-year follow-up study. Exp Hematol 2002;30(7):659–69.
21. Dale DC, Bolyard AA, Schwinzer BG, et al. The Severe Chronic Neutropenia International Registry: 10-year follow-up report. Support Cancer Ther 2006;3(4): 220–31.
22. Xia J, Miller CA, Baty J, et al. Somatic mutations and clonal hematopoiesis in congenital neutropenia. Blood 2018;131(4):408–16.
23. Burroughs LM, Shimamura A, Talano JA, et al. Allogeneic hematopoietic cell transplantation using treosulfan-based conditioning for treatment of marrow failure disorders. Biol Blood Marrow Transplant 2017;23(10):1669–77.
24. Beaussant Cohen S, Fenneteau O, Plouvier E, et al. Description and outcome of a cohort of 8 patients with WHIM syndrome from the French Severe Chronic Neutropenia Registry. Orphanet J Rare Dis 2012;7:71.
25. Hernandez PA, Gorlin RJ, Lukens JN, et al. Mutations in the chemokine receptor gene CXCR4 are associated with WHIM syndrome, a combined immunodeficiency disease. Nat Genet 2003;34(1):70–4.
26. Balabanian K, Lagane B, Pablos JL, et al. WHIM syndromes with different genetic anomalies are accounted for by impaired CXCR4 desensitization to CXCL12. Blood 2005;105(6):2449–57.
27. Bachelerie F. CXCL12/CXCR4-axis dysfunctions: markers of the rare immunodeficiency disorder WHIM syndrome. Dis Markers 2010;29(3–4):189–98.
28. Latger-Cannard V, Bensoussan D, Bordigoni P. The WHIM syndrome shows a peculiar dysgranulopoiesis: myelokathexis. Br J Haematol 2006;132(6):669.
29. Aprikyan AA, Liles WC, Park JR, et al. Myelokathexis, a congenital disorder of severe neutropenia characterized by accelerated apoptosis and defective expression of bcl-x in neutrophil precursors. Blood 2000;95(1):320–7.
30. Heusinkveld LE, Yim E, Yang A, et al. Pathogenesis, diagnosis and therapeutic strategies in WHIM syndrome immunodeficiency. Expert Opin Orphan Drugs 2017;5(10):813–25.
31. Badolato R, Donadieu J. How I treat warts, hypogammaglobulinemia, infections, and myelokathexis syndrome. Blood 2017;130(23):2491–8.
32. Brinkmann V, Reichard U, Goosmann C, et al. Neutrophil extracellular traps kill bacteria. Science 2004;303(5663):1532–5.
33. Winkelstein JA, Marino MC, Johnston RB Jr, et al. Chronic granulomatous disease. Report on a national registry of 368 patients. Medicine 2000;79(3):155–69.
34. Marciano BE, Spalding C, Fitzgerald A, et al. Common severe infections in chronic granulomatous disease. Clin Infect Dis 2015;60(8):1176–83.
35. Kuhns DB, Alvord WG, Heller T, et al. Residual NADPH oxidase and survival in chronic granulomatous disease. N Engl J Med 2010;363(27):2600–10.
36. Magnani A, Brosselin P, Beaute J, et al. Inflammatory manifestations in a single-center cohort of patients with chronic granulomatous disease. J Allergy Clin Immunol 2014;134(3):655–62.e8.
37. Marciano BE, Rosenzweig SD, Kleiner DE, et al. Gastrointestinal involvement in chronic granulomatous disease. Pediatrics 2004;114(2):462–8.
38. Gallin JI, Alling DW, Malech HL, et al. Itraconazole to prevent fungal infections in chronic granulomatous disease. N Engl J Med 2003;348(24):2416–22.

39. A controlled trial of interferon gamma to prevent infection in chronic granulomatous disease. The International Chronic Granulomatous Disease Cooperative Study Group. N Engl J Med 1991;324(8):509–16.

40. Gungor T, Teira P, Slatter M, et al. Reduced-intensity conditioning and HLA-matched haemopoietic stem-cell transplantation in patients with chronic granulomatous disease: a prospective multicentre study. Lancet 2014;383(9915): 436–48.

41. Boxer LA, Hedley-Whyte ET, Stossel TP. Neutrophil actin dysfunction and abnormal neutrophil behavior. N Engl J Med 1974;291(21):1093–9.

42. Harris ES, Weyrich AS, Zimmerman GA. Lessons from rare maladies: leukocyte adhesion deficiency syndromes. Curr Opin Hematol 2013;20(1):16–25.

43. Rotrosen D, Gallin JI. Disorders of phagocyte function. Annu Rev Immunol 1987; 5:127–50.

44. Moutsopoulos NM, Konkel J, Sarmadi M, et al. Defective neutrophil recruitment in leukocyte adhesion deficiency type I disease causes local IL-17-driven inflammatory bone loss. Sci Transl Med 2014;6(229):229ra240.

45. Glocker EO, Hennigs A, Nabavi M, et al. A homozygous CARD9 mutation in a family with susceptibility to fungal infections. N Engl J Med 2009;361(18): 1727–35.

46. Netea MG, Marodi L. Innate immune mechanisms for recognition and uptake of *Candida* species. Trends Immunol 2010;31(9):346–53.

47. Skokowa J, Welte K. Defective G-CSFR signaling pathways in congenital neutropenia. Hematol Oncol Clin North Am 2013;27(1):75–88, viii.

48. Klein C, Grudzien M, Appaswamy G, et al. HAX1 deficiency causes autosomal recessive severe congenital neutropenia (Kostmann disease). Nat Genet 2007; 39(1):86–92.

49. Boztug K, Jarvinen PM, Salzer E, et al. JAGN1 deficiency causes aberrant myeloid cell homeostasis and congenital neutropenia. Nat Genet 2014;46(9): 1021–7.

50. Boztug K, Rosenberg PS, Dorda M, et al. Extended spectrum of human glucose-6-phosphatase catalytic subunit 3 deficiency: novel genotypes and phenotypic variability in severe congenital neutropenia. J Pediatr 2012;160(4):679–83.e2.

51. Desplantes C, Fremond ML, Beaupain B, et al. Clinical spectrum and long-term follow-up of 14 cases with G6PC3 mutations from the French Severe Congenital Neutropenia Registry. Orphanet J Rare Dis 2014;9:183.

52. Makaryan V, Rosenthal EA, Bolyard AA, et al. TCIRG1-associated congenital neutropenia. Hum Mutat 2014;35(7):824–7.

53. Hoenig M, Pannicke U, Gaspar HB, et al. Recent advances in understanding the pathogenesis and management of reticular dysgenesis. Br J Haematol 2018; 180(5):644–53.

54. Vilboux T, Lev A, Malicdan MC, et al. A congenital neutrophil defect syndrome associated with mutations in VPS45. N Engl J Med 2013;369(1):54–65.

55. Aprikyan AA, Khuchua Z. Advances in the understanding of Barth syndrome. Br J Haematol 2013;161(3):330–8.

56. Winkelstein JA, Marino MC, Lederman HM, et al. X-linked agammaglobulinemia: report on a United States registry of 201 patients. Medicine 2006;85(4):193–202.

57. Kostjukovits S, Klemetti P, Valta H, et al. Analysis of clinical and immunologic phenotype in a large cohort of children and adults with cartilage-hair hypoplasia. J Allergy Clin Immunol 2017;140(2):612–4.e5.

58. Makitie O, Rajantie J, Kaitila I. Anaemia and macrocytosis–unrecognized features in cartilage-hair hypoplasia. Acta Paediatr 1992;81(12):1026–9.

59. Taskinen M, Ranki A, Pukkala E, et al. Extended follow-up of the Finnish cartilage-hair hypoplasia cohort confirms high incidence of non-Hodgkin lymphoma and basal cell carcinoma. Am J Med Genet A 2008;146a(18):2370–5.

60. Toro C, Nicoli ER, Malicdan MC, et al. Chediak-Higashi syndrome. In: Adam MP, Ardinger HH, Pagon RA, et al, editors. GeneReviews. Seattle (WA): University of Washington, Seattle; 1993. GeneReviews is a registered trademark of the University of Washington, Seattle. All rights reserved.

61. Wortmann SB, Wevers RA, de Brouwer APM. CLPB deficiency. In: Adam MP, Ardinger HH, Pagon RA, et al, editors. GeneReviews. Seattle (WA): University of Washington, Seattle; 1993. GeneReviews is a registered trademark of the University of Washington, Seattle. All rights reserved.

62. Wortmann SB, Zietkiewicz S, Kousi M, et al. CLPB mutations cause 3-methylglutaconic aciduria, progressive brain atrophy, intellectual disability, congenital neutropenia, cataracts, movement disorder. Am J Hum Genet 2015;96(2):245–57.

63. Wang L, Clericuzio C, Larizza L. Poikiloderma with neutropenia. In: Adam MP, Ardinger HH, Pagon RA, et al, editors. GeneReviews. Seattle (WA): University of Washington, Seattle; 1993. GeneReviews is a registered trademark of the University of Washington, Seattle. All rights reserved.

64. Kivitie-Kallio S, Norio R. Cohen syndrome: essential features, natural history, and heterogeneity. Am J Med Genet 2001;102(2):125–35.

65. Michniacki TF, Hannibal M, Ross CW, et al. Hematologic manifestations of deficiency of adenosine deaminase 2 (DADA2) and response to tumor necrosis factor inhibition in DADA2-associated bone marrow failure. J Clin Immunol 2018; 38(2):166–73.

66. Meyts I, Aksentijevich I. Deficiency of adenosine deaminase 2 (DADA2): updates on the phenotype, genetics, pathogenesis, and treatment. J Clin Immunol 2018; 38(5):569–78.

67. Tummala H, Walne AJ, Williams M, et al. DNAJC21 mutations link a cancer-prone bone marrow failure syndrome to corruption in 60S ribosome subunit maturation. Am J Hum Genet 2016;99(1):115–24.

68. D'Amours G, Lopes F, Gauthier J, et al. Refining the phenotype associated with biallelic DNAJC21 mutations. Clin Genet 2018;94(2):252–8.

69. Spinner MA, Sanchez LA, Hsu AP, et al. GATA2 deficiency: a protean disorder of hematopoiesis, lymphatics, and immunity. Blood 2014;123(6):809–21.

70. Visser G, Rake JP, Fernandes J, et al. Neutropenia, neutrophil dysfunction, and inflammatory bowel disease in glycogen storage disease type Ib: results of the European Study on Glycogen Storage Disease type I. J Pediatr 2000;137(2): 187–91.

71. Rake JP, Visser G, Labrune P, et al. Glycogen storage disease type I: diagnosis, management, clinical course and outcome. Results of the European Study on Glycogen Storage Disease Type I (ESGSD I). Eur J Pediatr 2002;161(Suppl 1): S20–34.

72. Mancini AJ, Chan LS, Paller AS. Partial albinism with immunodeficiency: Griscelli syndrome: report of a case and review of the literature. J Am Acad Dermatol 1998;38(2 Pt 2):295–300.

73. de Boer M, van Leeuwen K, Geissler J, et al. Hermansky-Pudlak syndrome type 2: aberrant pre-mRNA splicing and mislocalization of granule proteins in neutrophils. Hum Mutat 2017;38(10):1402–11.

74. de la Morena MT. Clinical phenotypes of Hyper-IgM syndromes. J Allergy Clin Immunol Pract 2016;4(6):1023–36.

75. Bohn G, Allroth A, Brandes G, et al. A novel human primary immunodeficiency syndrome caused by deficiency of the endosomal adaptor protein p14. Nat Med 2007;13(1):38–45.
76. Farruggia P, Di Cataldo A, Pinto RM, et al. Pearson syndrome: a retrospective cohort study from the Marrow Failure Study Group of A.I.E.O.P. (Associazione Italiana Emato-Oncologia Pediatrica). JIMD Rep 2016;26:37–43.
77. Stray-Pedersen A, Backe PH, Sorte HS, et al. PGM3 mutations cause a congenital disorder of glycosylation with severe immunodeficiency and skeletal dysplasia. Am J Hum Genet 2014;95(1):96–107.
78. Abdollahpour H, Appaswamy G, Kotlarz D, et al. The phenotype of human STK4 deficiency. Blood 2012;119(15):3450–7.
79. Monagle PT, Tauro GP. Long-term follow up of patients with transcobalamin II deficiency. Arch Dis Child 1995;72(3):237–8.
80. Julier C, Nicolino M. Wolcott-Rallison syndrome. Orphanet J Rare Dis 2010;5:29.
81. Devriendt K, Kim AS, Mathijs G, et al. Constitutively activating mutation in WASP causes X-linked severe congenital neutropenia. Nat Genet 2001;27(3):313–7.
82. Ancliff PJ, Blundell MP, Cory GO, et al. Two novel activating mutations in the Wiskott-Aldrich syndrome protein result in congenital neutropenia. Blood 2006; 108(7):2182–9.
83. Drewniak A, Gazendam RP, Tool AT, et al. Invasive fungal infection and impaired neutrophil killing in human CARD9 deficiency. Blood 2013;121(13):2385–92.
84. Root RK, Rosenthal AS, Balestra DJ. Abnormal bactericidal, metabolic, and lysosomal functions of Chediak-Higashi Syndrome leukocytes. J Clin Invest 1972; 51(3):649–65.
85. Bianchi M, Hakkim A, Brinkmann V, et al. Restoration of NET formation by gene therapy in CGD controls aspergillosis. Blood 2009;114(13):2619–22.
86. Hartl D, Lehmann N, Hoffmann F, et al. Dysregulation of innate immune receptors on neutrophils in chronic granulomatous disease. J Allergy Clin Immunol 2008; 121(2):375–82.e9.
87. Singh A, Zarember KA, Kuhns DB, et al. Impaired priming and activation of the neutrophil NADPH oxidase in patients with IRAK4 or NEMO deficiency. J Immunol 2009;182(10):6410–7.
88. Bigley V, Maisuria S, Cytlak U, et al. Biallelic interferon regulatory factor 8 mutation: a complex immunodeficiency syndrome with dendritic cell deficiency, monocytopenia, and immune dysregulation. J Allergy Clin Immunol 2018;141(6): 2234–48.
89. Hill HR, Ochs HD, Quie PG, et al. Defect in neutrophil granulocyte chemotaxis in Job's syndrome of recurrent "cold" staphylococcal abscesses. Lancet 1974; 2(7881):617–9.
90. Woellner C, Gertz EM, Schaffer AA, et al. Mutations in STAT3 and diagnostic guidelines for hyper-IgE syndrome. J Allergy Clin Immunol 2010;125(2): 424–32.e8.
91. Etzioni A. Genetic etiologies of leukocyte adhesion defects. Curr Opin Immunol 2009;21(5):481–6.
92. Lanza F. Clinical manifestation of myeloperoxidase deficiency. J Mol Med 1998; 76(10):676–81.
93. Picard C, von Bernuth H, Ghandil P, et al. Clinical features and outcome of patients with IRAK-4 and MyD88 deficiency. Medicine 2010;89(6):403–25.
94. Sreeramulu B, Shyam ND, Ajay P, et al. Papillon-Lefevre syndrome: clinical presentation and management options. Clin Cosmet Investig Dent 2015;7:75–81.

95. Gu Y, Jia B, Yang FC, et al. Biochemical and biological characterization of a human Rac2 GTPase mutant associated with phagocytic immunodeficiency. J Biol Chem 2001;276(19):15929–38.

96. Gallin JI, Fletcher MP, Seligmann BE, et al. Human neutrophil-specific granule deficiency: a model to assess the role of neutrophil-specific granules in the evolution of the inflammatory response. Blood 1982;59(6):1317–29.

97. Ochs HD, Slichter SJ, Harker LA, et al. The Wiskott-Aldrich syndrome: studies of lymphocytes, granulocytes, and platelets. Blood 1980;55(2):243–52.

Moving?

Make sure your subscription moves with you!

To notify us of your new address, find your **Clinics Account Number** (located on your mailing label above your name), and contact customer service at:

Email: journalscustomerservice-usa@elsevier.com

800-654-2452 (subscribers in the U.S. & Canada)
314-447-8871 (subscribers outside of the U.S. & Canada)

Fax number: 314-447-8029

Elsevier Health Sciences Division
Subscription Customer Service
3251 Riverport Lane
Maryland Heights, MO 63043

*To ensure uninterrupted delivery of your subscription, please notify us at least 4 weeks in advance of move.